Multidisciplinary Approach to Osteoporosis

Andrea Lenzi • Silvia Migliaccio
Editors

Multidisciplinary Approach to Osteoporosis

From Assessment to Treatment

Springer

Editors
Andrea Lenzi
Department of Experimental Medicine
Sapienza University of Rome
Rome
Italy

Silvia Migliaccio
Department of Movement, Human and Health Sciences
Foro Italico University of Rome
Rome
Italy

ISBN 978-3-319-75108-5 ISBN 978-3-319-75110-8 (eBook)
https://doi.org/10.1007/978-3-319-75110-8

Library of Congress Control Number: 2018949650

This Springer imprint is published by the registered company Springer Nature Switzerland AG
The registered company address is: Gewerbestrasse 11, 6330 Cham, Switzerland

Preface

Introduction to Interdisciplinary Approach to Osteoporosis: Why Is It So Important?

Osteoporosis is a skeletal metabolic disorder that has reached epidemic extents all over the industrialized world. Recent epidemiological studies confirm the tendency to a dramatic increase of individuals affected by osteoporosis and fragility fractures. Indeed, during the last decades, for the increase of life expectancy, this disease has become a major health threat around the world. Age, both in male and female population, increases the risk of developing osteoporosis, which affects millions of women, but lately, also men. Age-related changes in body composition, metabolic factors, and hormonal levels, accompanied by a decline in physical activity, may all provide mechanisms for the propensity to lose muscle mass, gain fat mass, and also develop bone loss.

Since many factors, such as genetic, environmental, nutritional, and hormonal, play an important role in determining this disorder, attention must be given to this health problem by researchers, politicians, the media, and the public in order to approach this skeletal alteration in a correct manner. In fact, osteoporosis is one of the most common chronic disorders in the industrialized societies, with an important impact on individual lives as well as on health economics (medical expenses, lost income as a result of disability, and complications of fragility fractures), and therefore, this skeletal disorder has become a major factor in health care planning systems due to the high socioeconomic costs.

Most reports agree that, among other factors, lack of physical activity and non-equilibrated nutrition play a role in the development of bone loss, altered skeletal homeostasis, and, thus, skeletal fragility.

The genetic basis of osteoporosis has been studied analyzing the role of different gene products, and an increase in knowledge suggests the role of different cytokines, hormones, and their receptors, indicating that genetic factors might play an important role in osteoporosis development besides all other known factors.

Thus, it appears clear that osteoporosis, being a multifactorial chronic skeletal disease, needs an interdisciplinary approach in order to accomplish all the needs of patients affected by osteoporosis and fragility fractures.

Indeed, many programs and advice are starting to be offered to the public. Many educational programs centered on nutritional intervention, physical activity, and pharmacological therapy are considered vital to improve the knowledge of this disease in order to reduce fragility fractures and to diminish disability and mortality and to improve quality of life of individuals affected by osteoporosis.

In this book, the authors' contributions address the spectrum of the multidisciplinary, and interdisciplinary, approach to osteoporosis, ranging from physiological characteristics to epidemiology, to clinical characteristics and pharmacological approaches. Metabolic and endocrinological aspects of obesity are analyzed in depth, considering the role of thyroid, adrenal, and ovarian functions, the interaction between osteoporosis and obesity or sarcopenia or kidney or rheumatological diseases. Clinical aspects are considered, starting from the multidisciplinary evaluation (clinical, nutritional, functional) through the different interventions (therapeutic education and physical activity and training prescription, prescription medications), up to the interdisciplinary management of osteoporosis.

The involvement of experts in nutrition, kidney diseases, endocrinology and andrology, rheumatology, exercise and sports medicine, and orthopedic surgery explains, the multidisciplinary approach that should characterize the clinical care of the patient affected by osteoporosis.

The experts of the different disciplines, who have been involved in this editorial project, have made every effort to produce manuscripts rich in evidence-based medicine contents, but also basic research, highlighting the importance of a translational approach "from the bench to the bedside" pointing viewpoints from multiple disciplines and the multilayered issues involved in the care of patients affected by osteoporosis.

The book will be useful to physicians, scientists, postgraduate students, and students of various disciplines dealing with osteoporosis and fragility fractures.

Rome, Italy Andrea Lenzi
Rome, Italy Silvia Migliaccio

Contents

1 **Anatomy and Physiology of Skeletal Tissue: The Bone Cells** 1
Giacomina Brunetti, Graziana Colaianni, Silvia Colucci, and Maria Grano

2 **Genetics of Osteoporosis** 25
Francesca Marini, Laura Masi, Gemma Marcucci, Luisella Cianferotti, and Maria Luisa Brandi

3 **Osteoporosis Diagnosis** 45
Claudio Marcocci and Federica Saponaro

4 **Functional Evaluation of the Subjects with Skeletal Alterations** 59
Giovanni Iolascon, Alessandro de Sire, Marco Paoletta, Antimo Moretti, and Francesca Gimigliano

Part I Endocrinologicic and Metabolic Regulation

5 **Skeletal Alterations and Parathyroid Function** 75
Elisabetta Romagnoli and Vincenzo Carnevale

6 **GH/IGF-I and Bone** 83
Stefano Frara, Filippo Maffezzoni, Mauro Doga, Anna Maria Formenti, Gherardo Mazziotti, and Andrea Giustina

7 **Adrenal Function and Skeletal Regulation** 107
Iacopo Chiodini, Claudia Battista, Elisa Cairoli, Cristina Eller-Vainicher, Valentina Morelli, Serena Palmieri, Antonio Stefano Salcuni, and Alfredo Scillitani

8 **Skeletal Tissue and Ovarian Function: Puberty and Menopause** 129
Annamaria Colao, Carolina Di Somma, and Volha V. Zhukouskaya

9 **Obesity and Osteoporosis: Is the Paradigm Changing?** 143
Emanuela A. Greco, Rachele Fornari, Andrea Lenzi, and Silvia Migliaccio

10 Bone and Diabetes . . . 153
Andrea Palermo, Anda Mihaela Naciu, Gaia Tabacco, Luca D'Onofrio, and Nicola Napoli

11 Renal Diseases and Skeletal Health . . . 183
Sandro Mazzaferro, Silverio Rotondi, Lida Tartaglione, Natalia De Martino, Cristiana Leonangeli, and Marzia Pasquali

12 Osteoporosis and Cardiovascular Risk . . . 211
Giancarlo Isaia, Lorenzo Marchese, Margherita Marchetti, and Mario Bo

13 Osteoporosis in Men . . . 223
Elena Nebot Valenzuela and Peter Pietschmann

14 Rheumatic Diseases and Osteoporosis . . . 237
Ombretta Di Munno, Nazzarena Malavolta, and Giovanni Minisola

Part II Prevention and Treatment

15 Nutrition and Skeletal Health . . . 259
Chiara Marocco, Rachele Fornari, Andrea Lenzi, and Emanuela A. Greco

16 Different Physical Activity Protocols in the Subjects Affected by Osteoporosis . . . 277
Gian Pietro Emerenziani, Emanuela A. Greco, Laura Guidetti, and Carlo Baldari

17 Pharmacological Therapy: Past, Present, and Future . . . 285
Silvia Migliaccio, Andrea Lenzi, and Emanuela A. Greco

18 Surgical Therapy: Vertebro-Cifoplastic: – Pros and Cons . . . 297
Umberto Tarantino, Giuseppina Resmini, Alessando Provenza, Eleonora Piccirilli, Maurizio Feola, and Riccardo Iundusi

19 Rehabilitation Therapy After Surgery in Osteoporotic Patients . . . 313
Francesca Gimigliano, Alessandro de Sire, Antimo Moretti, Claudio Curci, and Giovanni Iolascon

Index . . . 325

Anatomy and Physiology of Skeletal Tissue: The Bone Cells

1

Giacomina Brunetti, Graziana Colaianni, Silvia Colucci, and Maria Grano

1.1 Introduction

The skeleton is a hard structure formed by a set of bones that support the human body. According to their shape, the bones can be classified into four groups: long bones, short bones, flat bones, and irregular bones. Long bones, the major bones of limbs, are longer than they are wide and consist of an elongated central hollow shaft, known as diaphysis, and two expanded ends, known as epiphysis. The part between the diaphysis and the epiphysis is called metaphysis. The inner portion of the bone includes a cavity, known as marrow or medullary cavity, filled with bone marrow. Short bones are almost equivalent in length and diameter (i.e., the carpal bones of the hand); flat bones are skinny and plate-like (i.e., the skull and the sternum); irregular bones have a different shape with respect to the previously described three groups of bones (i.e., a vertebra).

Bone exists in two main forms due to the arrangement of collagen fibers: woven bone and lamellar bone. Woven bone is an immature form characterized by a disorganized disposition of collagen fibers, thereby resulting in a weaker structure. Lamellar bone is the mature form and displays a regular parallel alignment of collagen fibrils arranged in lamellae.

The mature bone tissue is structurally divided into two types: the cortical/compact bone and the spongy trabecular bone. Cortical bone is dense and solid and surrounds the marrow cavity, whereas trabecular bone is composed of a network of trabecular plates and rods strewed in the bone marrow compartment. Mature

G. Brunetti · S. Colucci
Department of Basic and Medical Sciences, Neurosciences and Sense Organs, Section of Human Anatomy and Histology, University of Bari, Bari, Italy

G. Colaianni · M. Grano (✉)
Department of Emergency and Organ Transplantation, Section of Human Anatomy and Histology, University of Bari, Bari, Italy
e-mail: maria.grano@uniba.it

A. Lenzi, S. Migliaccio (eds.), *Multidisciplinary Approach to Osteoporosis*,
https://doi.org/10.1007/978-3-319-75110-8_1

cortical bone is mainly composed of cylindrical units known as osteons or Haversian systems, which are formed by concentric lamellae of bone matrix containing a central neurovascular canal.

As all the other connective tissue, the bone consists of an extracellular matrix composed of an inorganic and organic part and a cellular component, consisting of osteoclasts (OCs), osteoblasts (OBs), and osteocytes. The major component of the inorganic matrix is hydroxyapatite, whereas the organic part includes primarily collagen type 1 but also other non-collagenic proteins, such as osteopontin, osteocalcin, and proteoglycans.

1.2 The Functions of the Bone

The bone is currently considered a multifunctional tissue. Indeed, it plays roles in mechanical support, provides a structure for the attachment of muscles, and allows body movements. The bone also exerts a protection for different organs, especially in vital areas such as the trunk, in which the ribcage shields the lungs and the heart or the vertebrae protect the spinal cord, or also cranial bones which kept the brain safe. Furthermore, the bone stores several minerals, such as calcium and phosphorus, which, when required, are released from the bone in the blood taking part in mineral homeostasis. In addition, the bone plays a role in hematopoiesis since all cellular blood components are derived from hematopoietic stem cells present in the bone marrow, the soft tissue hosted inside the cavity of the long bones and trabecular spaces, and also acts as energy storage due to yellow marrow, which, containing lipids, represents an energy reservoir. More recently, it has become clear that the bone can also display an endocrine function, as it regulates not only itself but also other organs through the two most well-known and well-studied molecules: osteocalcin (OCN) and fibroblast growth factor 23 (FGF23) [1].

Exclusively, the bone renews itself throughout the life through the physiological process known as bone remodeling consisting in the balanced activity of OCs, the resorptive cells of the bone, and OBs, the bone-building cells. Recently, more and more evidences have indicated that the osteocytes, the most abundant bone cell type embedded in the mineralized matrix, orchestrate bone remodeling.

Here we will address the current knowledge about bone cells.

1.3 Osteoclasts

OCs, generated by fusion of myeloid precursors [2], are multinucleated cells present in physiological condition on bone surfaces when extracellular matrix degradation occurs. OCs have an exclusive cytoskeletal organization and membrane polarization that allows them to isolate the bone-apposed extracellular space, "the Howship's lacunae," where bone resorption takes place. Through their resorption activity OCs absolve to numerous functions. First of all, they participate to renew the bone in order to maintain its homeostasis. Secondly, since the bone is the major organ for the calcium storage, OCs are sensitive to numerous signal regulating calcium release from the bone, such as parathyroid hormone and 1,25(OH)2 vitamin D3. Thirdly, through bone-resorbing activity, OCs are responsible of the release of growth factors stored in the bone matrix including insulin-like growth factor-1 (IGF-1) and transforming growth factor β (TGF-β) affecting the coupling of bone formation and resorption and targeting other cells in the bone microenvironment. Lastly, OCs maintain characteristics of other myeloid cells, such as cytokine release and antigen presentation, which give them the potential to influence immune responses.

Bone Resorption

OCs adhere to bone matrix by integrin αvβ3, expressed in specialized F-actin structures called podosomes; surround the portion of the bone to be digested and polarized in way that the cellular membrane in front of the bone is convoluted by the presence of microvilli, "the "ruffled border"; and hold the proton pump (V-ATPase) and Cl^- channel 7 (ClC7), whereas the basolateral membrane domain includes the $HCO3^-/Cl^-$ antiporter [2]. Cytoplasmic carbonic anhydrase type II (CAII) enzyme creates the protons to be released into the resorption Howship's lacuna under the cell. This "space" becomes separated from the rest of the extracellular space through the tight binding of αvβ3 to the bone matrix at the sealing zone. The β3 cytoplasmic domain recruits signaling proteins, inducing the binding of actin with different molecules (including vinculin, kindlin, talin, paxillin, and myosin IIA) and formation of the actin ring that labels the periphery of the ruffled membrane. Combined activity of ClC7 and V-ATPase determines elevated levels of HCl that acidifies the Howship's lacuna, leading to the solubilization of the inorganic compounds of the bone matrix. In parallel, acidified cytoplasmic vesicles containing lysosomal enzymes including cathepsin K and metalloprotease-9 are also transported toward the ruffled cell membrane and, ultimately, released in the lacunae to degrade the organic components of the bone matrix.

1.4 Osteoclastogenesis

The primary factors regulating OC differentiation are MCSF and RANKL, produced by stromal and OB lineage cells thereby providing support for this process [3, 4]. Beyond macrophage colony-stimulating factor (MCSF) and receptor activator of nuclear factor-κB ligand (RANKL), the normal bone marrow microenvironment also contains a wide variety of OC-regulating molecules, including cytokines, growth factors, and hormones which are discussed in detail below.

MCSF

MCSF is derived from osteoblastic cells and is involved in the growth and survival of the OCs through regulation of numerous pathways such as the mitogen-activated protein kinases (MAPKs), extracellular signal-regulated kinase (ERK), and Jun N-terminal kinase (JNK) [4], glycogen synthase kinase-3β/β-catenin [5], and mammalian target of rapamycin (mTOR) [6]. Moreover, MCSF also induces OC differentiation signals since it has been recently found to increase diacylglycerol levels through stimulation of phospholipase C-γ (PLC-γ), which in turn causes c-Fos activation [7]. The MCSF actions are mediated by binding with its receptor c-fms, and the importance of the growth factor and its receptor in osteoclastogenesis and bone phenotype came from data showing that null mutations in either the ligand or the receptor genes result in a severe osteopetrosis [8]. Recently, it has been demonstrated that c-fms can also interact with the newly identified interleukin-34 (IL-34) and that MCSF as well as IL-34 promote the expression of RANK, whose signaling pathways also promote osteoclastogenesis [9].

RANKL/RANK/OPG Axis

RANKL is another crucial factor required for the differentiation, survival, and function of OCs. Two decades ago the demonstrations that RANKL transgenic mice showed osteoporosis whereas mice knockout for RANKL or for the decoy receptor osteoprotegerin (OPG) are osteopetrotic [10] and osteoporotic [11], respectively, underline the crucial function of this pathway in osteoclastogenesis.

Furthermore, human osteoclast-poor osteopetrosis has been associated to inactivation or deficiency of RANKL [12]. Inactivation of *OPG* causes juvenile Paget's disease [13], a high-turnover bone disorder, whereas activating mutations of RANK generates different osteolytic diseases, such as familial expansile osteolysis [14].

Monocytes expressing RANK, a tumor necrosis factor (TNF) receptor family member, in the presence of RANKL fuse to differentiate into multinucleated OCs. RANKL–RANK interaction leads to the activation of numerous pathways including MAPKs (p38, JNK, ERK), mTOR, PI3K, NF-κB (canonical and alternative), and microphthalmia-associated transcription factor (MITF) [6, 15, 16].

Some of these pathways induce the expression of nuclear factor of activated T cells, cytoplasmic 1 (NFATc1), the key osteoclastogenic transcription factor [17], whose activation is also linked to the PLC-γ2/Ca^{2+} pathway. RANK signaling determines protein posttranslational modifications such as ubiquitination [18] (72), phosphorylation [19], and SUMOylation [20]. Ongoing studies also demonstrate a crucial role of epigenetic mechanisms in RANKL control of osteoclastogenesis [21, 22]. In fact, RANKL modulates the expression of several microRNAs [23]. RANKL also determines histone 3 (H3) lysine 4 trimethylation (H3K4me3, a mark of transcriptionally active chromatin) whereas mitigates H3K27me3 (a mark of silent chromatin) near the transcription start site of several genes encoding OC transcription factors, such as NFATc1 and NF-κB [24].

Recently, Luo et al. reported that leucine-rich repeat-containing G-protein-coupled receptor 4 (LGR4, also called GPR48) is another receptor for RANKL. LGR4 competes with RANK to bind RANKL and inhibited canonical RANK signaling during osteoclastogenesis [25]. RANKL binding to LGR4 activates the Gaq and GSK3-β signaling pathway, thereby inhibiting the expression and activity of NFATC1 during OC differentiation. Both total (Lgr4$^{-/-}$) and monocyte conditional knockout mice of Lgr4 (Lgr4 CKO) showed increased OC formation and activity. The same authors demonstrated that LGR4 extracellular domain therapeutically abrogated RANKL-induced bone loss in three mouse models of osteoporosis [25].

OSCAR, FcRγ, and DAP12

A third signal controlling osteoclastogenesis arises from ITAM adaptors including DNAX activation protein of 12 kDa (DAP12) [26] and Fc receptor γ (FcRγ). These cell surface molecules interact with co-receptors TREM2 and Sirpβ1 (DAP12) or OSCAR and PIR-A (FcRγ) in order to activate Ca^{2+}/NFATc1 through PLC-γ2 [27, 28]. In mice, deletion of either ITAM protein has no effect on bone mass, while deletion of both causes severe osteopetrosis. Other studies reported that the primary role of the ITAM-mediated signaling seems to be in the regulation of the OC cytoskeleton, with modest effect on osteoclastogenesis [26, 29]. Furthermore, loss of TREM2, the co-receptor for DAP12, increases OC formation, through β-catenin, indicative of a Ca^{2+}/NFATc1-independent effect [2]. Thus, ITAM signaling role in osteoclastogenesis requires further studies.

Tumor Necrosis Factor-α (TNF-α)

Already before the discovery of RANKL pro-osteoclastogenic role, TNF-α was recognized for its ability to stimulate bone resorption in vivo and in vitro [30, 31]. TNF-α stimulates RANKL and MCSF expression by osteoblastic cells and also binds directly OC precursors [32, 33]. Numerous signaling pathways activated by TNF-α and RANKL are very similar and together stimulate OC differentiation [34, 35]. However, the ability of TNF-α alone to induce osteoclastogenesis is quite low, due to little diversities in signaling pathway. In detail, RANK engages TRAF3, allowing the processing of p100 to p52, thereby removing significant brakes on the alternative NF-κB signaling pathway [36]. TNFR1 signaling augments p100 levels but not its transformation to p52.

Another molecule that negatively affect TNF-α pro- osteoclastogenic effect is RBP-J, a transcription factor which if it is removed leads to strong osteolysis in response to TNF-α [37]. In normal cells, small amounts of RANKL with TNF-α have a synergic on osteoclastogenesis. However, in conditions in which RANKL is severely excluded from the system, exposure of precursors to TNF-α prior to RANKL inhibits osteoclastogenesis [34]. Due to the presence of a death domain in TNFR1, TNFα stimulates pro-apoptotic pathways in addition to the pro-survival pathways that are downstream of classical NF-κB. Thus, the addition of TNF-α to OCs or their precursors causes apoptosis only when classical NF-κB is blocked. Thus, NF-κB signaling downstream of TNFα supplies a strong survival signal to OC lineage cells.

LIGHT

LIGHT (homologous to *L*ymphotoxins exhibiting Inducible expression and competing with herpes simplex virus *G*lycoprotein D for herpes virus entry mediator [*H*VEM], a receptor expressed by *T* lymphocytes) is a member of TNFSF (TNFSF14) expressed on activated T cells, natural killer cells, monocytes, granulocytes, spleen cells, and immature dendritic cells [38–40]. LIGHT can engage two membrane-bound TNFSF signaling receptors, HVEM and lymphotoxin beta receptor (LTβR). HVEM is expressed on endothelial, dendritic, natural killer, and T and B cells [41, 42], while LTβR is expressed on fibroblast, monocyte, endothelial, epithelial, and stromal cells [43]. Following the interaction of LIGHT with HVEM or LTβR resulted in cytokine production and cell survival or proliferation [44–47]. The LIGHT–LTβR interaction can also lead to cell death [48, 49]. Through the interaction with HVEM, LIGHT is described as a potent T cell co-stimulatory molecule [41, 50, 51]; its constitutive expression on T cells causes activation and expansion of these cells, favoring autoimmune disease development [52, 53]. LIGHT could also bind a soluble receptor decoy receptor 3 (DcR3), which is known to be involved in OC formation [54]. Moreover, LIGHT has been implicated in osteolytic rheumatoid arthritis and multiple myeloma [55, 56], although conflicting results have been reported about the role of LIGHT on OC formation [55–59]. In particular, Hishida et al. reported no OC differentiation from peripheral blood (PB) $CD14^+$ monocytes treated with LIGHT [55], whereas our previous work in agreement with what demonstrated by Edwards et al. and Hemingway et al. showed a LIGHT pro-osteoclastogenic effect [56–59]. However, all the cited authors concordantly reported that LIGHT and RANKL synergically stimulated OC formation [55–59].

Interleukin-17 (IL-17)

Interleukins are known to affect OC differentiation [60, 61]. Recently, IL-17 attracted numerous scientists overall for the therapeutic implications. IL-17 is expressed by a type of human T-helper cell (Th17) [61]. This cytokine plays a crucial role in inflammation and the development of autoimmune diseases such as rheumatoid arthritis; however, its mechanism of action in the development of bone erosions, especially in relation to other known key cytokines such as IL-1, TNF, and RANKL, remains unclear.

IL-17 has been demonstrated to be implicated in osteoclastogenesis augmentation in inflammation by increasing the release of RANKL, which may synergize with IL-1 and TNF [62].

1.5 Osteoblasts

OBs differentiate from mesenchymal stem cells (MSCs), sharing their origin with other cells of connective tissues such as fibroblasts, adipocytes, and chondrocytes. They represent only 5% of total bone resident cells that are mainly constituted by osteocytes. OBs have the crucial function of building the bone [63] but also of regulating OC differentiation through the production of MCSF, RANKL, and OPG [3, 64].

Osteoblastogenesis is defined by several steps: lineage commitment, proliferative expansion, synthesis and mineralization of bone matrix, and differentiation in osteocytes. All these stages are signed by specific activation of transcription factors and sequential gene transcription thereby determining the expression of the typical OB markers. The key transcription factors involved in osteoclastogenesis are RUNX2 and Osterix, whereas the typical OB markers include collagen I (COLL I), alkaline phosphatase (ALP), bone sialoprotein, osteonectin, osteopontin, and OCN.

1.6 Transcription Factors Affecting Osteoblastogenesis

Runt domain-containing transcription factor (Runx2) represents a master switch for osteoblastogenesis. Runx2 levels progressively enhance during osteoblastogenesis, reaching the maximum expression in complete differentiated OBs. *Runx2* homozygous deletion in mice determined a total lack of OBs [65], whereas *Runx2* haploinsufficiency in mice or in humans led to hypoplastic clavicles and delayed closure of the fontanelles, defects that are typical of cleidocranial dysplasia in humans [66–68]. RUNX2 is necessary for the suitable activity of mature OBs, including the synthesis of bone matrix [69]. In fact Runx2 target genes include both genes expressed by immature and differentiated OBs, such as TGF-β receptor, ALP, COLL I, OPN, OCN, and collagenase [70].

Osterix (OSX)

OSX, transcription factor, is required downstream of RUNX2 and thereby necessary for OB differentiation. In mouse embryos OSX deletion led to OB absence, although RUNX2 is expressed [71]. These findings, together with the demonstration that OSX levels were undetectable in RUNX2-null mice [71], suggested that OSX works downstream of RUNX2 during osteoblastogenesis. OSX is essential both during embryogenesis and for postnatal OB and osteocyte differentiation and activity [72].

Activating Transcription Factor 4 (ATF4)
ATF4, a member of the basic Leu zipper (bZIP) family of transcription factors, has a key role in mature OB lineage cells. Alteration of ATF4 activity has been associated with the skeletal abnormalities observed in Coffin–Lowry syndrome patients [73, 74]. ATF4 directly regulates the expression of the bone matrix protein OCN and of RANKL. ATF4 also is involved in the amino acid import to guarantee a suitable protein synthesis by OBs [73].

Activating Protein 1 (AP1)
AP1 is a transcription factor which consists of different dimers of proteins belonging to Fos (c-Fos, FosB, Fra-1, and Fra-2) and Jun families (c-Jun, JunB, and JunD) [75]. Conditional deletion of *Fra-1* in mice resulted in osteopenia that seems to be due to the reduced expression of OCN and COLL I [76]. Transgenic overexpression of FRA1 determined high bone mass due to increased osteoblastogenesis [73–80]. Moreover, a direct transcriptional control of *OCN* and *Coll I* by Fra-2 in human subjects has been reported [77, 78]. Additionally, ΔFOSB transgenic mice, an isoform of FOSB, increased bone mass through stimulation of OB formation and activity [79, 80].

1.7 Molecules Affecting Osteoblastogenesis

The WNT family of glycoproteins has crucial functions in the regulation of osteoblastogenesis. Following the binding to different transmembrane receptor, WNT glycoproteins trigger several intracellular pathways that may be β-catenin dependent or independent [81, 82].

In β-catenin-dependent WNT signaling, the glycoproteins (WNT1, WNT3, WNT3A, WNT8, WNT9A, or WNT10B) engage frizzled receptors and their co-receptors low-density lipoprotein receptor-related protein 5 (LRP5) or LRP6 leading to the activation of a cascade of intracellular mediators that stabilize cytosolic β-catenin [83]. Thus, β-catenin translocates into the nucleus, interacts with lymphoid enhancer-binding factor 1 (LEF1) and T cell factor 1 (TCF1), TCF3, and TCF4 transcription factors, and promotes the transcription of osteoblastic genes. Wnt pathway is tightly regulated by numerous secreted antagonists that are soluble frizzled-related proteins (sFRPs), which interfere with Wnt/frizzled receptor binding or Dickkopf (DKK) proteins and sclerostin, which bind the co-receptor LRP5/6. Indeed, loss-of-function mutations in *LRP5* gene cause osteoporosis–pseudoglioma syndrome [84]. Mutations in LRP5 cause high bone mass syndrome [85–89]. Whereas, mutations in *SOST* (which encodes sclerostin) result in sclerosteosis or Van Buchem disease, respectively [90–93]. Genetic deletion of β-catenin in embryonic mesenchymal progenitors abolishes mature OB generation [94–97].

Noncanonical Wnt glycoproteins such as WNT5A, WNT5B, WNT6, WNT7B, WNT11, and WNT16 can trigger the planar cell polarity (PCP) pathway or the Wnt/Ca^{2+} signaling. The PCP pathway affects cell orientation in tissues as well as cell mobility, shape, differentiation, and communication. WNT5A is fundamental for controlling the PCP pathway through a DSH, Ras homolog gene family member (RhoB) and the small GTPase Rab4, activating kinases such as the c-Jun N-terminal kinase (JNK) controlling cytoskeletal rearrangements [98, 99]. The Wnt/Ca^{2+} pathway triggers the activation of phospholipase C with consequent release of calcium that sequentially stimulates NFAT [100, 101]. Calcium signaling is engaged for cell fate and cell migration.

WNT5A was first classified as a noncanonical Wnt that activates β-catenin-independent pathways. However, recent studies demonstrated that the downstream signaling of WNT5A can affect canonical β-catenin-dependent signaling [102]. Indeed depending on the receptor availability, noncanonical Wnts such as WNT5A or WNT16 can trigger or even antagonize alternative pathways [102, 103]. Thus, the division between canonical and noncanonical signaling pathways is becoming progressively more imprecise.

BMP Signaling

BMPs, a TGFβ superfamily member, bind to receptor complexes composed of heterotetramers of type I and type II Ser/Thr kinase receptors and activate SMADs (SMAD1, SMAD5, or SMAD8). The phosphorylated SMADs form a complex with SMAD4 and translocate into the nucleus to regulate gene expression. Genetic studies have shown that BMP2 and BMP4 signaling is required for differentiation to mature OBs. Furthermore, mice lacking only BMP2 in the limb mesenchyme formed bone during embryogenesis but exhibited a clear defect in bone mineral density shortly after birth, resulting in frequent fractures that failed to heal [104]. Deletion of BMP receptor 1A (BMPR1A) in pre-osteoblasts and OBs, either in utero or postnatally, resulted in an unexpected increase in bone mass [105–107]. These studies indicated that, although BMPR1A loss decreased bone formation, it also reduced bone resorption to a greater extent, resulting in a net increase in bone mass. Thus, BMP signaling in OB lineage cells seems to also have an important role in regulating OCs. In addition to its role in OB differentiation, BMP signaling regulates the function of mature OBs. Deletion of BMPR1A in mature OBs decreased OB function [108], whereas overexpression of noggin, a secreted inhibitor for BMPs, caused a reduction in OB function and a lower bone mass in mice postnatally [109]. Similarly, deletion of SMAD4 in mature OBs impaired OB activity [110]. Interestingly, BMP3 may counteract BMP2 and BMP4 activity to maintain a proper bone mass in vivo, as BMP3 knockout mice had increase trabecular bone respect to wild-type mice.

Semaphorins

Semaphorins emerged as a family of cell surface attached or secreted proteins. The semaphorins are grouped into eight major classes [111]: the first seven are ordered by number, from class 1 to class 7; the eighth group is class V (V stands for virus). Classes 1 and 2 are found in invertebrates only, while classes 3, 4, 6, and 7 are found in vertebrates only. Class 5 is found in both vertebrates and invertebrates, and class V is specific to viruses. Most semaphorins use receptors in the group of proteins known as plexins. Class 3 semaphorins signal through heterocomplexes of neuropilins, class A plexins, and cell adhesion molecules; class 7 semaphorin use integrins as their receptors. Recently, it emerged the role of semaphorins in the regulation of bone cell activity. In detail, Sema3A is abundantly expressed in bone, and cell-based assays showed that Sema3A affected OB differentiation [112]. Semaphorin 3A (Sema3A) has an osteoprotective effect by both inhibiting bone resorption and promoting bone formation. The binding of Sema3A to neuropilin-1 (Nrp1) suppressed RANKL-induced osteoclastogenesis. Furthermore, Sema3A and Nrp1 binding promotes osteoblastogenesis and suppresses adipogenesis through canonical Wnt/β-catenin pathway [112]. In mice Sema3A injection augmented bone volume and accelerated bone regeneration. Further studies showed that osteoblast-specific Sema3A-deficient mice had normal bone mass [113]. In contrast, mice lacking Sema3A in neurons had low bone mass, comparable to Sema3a-KO mice, signifying that neuron-derived Sema3A is responsible for the observed bone alterations independent of the local effect of Sema3A in the bone [113].

OCs express semaphorin 4D (Sema4D), which strongly suppresses bone formation [114]. On OBs the binding of Sema4D to its receptor plexin-B1 resulted in the suppression of IGF-1 signaling and by modulating OB motility. *Sema4d−/−* mice and *Plxnb1−/−* mice specifically in OBs showed increased bone mass due to augmented bone formation. Notably, mice treatment with Sema4D neutralizing antibody prevented bone loss in postmenopausal osteoporosis murine model.

Semaphorin 7A (SEMA7A) has been shown to play a crucial role in the activation of monocyte/macrophages, thus contributing to osteoclastogenesis [115]. Polymorphisms of the *SEMA7A* gene were associated with low bone mineral density of the lumbar spine and femoral neck and with risk of vertebral fracture [116].

Semaphorin 3B (SEMA3B) has been identified as a 1,25(OH)(2)D(3)-stimulated gene in osteoblastic cells. Moreover, during OB differentiation SEMA3B gene expression increased. Transgenic SEMA3B mice showed reduced bone mineral density and altered trabecular bone, due to increased OC numbers and activity [117].

Collectively, these studies support the key role of semaphorins in the regulation of skeletal homeostasis.

Lipocalin-2

Lipocalin-2 (LCN2) is a 25-kD adipokine belonging to a large superfamily of proteins that bind and transport lipids and other hydrophobic molecules. In mice subjected to experimentally induced mechanical unloading, *Lcn2* expression was upregulated in the long bones [118]. In primary OBs transfected with LCN2-expression-vector (OBs-Lcn2), the levels of *Runx2*, *Osterix*, and *Alp* were downregulated, whereas *IL-6* mRNA and the *Rankl/Opg* ratio were p-regulated. These findings suggest that LCN2 directly affect osteoblastogenesis and indirectly osteoclastogenesis [118].

The Myokine Irisin

Irisin was originally identified as hormone-like myokine, secreted from skeletal muscle in response to exercise both in mice and humans, and able to induce the so-called browning response in white adipose tissue [119]. However, latest evidence has questioned the primary biological role of irisin, demonstrating that irisin also targets bone tissue directly, driving positive effects on cortical mineral density and improving bone strength and geometry in mice [120]. This study highlighted a new biological significance of irisin as one of the molecules responsible for the yet poorly characterized bone-muscle unit and suggested that irisin might be the link between physical exercise and healthy bone. The effect of irisin on the bone is mainly exerted on OB lineage by enhancing differentiation and activity of bone-forming cells, through the upregulation of the Atf4. The increased differentiation and activity of OBs were also proved by the enhancement of ALP-positive colonies and nodules of mineralized matrix. Consistently, the expression of ALP and COLL I mRNA were upregulated by irisin treatment in vitro [120, 121]. Although its receptor has not been identified yet, the action of irisin on OB is receptor mediated, as demonstrated by the activation of the MAP kinases Erk and p38 upon r-irisin administration in vitro [120–122].

In vivo data also showed higher Atf4 expression in bone marrow of irisin-treated mice, suggesting a substantial commitment of OB precursor toward osteogenesis. In addition, long bones of r-irisin-treated mice expressed high level of osteopontin, one of the most abundant protein of bone matrix that is also known to be a mechanically responsive molecule [123], and strongly reduced expression of sclerostin, one of the inhibitors of the bone anabolic Wnt pathway [124].

1.8 Osteocytes

Osteocytes, the most abundant cells in the bone, are essential for the maintenance of skeletal homeostasis. Osteocytes orchestrate bone formation during growth and the preservation of a healthy skeletal frame for locomotion. These cells modulate OB and OC activity by releasing factors that allow the skeleton to respond to mechanical needs and hormonal variation. Osteocytes participate to bone endocrine functions by producing hormones that influence other tissues/organs and control mineral metabolism as well as hematopoiesis.

1.9 Osteocytogenesis

About 5–20% of OBs resident on the bone surface are progressively surrounded by the bone matrix proteins they secrete and became osteocytes [125, 126]. This differentiation process is delineated by changes in gene expression and is associated to functional and morphological changes. The active OBs have cuboidal shape, large nucleus located near the basal membrane of the cell, and copious endoplasmic reticulum and Golgi apparatus. During osteocytogenesis, organelle number strongly declines, and the nuclear-to-cytoplasm volume ratio enhances as cells attain a star-like morphology. The cytoplasmic processes of osteocytes are localized in the canaliculi of the mineralized bone and interact with adjacent osteocytes, cells on the bone surface, and endothelial cells of blood vessels. This wide lacunar–canalicular system is preserved by osteocyte capability to remodel their neighboring space. The osteocyte lacunar–canalicular system also permits the diffusion of osteocyte-produced molecules among all the cells of the bone and the bone marrow. Genes that are modulated during osteocytogenesis can be divided, based on their function, into three groups: genes associated to dendritic morphology and canaliculi formation, genes linked to phosphate metabolism and matrix mineralization, and genes modulating bone formation or resorption.

1.9.1 Development and Maintenance of the Osteocytic Network

The differentiation from OBs to osteocytes is mediated by several proteins controlling the development of dendrites and the mineralization and matrix degradation to guarantee the proper formation of the lacunar–canaliculi system.

Podoplanin

Podoplanin is expressed in newly embedded osteocytes, but not in mature osteocytes or in OBs on the bone surface, thereby podoplanin is a marker of early osteocyte differentiation [127]. Podoplanin expression is necessary for elongation of the dendrite and is augmented by mechanical stimulation both in vitro and in vivo. Podoplanin interacts with CD44, and their expression has been linked with dendrite branching of the osteocytes [128, 129]. Osteocytic dendrites also have α-actinin and fimbrin, key proteins for cytoskeletal organization of osteocytes isolated from chicken [130, 131].

Dentin Matrix Acidic Phosphoprotein-1 (DMP-1)

DMP-1 is expressed in mature OBs, and its expression enhances as OBs differentiate toward osteocytes [132]. DMP-1 is necessary for suitable osteocyte maturation. Indeed, in mice lacking DMP1 osteocytes expressed elevated levels of osteoblastic and early osteocytic genes (such as those podoplanin) and low levels of sclerostin (a marker of mature osteocytes) [133]. Additionally, these mice have defective mineralization and disorganized osteocytic lacunar–canalicular system.

MMPs

The expression of MMPs also progressively increases as OBs differentiate into osteocytes. In osteocytogenesis MMP role can be associated to their function to cleave collagen in the matrix surrounding osteocytes, thereby allowing the formation of canaliculi through which osteocytes extend cytoplasmic projections. Consistently, in mice MMP-14 deletion led to few or absent osteocytic processes [134]. Moreover, MMP-13 is required to maintain osteocyte viability [135].

Connexin 43 (CX43)

CX43, critical protein for the activity of the osteocyte network, forms gap junction channels between communicating cells; CX43 also forms hemichannels connecting cells with the extracellular environment. In mice CX43 deletion from osteocytes reduces their viability and determines modifications in long bone geometry [136–138]. In vitro CX43 knockdown leads to cells that die spontaneously and express an increased RANKL/OPG ratio [138]. Furthermore, in CX43 knockout mice, OCs are localized on bone surfaces neighboring to areas where apoptotic osteocytes accumulate, suggesting that signals by dying osteocytes are crucial for OC recruitment.

1.9.2 Phosphate Metabolism and Matrix Mineralization

During osteocytogenesis the genes of the phosphate metabolism and matrix mineralization are highly expressed 35. These genes include fibroblast growth factor 23 (FGF23), DMP-1, matrix extracellular phosphoglycoprotein (MEPE), phosphate-regulating neutral endopeptidase (PHEX), and fetuin-A. FGF23 is expressed by osteocytes and affects phosphate metabolism by targeting the kidney. FGF23 interacts with FGF receptors and klotho co-receptor in the renal proximal tubule, which results into inhibition of renal phosphate reabsorption [139]. Fgf23 knockout mice showed hyperphosphatemia, decreased BMD, reduced bone formation, and accumulation of unmineralized osteoid [140].

FGF23 also works in an autocrine and/or paracrine way in osteocytes and other bone cells, as FGF receptor 1 (FGFR1) and klotho are also present on these cells. Other osteocyte-produced molecules affect FGF23 expression and/or function and consequently indirectly influence phosphate metabolism. Indeed, in humans inactivating mutations in DMP1 or PHEX lead to high levels of FGF23 and hypophosphatemia [141].

DMP-1 is necessary for correct bone mineralization, whereas MEPE is an inhibitor of the mineralization whose deletion in mice leads to increased bone mineral density [142]. DMP-1 and MEPE expression is increased by loading, and these proteins might mediate the local outcomes of mechanical stimulation in the matrix neighboring osteocytes [143]. Enzymatic degradation of MEPE generates a peptide that blocks mineralization both in vitro and in vivo [144]. PHEX is a metalloendopeptidase that interacts with MEPE and its peptide. Phex knockout mice develops osteomalacia and an altered osteocytic lacuna–canalicular system [145].

The liver protein fetuin-A, bone mineralization and calcification inhibitor, has been found in the bone and is more expressed by osteocytes compared with OBs [146]. Fetuin-A might be involved in the formation of dendrites by slowing matrix calcification of the surroundings developing osteocytes. Thus, phosphate metabolism regulation results from highly interconnected functions of these osteocytic proteins, because changes in the levels of one of them modifies the expression of the others, thereby generating a cascade of events that finally affects bone mineralization.

1.9.3 Regulation of Bone Formation and Resorption

Wnt Signaling

The Wnt antagonist DKK-1 is expressed in OBs and at higher levels in osteocytes [147]. Another Wnt inhibitor, secreted frizzled-related protein-1 (SFRP-1), is present in early osteocytes, and its expression decreases in mature osteocytes [148]. Another Wnt signaling antagonist, sclerostin, is primarily expressed in mature osteocytes and not in early osteocytes or OBs [149]. Sclerostin also binds to LRP4, which is required for the inhibitory action of sclerostin on Wnt–βcatenin signaling [150]. Importantly, osteocyte-targeted deletion of Lrp5 or overexpression of high bone mass LRP5 mutants in osteocytes repeats the low or high bone mass phenotypes displayed by mice or humans with the genetic modifications in all cells [151], suggesting that activation of the Wnt pathway in osteocytes is sufficient to achieve bone formation downstream of LRP5 [86, 151].

Osteocalcin (OCN), the most abundant non-collagenous protein present in the bone, is an inhibitor of bone formation, as evidenced by the high bone mass in the absence of defective bone mineralization or bone resorption in mice. OCN is a marker of OBs. However, in mice OCN is expressed at higher levels in osteocytes than in OBs [152], and osteocytes are more abundant than OBs. Osteocytes with the OBs, therefore, possibly contribute to the pool of OCN in the circulation. Studies in mice have also demonstrated that OCN in its undercarboxylated form can modulate insulin secretion by pancreatic β-cells, insulin sensitivity and glucose uptake in muscle, and fat metabolism [153].

RANKL

Osteocytes also secrete RANKL. In studies using genetically modified mice, deletion of *RANKL* from osteocytes renders mice osteopetrotic, due to a reduced number of OCs, decreased bone resorption, and a progressive increase in bone mass [154], which suggests that osteocytes are an important source of RANKL in the bone.

MCSF

Similar to MCSF knockout mice in all tissues, targeting deletion of MCSF in osteocytes led to reduced OC numbers and osteopetrosis, demonstrating that osteocytes are a key source of MCSF in the bone [155]. Osteocytes also express c-fms, the receptors for MCSF [147], and mice lacking osteocytic MCSF have osteocytes with abnormal morphology, a high prevalence of apoptosis, and reduced gap junctions [155]. These results suggest that osteocytes are both important source and target of MCSF.

OPG

The anti-osteoclastogenic molecule OPG is produced in both OBs and osteocytes, and OPG mRNA levels are more profuse in osteocytes than in OBs [156]. Moreover, OPG is a target of canonical Wnt signaling, and mice lacking β-catenin in OBs and/or osteocytes show in the same way reduced OPG levels, increased OC number, and low bone mass [156–158]. Therefore, the modulation of osteocytic OPG by canonical Wnt signaling has key role in bone resorption control.

References

1. Cappariello A, Ponzetti M, Rucci N. The "soft" side of the bone: unveiling its endocrine functions. Horm Mol Biol Clin Invest. 2016;28(1):5–20. https://doi.org/10.1515/hmbci-2016-0009.
2. Novack DV, Mbalaviele G. Osteoclasts-key players in skeletal health and disease. Microbiol Spectr. 2016;4(3). https://doi.org/10.1128/microbiolspec.MCHD-0011-2015.
3. Takahashi N, Akatsu Y, Udawa N, et al. Osteoblastic cells are involved in osteoclast formation. Endocrinology. 1988;123:2600–2. https://doi.org/10.1210/endo-123-5-2600.

4. Udafawa N, Takahashi N, Akatsu T, et al. Origin of osteoclasts: mature monocytes and macrophages are capable of differentiating into osteoclasts under a suitable microenviroment prepared by bone marrow-derived stromal cells. Proc Natl Acad Sci U S A. 1990;87:7260–4.
5. Stanley ER, Chitu V. CSF-1 receptor signalling in myeloid cells. Cold Spring Harb Perspect Biol. 2014;6:a021857. https://doi.org/10.1101/cshperspect.a021857.
6. Glantschnig H, Fisher JE, Wsolowski G, et al. M-CSF, TNFa and RANK ligand promote osteoclast survival by signalling hrough mTOR/S6 kinase. Cell Death Differ. 2003;10:1165–77. https://doi.org/10.1038/sj.cdd.4401285.
7. Zamani A, Decker C, Cremasco V, et al. Diacylglycerol kinase ζ (DGKζ) is a critical regulator of bone homeostasis via modulation of c-Fos levels in osteoclasts. J Bone Miner Res. 2015;30:1852–63. https://doi.org/10.1002/jbmr.2533.
8. Li J, Chen L, Zhu L, Pollard JW. Conditional deletion of the colony stimulating factor-1 receptor (c-fms proto-oncogene) in mice. Genesis. 2006;44:328–35. https://doi.org/10.1002/dvg.20219.
9. Chen Z, Buki K, Vaananen HK. The critical role of IL-34 in osteoclastogenesis. PLoS One. 2011;6:e18689. https://doi.org/10.1371/journal.pone.0018689.
10. Kong YY, Yoshida H, Sarosi I, et al. OPGL is a key regulator of osteoclastogenesis, lymphocyte development and lymph-node organogenesis. Nature. 1999;397:315–23. https://doi.org/10.1038/16852.
11. Bucay N, Sarosi I, Duncstan CR, et al. Osteoprotegerin-deficient mice develop eartly onset osteoporosis and arterial calcification. Genes Dev. 1998;12:1260–8.
12. Whyte MP, Tau C, McAlister W, et al. Juvenile Paget's disease with heterozygous duplication within TNFRSF11A encoding RANKL. Bone. 2014;68:153–61. https://doi.org/10.1016/j.bone.2014.07.019.
13. Brunetti G, Marzano F, Colucci S, Ventura A, et al. Genotype-phenotype correlation in juvenile paget disease: role of molecular alterations of the TNFRSF11B gene. Endocrine. 2012;42(2):266–71. https://doi.org/10.1007/s12020-012-9705-0.
14. Hughes AE, Ralston SH, Marken J, et al. Mutations in TNFRSF11A, affectiong the signal peptide of RANK, cause familial expansile osteolysis. Nat Genet. 2000;24:45–8. https://doi.org/10.1038/71667.
15. Novack DV, Teitelbaum SL. The osteoclast: friend or foe? Annu Rev Pathol. 2008;3:457–84. https://doi.org/10.1146/annurev.pathmechdis.3.121806.151431.
16. Smink JJ, Bégay V, Schoenmaker T, et al. Transcription facton C/EBPb isoform ratio regulates osteoclastogenesis through MafB. EMBO J. 2009;28:1769–81. https://doi.org/10.1038/emboj.2009.127.
17. Takayanagi H, Kim S, Koga T, et al. Induction and activation of the transcription factor NFATc1 (NFAT2) instegrate RANKL signalling in terminal differentiation of osteoclasts. Dev Cell. 2002;3:889–901. https://doi.org/10.1016/S1534-5807(02)00369-6.
18. Alhawagri M, Yamanaka Y, Ballard D, et al. Lysine392, a K63-linked ubiquination site in NEMO mediates inglammatory osteoclastogenesis and osteolysis. J Orthop Res. 2012;30:554–60. https://doi.org/10.1002/jor.21555.
19. Mao D, Epple H, Uthgenannt B, et al. PLCy2 regulates osteoclastogenesis via its interaction with ITAM proteins and GAB2. J Clin Invest. 2006;116:2869–79. https://doi.org/10.1172/JCI28775.
20. Bronisz A, Carey HA, Godlewski J, et al. The multifunctional protein fusd in sarcoma (FUS) is a coactivator of microphtalmia-associated transcription factor (MITF). J Biol Chem. 2014;289:326–34. https://doi.org/10.1074/jbc.M113.493874.
21. Yasui T, Hirose J, Aburatani H, et al. Epigenetic regulation of osteoclast differentiation. Ann N Y Acad Sci. 2011;1240:7–13. https://doi.org/10.1111/j.1749-6632.2011.06245.x.
22. Kim JH, Kim N. Reguation of NFATc1 in osteoclast differentiation. J Bone Metab. 2014;21:233–41. https://doi.org/10.11005/jbm.2014.21.4.233.
23. Mizoguchi F, Izu Y, Hayata T, et al. Osteoclast-specific Dicer gene deficiency suppresses osteoclastic bone resorption. J Cell Biochem. 2010;109:866–75. https://doi.org/10.1002/jcb.22228.

24. Yasui T, Hirose J, Tsutsumi S, et al. Epigenetic regulation of osteoclast differentiation: possible involvement of Jmjd3 in the histone demethylation of Nfact1. J Bone Miner Res. 2011;26:2665–71. https://doi.org/10.1002/jbmr.464.
25. Luo J, Yang Z, Ma Y, et al. LGR4 is a receptor for RANKL and negatively regulates osteoclast differentiation and bone resorption. Nat Med. 2016;22(5):539–46. https://doi.org/10.1038/nm.4076.
26. Zou W, Reeve JL, Iu Y, et al. DAP12 couples c-Fms activation to the osteoclast cytoskeleton by recruitment of Syk. Mol Cell. 2008;31:422–31. https://doi.org/10.1016/j.molcel.2008.06.023.
27. Mòcsai A, Humpherey MB, Van Ziffle JAG, et al. The immunomodulatory adapter proteins DAP12 and Fc receptor y-chain (FcRy) regulate development of functional osteoclasts through the Syk tyrosine kinase. Proc Natl Acad Sci U S A. 2004;101:6158–63. https://doi.org/10.1073/pnas.0401602101.
28. Koga T, Inui M, Inour L, et al. Costimulatory signals mediated by the ITAM motif cooperate with RANKL for bone homeostasis. Nature. 2004;428:758–63. https://doi.org/10.1038/nature02444.
29. Zou W, Teitelbaum SL. Absence of Dap12 and the avb3 integrin causes severe ostepetrosis. J Cell Biol. 2015;208:125–36. https://doi.org/10.1083/jcb.201410123.
30. Johnson RA, Boyce BF, Mundy GR, et al. Tumors producing human necrosis factor induce hypercalcemia and osteoclastic bone resorption in nude mice. Endocrinology. 1989;124:1424–7.
31. Pfeilschifter J, Chenu C, Bird A, et al. Interleukin-1 and tumor necrosis factor stimulate the formation of human osteoclastlike cells in vitro. J Bone Miner Res. 1989;4:113–8. https://doi.org/10.1002/jbmr.5650040116.
32. Azuma Y, Kaji L, Katogi R, et al. Tumor necrosis factor-a induces differentiation of and bone resorption by osteoclasts. J Biol Chem. 2000;275:4858–64. https://doi.org/10.1074/jbc.275.7.4858.
33. Kudo O, Fujikawa Y, Itonaga I, et al. Proinflammatory cytokine (TNFa/IL-1alpha) induction of human osteoclast formation. J Pathol. 2002;198:220–7. https://doi.org/10.1002/path.1190.
34. Lam J, Takeshita S, Barker JE, et al. TNF-a induces osteoclastogenesis by direct stimulation of macrophages exposed to permissive levels of RANK ligand. J Clin Invest. 2000;106:1481–8. https://doi.org/10.1172/JCI11176.
35. O'Gradaigh D, Ireland D, Bord S, et al. Joint erosion in rheumatoid arthritis: interactions between tumour necrosis factor a, interleukin 1, and receptor activator of nuclear factor kB ligand (RANKL) regulate osteoclasts. Ann Rheum Dis. 2004;63:354–9. https://doi.org/10.1136/ard.2003.008458.
36. Novack DV, Yin L, Hagen-Stapleton A, et al. The IkB function of NF-kB2 p100 controls stimulated osteoclatogenesis. J Exp Med. 2003;198:771–81. https://doi.org/10.1084/jem.20030116.
37. Zhao B, Grimes SN, Li S, et al. TNF-induced osteoclastogensis and inflammatory bone resorption are inhibited by transcription factor RBP-J. J Exp Med. 2012;209:319–34. https://doi.org/10.1084/jem.20111566.
38. Mauri DN, Ebner R, Montgomery RI, et al. LIGHT, a new member of the TNF superfamily, and lymphotoxin α are ligands for herpesvirus entry mediator. Immunity. 1998;8:21–30. https://doi.org/10.1016/S1074-7613(00)80455-0.
39. Tamada K, Shimozaki K, Chapoval AI, et al. LIGHT, a TNF-like molecule, costimulates T cell proliferation and is required for dendritic cell-mediated allogeneic T cell response. J Immunol. 2000;164:4105–10. https://doi.org/10.4049/jimmunol.164.8.4105.
40. Holmes TD, Wilson EB, Black EV, et al. Licensed human natural killer cells aid dendritic cell maturation via TNFSF14/LIGHT. Proc Natl Acad Sci U S A. 2014;111(52):E5688–96. https://doi.org/10.1073/pnas.1411072112.
41. Harrop JA, Reddy M, Dede K, et al. Antibodies to TR2 (herpesvirus entry mediator), a new member of the TNF receptor superfamily, block T cell proliferation, expression of activation markers, and production of cytokines. J Immunol. 1998;161:1786–94.

42. Kwon BS, Tan KB, Ni J, et al. A newly identified member of the tumor necrosis factor receptor superfamily with a wide tissue distribution and involvement in lymphocyte activation. J Biol Chem. 1997;272:14272–6. https://doi.org/10.1074/jbc.272.22.14272.
43. Browning JL, Miatkowski K, Sizing I, et al. Signaling through the lymphotoxin β receptor induces the death of some adenocarcinoma tumor lines. J Exp Med. 1996;183:867–78.
44. Harrop JA, McDonnell PC, Brigham-Burke M, et al. Herpesvirus entry mediator ligand (HVEM-L), a novel ligand for HVEM/TR2, stimulates proliferation of T cells and inhibits HT29 cell growth. J Biol Chem. 1998;273:27548–56. https://doi.org/10.1074/jbc.273.42.27548.
45. Hsu H, Solovyev I, Colombero A, et al. ATAR, a novel tumor necrosis factor receptor family member, signals through TRAF2 and TRAF5. J Biol Chem. 1997;272:13471–4. https://doi.org/10.1074/jbc.272.21.13471.
46. Marsters SA, Ayres TM, Skubatch M, et al. Herpesvirus entry mediator, a member of the tumor necrosis factor receptor (TNFR) family, interacts with members of the TNFR-associated factor family and activates the transcription factors NF-kappaB and AP-1. J Biol Chem. 1997;272:14029–32. https://doi.org/10.1074/jbc.272.22.14029.
47. Arch RH, Gedrich RW, Thompson CB. Tumor necrosis factor receptor-associated factors (TRAFs)—a family of adapter proteins that regulates life and death. Genes Dev. 1998;12:2821–30. https://doi.org/10.1101/gad.12.18.2821.
48. Zhai Y, Guo R, Hsu TL, et al. LIGHT, a novel ligand for lymphotoxin beta receptor and TR2/HVEM induces apoptosis and suppresses in vivo tumor formation via gene transfer. J Clin Invest. 1998;102:1142–51. https://doi.org/10.1172/JCI3492.
49. Rooney IA, Butrovich KD, Glass AA, et al. The lymphotoxin-beta receptor is necessary and sufficient for LIGHT-mediated apoptosis of tumor cells. J Biol Chem. 2000;275:14307–15. https://doi.org/10.1074/jbc.275.19.14307.
50. Granger SW, Rickert S. LIGHT-HVEM signaling and the regulation of T cell-mediated immunity. Cytokine Growth Factor Rev. 2003;14:289–96. https://doi.org/10.1172/JCI11176.
51. Tamada K, Shimozaki K, Chapoval AI, et al. Modulation of T-cell-mediated immunity in tumor and graft-versus-host disease models through the LIGHT co-stimulatory pathway. Nat Med. 2000;6:283–9. https://doi.org/10.1038/73136.
52. Shaikh RB, Santee S, Granger SW, et al. Constitutive expression of LIGHT on T cells leads to lymphocyte activation, inflammation, and tissue destruction. J Immunol. 2001;167:6330–7. https://doi.org/10.4049/jimmunol.167.11.6330.
53. Wang J, Lo JC, Foster A, et al. The regulation of T cell homeostasis and autoimmunity by T cell-derived LIGHT. J Clin Invest. 2001;108:1771–80. https://doi.org/10.1172/JCI13827.
54. Colucci S, Brunetti G, Mori G, et al. Soluble decoy receptor 3 modulates the survival and formation of osteoclasts from multiple myeloma bone disease patients. Leukemia. 2009;23(11):2139–46. https://doi.org/10.1038/leu.2009.136.
55. Ishida S, Yamane S, Nakano S, et al. The interaction of monocytes with rheumatoid synovial cells is a key step in LIGHT-mediated inflammatory bone destruction. Immunology. 2009;128:e315–24. https://doi.org/10.1111/j.1365-2567.2008.02965.x.
56. Edwards JR, Sun SG, Locklin R, et al. LIGHT (TNFSF14), a novel mediator of bone resorption, is elevated in rheumatoid arthritis. Arthritis Rheum. 2006;54:1451–62. https://doi.org/10.1002/art.21821.
57. Hemingway F, Kashima TG, Knowles HJ, et al. Investigation of osteoclastogenic signalling of the RANKL substitute LIGHT. Exp Mol Pathol. 2013;94:380–5. https://doi.org/10.1016/j.yexmp.2013.01.003.
58. Brunetti G, Rizzi R, Oranger A, et al. LIGHT/TNFSF14 increases osteoclastogenesis and decreases osteoblastogenesis in multiple myeloma-bone disease. Oncotarget. 2014;5(24):12950–67. https://doi.org/10.18632/oncotarget.2633.
59. Brunetti G, Faienza MF, Colaianni G, et al. Impairment of Bone Remodeling in LIGHT/TNFSF14-Deficient Mice. J Bone Miner Res. 2018;33:704–19. https://doi.org/10.1002/jbmr.3345.

60. Colucci S, Mori G, Brunetti G, et al. Interleukin-7 production by B lymphocytes affects the T cell-dependent osteoclast formation in an in vitro model derived from human periodontitis patients. Int J Immunopathol Pharmacol. 2005;18(3 Suppl):13–9.
61. Yao Z, Painter SL, Fanslow WC, et al. Human IL-17: a novel cytokine derived from T cells. J Immunol. 1995;155:5483–6.
62. Lubberts E, Koenders M, van den Berg WB. The role of T cell interleukin-17 in conducting destructive arthritis: lessons from animal models. Arthritis Res Ther. 2005;7:29–37. https://doi.org/10.1186/ar1478.
63. Long F. Building strong bones: molecular regulation of the osteoblast lineage. Nat Rev Mol Cell Biol. 2011;13(1):27–38. https://doi.org/10.1038/nrm3254.
64. Yasuda H, Shima N, Nakagawa N, et al. Osteoclast differentiation factor is a ligand for osteoprotegerin/osteoclastogenesis-inhibitory factor and is identical to TRANCE/RANKL. Proc Natl Acad Sci U S A. 1998;95:3597–602.
65. Komori T, Yagi H, Nomura S, et al. Targeted disruption of Cbfa1 results in a complete lack of bone formation owing to maturational arrest of osteoblasts. Cell. 1997;89:755–64. https://doi.org/10.1016/S0092-8674(00)80258-5.
66. Mundlos S, Otto F, Mundlos C, et al. Mutations involving the transcription factor CBFA1 cause cleidocranial dysplasia. Cell. 1997;89:773–9. https://doi.org/10.1016/S0092-8674(00)80260-3.
67. Lee B, Thirunavukkarasu K, Zhou L, et al. Missense mutations abolishing DNA binding of the osteoblast-specific transcription factor OSF2/CBFA1 in cleidocranial dysplasia. Nat Genet. 1997;16:307–10. https://doi.org/10.1038/ng0797-307.
68. Faienza MF, Ventura A, Piacente L, et al. Osteoclastogenic potential of peripheral blood mononuclear cells in cleidocranial dysplasia. Int J Med Sci. 2014;11(4):356–64. https://doi.org/10.7150/ijms.7793.
69. Ducy P, Starbuck M, Priemel M, et al. A Cbfa1-dependent genetic pathway controls bone formation beyond embryonic development. Genes Dev. 1999;13:1025–36.
70. Lian JB, Javed A, Zaidi SK, et al. Regulatory controls for osteoblast growth and differentiation: role of Runx/Cbfa/AML factors. Crit Rev Eukaryot Gene Expr. 2004;14(1-2):1–41. https://doi.org/10.1615/CritRevEukaryotGeneExpr.v14.i12.10.
71. Nakashima K, Zhou X, Kunkel G, et al. The novel zinc finger-containing transcription factor osterix is required for osteoblast differentiation and bone formation. Cell. 2002;108:17–29. https://doi.org/10.1016/S0092-8674(01)00622-5.
72. Zhou X, Zhang Z, Feng JQ, et al. Multiple functions of Osterix are required for bone growth and homeostasis in postnatal mice. Proc Natl Acad Sci U S A. 2010;107:12919–24. https://doi.org/10.1073/pnas.0912855107.
73. Yang X, Matsuda K, Bialek P, et al. ATF4 is a substrate of RSK2 and an essential regulator of osteoblast biology; implication for Coffin–Lowry Syndrome. Cell. 2004;117:387–98. https://doi.org/10.1016/S0092-8674(04)00344-7.
74. Elefteriou F, Benson MD, Sowa H, et al. ATF4 mediation of NF1 functions in osteoblast reveals a nutritional basis for congenital skeletal dysplasiae. Cell Metab. 2006;4:441–51. https://doi.org/10.1016/j.cmet.2006.10.010.
75. Eferl R, Wagner EF. AP-1: a double-edged sword in tumorigenesis. Nat Rev Cancer. 2003;3:859–68. https://doi.org/10.1038/nrc1209.
76. Eferl R, Hoebertz A, Schilling AF, et al. The Fos-related antigen Fra-1 is an activator of bone matrix formation. EMBO J. 2004;23:2789–99. https://doi.org/10.1038/sj.emboj.7600282.
77. Bozec A, Bakiri L, Jimenez M, et al. Fra-2/AP-1 controls bone formation by regulating osteoblast differentiation and collagen production. J Cell Biol. 2010;190:1093–106. https://doi.org/10.1083/jcb.201002111.
78. Jochum W, David JP, Elliott C, et al. Increased bone formation and osteosclerosis in mice overexpressing the transcription factor Fra-1. Nat Med. 2000;6:980–4. https://doi.org/10.1038/79676.
79. Kveiborg M, Sabatakos G, Chiusaroli R, et al. ΔFosB induces osteosclerosis and decreases adipogenesis by two independent cellautonomous mechanisms. Mol Cell Biol. 2004;24:2820–30. https://doi.org/10.1128/MCB.24.7.2820-2830.2004.

80. Sabatakos G, Sims NA, Chen J, et al. Overexpression of ΔFosB transcription factor(s) increases bone formation and inhibits adipogenesis. Nat Med. 2000;6:985–90. https://doi.org/10.1038/79683.
81. Huelsken J, Birchmeier W. New aspects of Wnt signaling pathways in higher vertebrates. Curr Opin Genet Dev. 2001;11:547–53. https://doi.org/10.1016/S0959-437X(00)00231-8.
82. Veeman MT, Axelrod JD, Moon RT. A second canon. Functions and mechanisms of β-catenin-independent Wnt signaling. Dev Cell. 2003;5:367–77. https://doi.org/10.1016/S1534-5807(03)00266-1.
83. Wu X, Tu X, Joeng KS, et al. Rac1 activation controls nuclear localization of β-catenin during canonical Wnt signaling. Cell. 2008;133:340–53. https://doi.org/10.1016/j.cell.2008.01.052.
84. Gong Y, Slee RB, Fukai N, et al. LDL receptor-related protein 5 (LRP5) affects bone accrual and eye development. Cell. 2001;107:513–23. https://doi.org/10.1016/S0092-8674(01)00571-2.
85. Boyden LM, Mao J, Belsky J, et al. High bone density due to a mutation in LDL-receptor-related protein 5. N Engl J Med. 2002;346:1513–21. https://doi.org/10.1056/NEJMoa013444.
86. Little RD, Carulli JP, Del Mastro RG, et al. A mutation in the LDL receptorrelated protein 5 gene results in the autosomal dominant high-bone-mass trait. Am J Hum Genet. 2002;70:11–9. https://doi.org/10.1086/338450.
87. Ai M, Holmen SL, Van Hul W, et al. Reduced affinity to and inhibition by DKK1 form a common mechanism by which high bone mass-associated missense mutations in LRP5 affect canonical Wnt signaling. Mol Cell Biol. 2005;25:4946–55. https://doi.org/10.1128/MCB.25.12.4946-4955.2005.
88. Semenov MV, He X. LRP5 mutations linked to high bone mass diseases cause reduced LRP5 binding and inhibition by SOST. J Biol Chem. 2006;281:38276–84. https://doi.org/10.1074/jbc.M609509200.
89. Ellies DL, Viviano B, McCarthy J, et al. Bone density ligand, Sclerostin, directly interacts with LRP5 but not LRP5G171V to modulate Wnt activity. J Bone Miner Res. 2006;21:1738–49. https://doi.org/10.1359/jbmr.060810.
90. Balemans W, Ebeling M, Patel N, et al. Increased bone density in sclerosteosis is due to the deficiency of a novel secreted protein (SOST). Hum Mol Genet. 2001;10:537–43. https://doi.org/10.1093/hmg/10.5.537.
91. Balemans W, Patel N, Ebeling M, et al. Identification of a 52 kb deletion downstream of the SOST gene in patients with van Buchem disease. J Med Genet. 2002;39:91–7. https://doi.org/10.1136/jmg.39.2.91.
92. Brunkow ME, Gardner JC, Van Ness J. Bone dysplasia sclerosteosis results from loss of the SOST gene product, a novel cystine knot-containing protein. Am J Hum Genet. 2001;68:577–89. https://doi.org/10.1086/318811.
93. Staehling-Hampton K, Proll S, Paeper BW, et al. A 52-kb deletion in the SOST-MEOX1 intergenic region on 17q12-q21 is associated with van Buchem disease in the Dutch population. Am J Med Genet. 2002;110:144–52. https://doi.org/10.1002/ajmg.10401.
94. Hu H, Hilton MJ, Tu X, et al. Sequential roles of Hedgehog and Wnt signaling in osteoblast development. Development. 2005;132:49–60. https://doi.org/10.1242/dev.01564.
95. Rodda SJ, McMahon AP. Distinct roles for Hedgehog and canonical Wnt signaling in specification, differentiation and maintenance of osteoblast progenitors. Development. 2006;133:3231–44. https://doi.org/10.1242/dev.02480.
96. Day TF, Guo X, Garrett-Beal L, et al. Wnt/β-catenin signaling in mesenchymal progenitors controls osteoblast and chondrocyte differentiation during vertebrate skeletogenesis. Dev Cell. 2005;8:739–50. https://doi.org/10.1016/j.devcel.2005.03.016.
97. Hill TP, Spater D, Taketo MM, et al. Canonical Wnt/β-catenin signaling prevents osteoblasts from differentiating into chondrocytes. Dev Cell. 2005;8:727–38. https://doi.org/10.1016/j.devcel.2005.02.013.
98. Qian D, Jones C, Rzadzinska A, et al. Wnt5a functions in planar cell polarity regulation in mice. Dev Biol. 2007;306(1):121–33. https://doi.org/10.1016/j.ydbio.2007.03.011.
99. Witze ES, Litman ES, Argast GM, et al. Wnt5a control of cell polarity and directional movement by polarized redistribution of adhesion receptors. Science. 2008;320(5874):365–9. https://doi.org/10.1126/science.1151250.

100. Gómez-Orte E, Sáenz-Narciso B, Moreno S, et al. Multiple functions of the noncanonical Wnt pathway. Trends Genet. 2013;29(9):545–53. https://doi.org/10.1016/j.tig.2013.06.003.
101. Lories RJ, Corr M, Lane NE. To Wnt or not to Wnt: the bone and joint health dilemma. Nat Rev Rheumatol. 2013;9(6):328–39. https://doi.org/10.1038/nrrheum.2013.25.
102. Mikels AJ, Nusse R. Purified Wnt5a protein activates or inhibits beta-catenin-TCF signaling depending on receptor context. PLoS Biol. 2006;4(4):e115. https://doi.org/10.1371/journal.pbio.0040115.
103. Benhaj K, Akcali KC, Ozturk M. Redundant expression of canonical Wnt ligands in human breast cancer cell lines. Oncol Rep. 2006;15(3):701–7. https://doi.org/10.3892/or.15.3.701.
104. Tsuji K, Bandyopadhyay A, Harfe BD, et al. BMP2 activity, although dispensable for bone formation, is required for the initiation of fracture healing. Nat Genet. 2006;38:1424–9. https://doi.org/10.1038/ng1916.
105. Kamiya N, Ye L, Kobayashi T, Mochida Y, et al. BMP signaling negatively regulates bone mass through sclerostin by inhibiting the canonical Wnt pathway. Development. 2008;135:3801–11. https://doi.org/10.1242/dev.025825.
106. Kamiya N, Ye L, Kobayashi T, et al. Disruption of BMP signaling in osteoblasts through type IA receptor (BMPRIA) increases bone mass. J Bone Miner Res. 2008;23:2007–17. https://doi.org/10.1359/jbmr.080809.
107. Kamiya N, Kobayashi T, Mochida Y, et al. Wnt inhibitors Dkk1 and Sost are downstream targets of BMP signaling through the type IA receptor (BMPRIA) in osteoblasts. J Bone Miner Res. 2010;25:200–10. https://doi.org/10.1359/jbmr.090806.
108. Mishina Y, Starbuck MW, Gentile MA, et al. Bone morphogenetic protein type IA receptor signaling regulates postnatal osteoblast function and bone remodeling. J Biol Chem. 2004;279:27560–6. https://doi.org/10.1074/jbc.M404222200.
109. Devlin RD, Du Z, Pereira RC, et al. Skeletal overexpression of noggin results in osteopenia and reduced bone formation. Endocrinology. 2003;144:1972–8. https://doi.org/10.1210/en.2002-220918.
110. Tan X, Weng T, Zhang J, et al. Smad4 is required for maintaining normal murine postnatal bone homeostasis. J Cell Sci. 2007;120:2162–70. https://doi.org/10.1242/jcs.03466.
111. Negishi-Koga T, Takayanagi H. Bone cell communication factors and Semaphorins. Bonekey Rep. 2012;1:183. https://doi.org/10.1038/bonekey.2012.183.
112. Hayashi M, Nakashima T, Taniguchi M, et al. Osteoprotection by semaphorin 3A. Nature. 2012;485(7396):69–74. https://doi.org/10.1038/nature11000.
113. Fukuda T, Takeda S, Xu R, et al. Sema3A regulates bone-mass accrual through sensory innervations. Nature. 2013;497(7450):490–3. https://doi.org/10.1038/nature12115.
114. Negishi-Koga T, Shinohara M, Komatsu N, et al. Suppression of bone formation by osteoclastic expression of semaphorin 4D. Nat Med. 2011;17(11):1473–80. https://doi.org/10.1038/nm.2489.
115. Holmes S, Downs AM, Fosberry A, et al. Sema7A is a potent monocyte stimulator. Scand J Immunol. 2002;56:270–5. https://doi.org/10.1046/j.1365-3083.2002.01129.x.
116. Koh JM, Oh B, Lee JY, et al. Association study of semaphorin 7a (sema7a) polymorphisms with bone mineral density and fracture risk in postmenopausal Korean women. J Hum Genet. 2006;51(2):112–7. https://doi.org/10.1007/s10038-005-0331-z.
117. Sutton AL, Zhang X, Dowd DR, et al. Semaphorin 3B is a 1,25-Dihydroxyvitamin D3-induced gene in osteoblasts that promotes osteoclastogenesis and induces osteopenia in mice. Mol Endocrinol. 2008;22(6):1370–81. https://doi.org/10.1210/me.2007-0363.
118. Rucci N, Capulli M, Piperni SG, Cappariello A, et al. Lipocalin 2: a new mechanoresponding gene regulating bone homeostasis. J Bone Miner Res. 2015;30(2):357–68. https://doi.org/10.1002/jbmr.2341.
119. Boström P, Wu J, Jedrychowski MP, et al. A PGC1-α-dependent myokine that drives brown-fat-like development of white fat and thermogenesis. Nature. 2012;481:463–8. https://doi.org/10.1038/nature10777.
120. Colaianni G, Cuscito C, Mongelli T, et al. The myokine irisin increases cortical bone mass. Proc Natl Acad Sci U S A. 2015;112:12157–62. https://doi.org/10.1038/bonekey.2015.134.

121. Colaianni G, Cuscito C, Mongelli T, et al. Irisin enhances osteoblast differentiation in vitro. Int J Endocrinol. 2014;2014:902186. https://doi.org/10.1155/2014/902186.
122. Qiao X, Nie Y, Ma Y, et al. Irisin promotes osteoblast proliferation and differentiation via activating the MAP kinase signaling pathways. Sci Rep. 2016;6:21053. https://doi.org/10.1038/srep21053.
123. Toma CD, Ashkar S, Gray ML, et al. Signal transduction of mechanical stimuli is dependent on microfilament integrity: identification of osteopontin as a mechanically induced gene in osteoblasts. J Bone Miner Res. 1997;12(10):1626–36. https://doi.org/10.1359/jbmr.1997.12.10.1626.
124. Lin C, Jiang X, Dai Z, et al. Sclerostin mediates bone response to mechanical unloading through antagonizing Wnt/beta-catenin signaling. J Bone Miner Res. 2009;24(10):1651–61. https://doi.org/10.1359/jbmr.090411.
125. Parfitt AM. The actions of parathyroid hormone on bone: relation to bone remodeling and turnover, calcium homeostasis, and metabolic bone disease. Part I of IV parts: mechanisms of calcium transfer between blood and bone and their cellular basis: morphological and kinetic approaches to bone turnover. Metabolism. 1976;25:809–44.
126. Martin RB, Burr DB, Sharkey NA. Skeletal tissue mechanics. New York: Springer; 1998.
127. Zhang K, Barragan-Adjemian C, Ye L, et al. E11/gp38 selective expression in osteocytes: regulation by mechanical strain and role in dendrite elongation. Mol Cell Biol. 2006;26:4539–52. https://doi.org/10.1128/MCB.02120-05.
128. Hughes DE, Salter DM, Simpson R. CD44 expression in human bone: a novel marker of osteocytic differentiation. J Bone Miner Res. 1994;9:39–44. https://doi.org/10.1002/jbmr.5650090106.
129. Ohizumi I, Harada N, Taniguchi K, et al. Association of CD44 with OTS-8 in tumor vascular endothelial cells. Biochim Biophys Acta. 2000;1497:197–203. https://doi.org/10.1016/S0167-4889(00)00063-X.
130. Tanaka-Kamioka K, Kamioka H, Ris H, et al. Osteocyte shape is dependent on actin filaments and osteocyte processes are unique actin-rich projections. J Bone Miner Res. 1998;13:1555–68. https://doi.org/10.1359/jbmr.1998.13.10.1555.
131. Kamioka H, Sugawara Y, Honjo T, et al. Terminal differentiation of osteoblasts to osteocytes is accompanied by dramatic changes in the distribution of actin-binding proteins. J Bone Miner Res. 2004;19:471–8. https://doi.org/10.1359/JBMR.040128.
132. Bellido T, Plotkin LI, Bruzzaniti A. In: Burr D, Allen M, editors. Bone cells in basic and applied bone biology. Waltham: Elsevier; 2014. p. 27–45.
133. Feng JQ, Ward LM, Liu S, et al. Loss of DMP1 causes rickets and osteomalacia and identifies a role for osteocytes in mineral metabolism. Nat Genet. 2006;38:1310–5. https://doi.org/10.1038/ng1905.
134. Holmbeck K, Bianco P, Pidoux I, et al. The metalloproteinase MT1-MMP is required for normal development and maintenance of osteocyte processes in bone. J Cell Sci. 2005;118:147–56. https://doi.org/10.1242/jcs.01581.
135. Zhao W, Byrne MH, Wang Y, et al. Osteocyte and osteoblast apoptosis and excessive bone deposition accompany failure of collagenase cleavage of collagen. J Clin Invest. 2000;106:941–9. https://doi.org/10.1172/JCI10158.
136. Qiu S, Rao DS, Palnitkar S, et al. Age and distance from the surface but not menopause reduce osteocyte density in human cancellous bone. Bone. 2002;31(2):313–8. https://doi.org/10.1016/S8756-3282(02)00819-0.
137. Almeida M, Han L, Martin-Millan M, et al. Skeletal involution by age-associated oxidative stress and its acceleration by loss of sex steroids. J Biol Chem. 2007;282(37):27285–97. https://doi.org/10.1074/jbc.M702810200.
138. Bivi N, Condon KW, Allen MR, et al. Cell autonomous requirement of connexin 43 for osteocyte survival: consequences for endocortical resorption and periosteal bone formation. J Bone Miner Res. 2012;27(2):374–89. https://doi.org/10.1002/jbmr.548.
139. Shimada T, Mizutani S, Muto T, et al. Cloning and characterization of FGF23 as a causative factor of tumor-induced osteomalacia. Proc Natl Acad Sci U S A. 2001;98(11):6500–5. https://doi.org/10.1073/pnas.101545198.

140. Sitara D, Razzaque MS, Hesse M, et al. Homozygous ablation of fibroblast growth factor-23 results in hyperphosphatemia and impaired skeletogenesis, and reverses hypophosphatemia in Phex-deficient mice. Matrix Biol. 2004;23(7):421–32. https://doi.org/10.1016/j.matbio.2004.09.007.
141. Feng JQ, Clinkenbeard EL, Yuan B, et al. Osteocyte regulation of phosphate homeostasis and bone mineralization underlies the pathophysiology of the heritable disorders of rickets and osteomalacia. Bone. 2013;54(2):213–21. https://doi.org/10.1016/j.bone.2013.01.046.
142. Gowen LC, Petersen DN, Mansolf AL, et al. Targeted disruption of the osteoblast/osteocyte factor 45 gene (OF45) results in increased bone formation and bone mass. J Biol Chem. 2003;278(3):1998–2007. https://doi.org/10.1074/jbc.M203250200.
143. Harris SE, Gluhak-Heinrich J, Harris MA, et al. DMP1 and MEPE expression are elevated in osteocytes after mechanical loading in vivo: theoretical role in controlling mineral quality in the perilacunar matrix. J Musculoskelet Neuronal Interact. 2007;7(4):313–5.
144. Rowe PS. Regulation of bone-renal mineral and energy metabolism: the PHEX, FGF23, DMP1, MEPE ASARM pathway. Crit Rev Eukaryot Gene Expr. 2012;22(1):61–86. https://doi.org/10.1615/CritRevEukarGeneExpr.v22.i1.50.
145. Yuan B, Takaiwa M, Clemens TL, et al. Aberrant Phex function in osteoblasts and osteocytes alone underlies murine X-linked hypophosphatemia. J Clin Invest. 2008;118(2):722–34. https://doi.org/10.1172/JCI32702.
146. Mattinzoli D, Rastaldi MP, Ikehata M, et al. FGF23-regulated production of Fetuin-A (AHSG) in osteocytes. Bone. 2016;83:35–47. https://doi.org/10.1016/j.bone.2015.10.008.
147. Paic F, Igwe JC, Nori R, et al. Identification of differentially expressed genes between osteoblasts and osteocytes. Bone. 2009;45(4):682–92. https://doi.org/10.1016/j.bone.2009.06.010.
148. Bodine PV, Billiard J, Moran RA, et al. The Wnt antagonist secreted frizzled-related protein-1 controls osteoblast and osteocyte apoptosis. J Cell Biochem. 2005;96(6):1212–30. https://doi.org/10.1002/jcb.20599.
149. Poole KE, van Bezooijen RL, Loveridge N, et al. Sclerostin is a delayed secreted product of osteocytes that inhibits bone formation. FASEB J. 2005;19(13):1842–4. https://doi.org/10.1096/fj.05-4221fje.
150. Leupin O, Piters E, Halleux C, et al. Bone overgrowth-associated mutations in the LRP4 gene impair sclerostin facilitator function. J Biol Chem. 2011;286(22):19489–500. https://doi.org/10.1074/jbc.M110.190330.
151. Cui Y, Niziolek PJ, MacDonald BT, et al. Lrp5 functions in bone to regulate bone mass. Nat Med. 2011;17(6):684–91. https://doi.org/10.1038/nm.2388.
152. Kato Y, Windle JJ, Koop BA, et al. Establishment of an osteocyte-like cell line, MLO-Y4. J Bone Miner Res. 1997;12(12):2014–23. https://doi.org/10.1359/jbmr.1997.12.12.2014.
153. Confavreux CB, Levine RL, Karsenty G. A paradigm of integrative physiology, the crosstalk between bone and energy metabolisms. Mol Cell Endocrinol. 2009;310(1-2):21–9. https://doi.org/10.1016/j.mce.2009.04.004.
154. Xiong J, Onal M, Jilka RL, et al. Evidence for osteocyte regulation of bone homeostasis through RANKL expression. Nat Med. 2011;17(10):1231–4. https://doi.org/10.1038/nm.2452.
155. Plotkin LI, Bellido T. Osteocytic signalling pathways as therapeutic targets for bone fragility. Nat Rev Endocrinol. 2016;12(10):593–605. https://doi.org/10.1038/nrendo.2016.71.
156. Kramer I, Halleux C, Keller H, et al. Osteocyte Wnt/beta-catenin signaling is required for normal bone homeostasis. Mol Cell Biol. 2010;30(12):3071–85. https://doi.org/10.1128/MCB.01428-09.
157. Holmen SL, Zylstra CR, Mukherjee A, et al. Essential role of beta-catenin in postnatal bone acquisition. J Biol Chem. 2005;280(22):21162–8. https://doi.org/10.1074/jbc.M501900200.
158. Glass DA, Bialek P, Ahn JD, et al. Canonical Wnt signaling in differentiated osteoblasts controls osteoclast differentiation. Dev Cell. 2005;8(5):751–64. https://doi.org/10.1016/j.devcel.2005.02.017.

Genetics of Osteoporosis

2

Francesca Marini, Laura Masi, Gemma Marcucci,
Luisella Cianferotti, and Maria Luisa Brandi

2.1 Introduction

Osteoporosis is a clinical condition of the skeleton, defined when value of bone mineral density (BMD) is lower than 2.5 standard deviations from the mean value of the young adult population (T-score values), usually measured at the lumbar spine (L1–L4) and femoral neck. Low bone mass is associated with deterioration in micro-architecture and geometry of the skeleton, and with a deregulated bone turnover, resulting in an excessive bone resorption and a reduced novel bone formation. The final clinical endpoints of osteoporosis are fragility fractures, mainly at the wrist, spine, and femoral neck that occur in about 30% of postmenopausal women and 12% of elderly men [1] and are responsible for the morbidity and mortality of the disease.

Bone strength is the parameter to measure the risk of fracture, and it is principally determined by the combination of BMD, bone size, and bone quality. For years BMD has been the only one measurable marker for assessing osteoporosis and fracture risk, and also today it is widely used to define the osteoporosis status. However, it is now well assessed that BMD value alone is not sufficient to determine the real risk of develop osteoporotic fracture, and other important parameters of bone quality (such as bone architecture and bone metabolism) have to be taken into account.

Osteoporosis risk depends by the failure to acquire the optimal bone mass peak during growth and by the capacity of maintain bone mass during the elderly and aspects that are both regulated by numerous dietary, lifestyle, hormonal, and genetic factors. Deficiency of calcium and/or vitamin D during childhood and adolescence may be responsible for the reduction of bone mass peak, while during the adulthood

F. Marini · L. Masi · G. Marcucci · L. Cianferotti · M. L. Brandi (✉)
Department of Surgery and Translational Medicine, University of Florence, Florence, Italy
e-mail: f.marini@dmi.unifi.it; laura.masi@aouc.unifi.it; luisella.cianferotti@unifi.it;
marialuisa.brandi@unifi.it

A. Lenzi, S. Migliaccio (eds.), *Multidisciplinary Approach to Osteoporosis*,
https://doi.org/10.1007/978-3-319-75110-8_2

and elderly may have a fundamental negative role in increasing bone mass loss. The rapid decrease of estrogens at menopause strongly contributes to a rapid bone loss in postmenopausal women, and it is one of the main causes of the higher incidence of osteoporosis in women.

Today, it is well assessed that osteoporosis is a multifactorial complex disorder whose pathogenesis is due to the interaction and synergic effects of various predisposing genetic determinants regulating bone and mineral metabolism, of "non-skeletal" risk factors that could influence the risk of falling (i.e., muscle strength, balance, and visual acuity), of environmental influences, and of dietary and lifestyle habits.

2.2 Genetic Contribution to Osteoporosis

Principal skeletal determinants of osteoporosis predisposition and fragility fracture risk, such as BMD, bone geometry, and bone metabolism, are all under strong genetic influences. Major advances in the knowledge of genetic aspects of osteoporosis and fracture risk have been made in the last two decades, and they have been principally derived by study on monogenic bone diseases, linkage analyses in osteoporotic pedigrees, association case-control and population-based studies for candidate genes, and experimental crosses in animal models.

Twin and family studies allowed to assess that about 60–85% of human BMD variability is under control of genetic factors [2, 3], and the heritability of other bone characteristics, such as bone geometry and bone turnover markers, ranges between 50 and 80% [4, 5]. Moreover, genetic factors demonstrated to regulate up to 80% of individual variability of bone mass peak acquisition [6], acting principally before puberty. Conversely, the effect of genetic influences on fracture risk is less than 30% [7], maybe because fracture is a more complex phenotype that is determined not only by bone density and quality but also by other non-skeletal conditions.

Several genes have been associated with bone mass and other determinants of bone quality and fracture risk, but each of them has demonstrated to exert only a relatively modest single effect on bone tissue, suggesting that osteoporosis is the result of the synergic effect of various predisposing genetic variants, within different genes, in association with environmental and lifestyle risk factors. To date, more than 100 candidate gene polymorphic variants have been tested for their association with BMD, fractures, and other bone-related quantitative trait loci (QTLs).

Briefly, we reported data about studies on major genes involved in osteoporosis and related phenotypes, discussing the effect of their polymorphic variants on bone mass, bone quality, and metabolism.

2.2.1 Lipoprotein Receptor-Related Protein 5 (*LRP5*) and Lipoprotein Receptor-Related Protein 6 (*LRP6*) Genes

These two genes are discussed together since they form a receptor complex with frizzled (Fz) to activate the transcriptional activity of the beta-catenin within the

Wnt signaling pathway that is involved in the regulation of osteoblast commitment, differentiation, and apoptosis, in the synthesis of bone matrix protein and mineralization process, as well as in the coupling to osteoclasts and induction of bone resorption [8]. Inactivating mutations of the *LRP5* gene are responsible for the osteoporosis pseudoglioma (OPPG), an autosomal recessive monogenic Mendelian disorder, characterized by severe early juvenile osteoporosis, very low bone mass, and fragility fractures. Conversely, activating mutations of the *LRP5* gene result in sclerosing bone dysplasias, clinical conditions characterized by an excessive bone mass. Due to its role in the development of these two rare inherited bone disorders, *LRP5* has been suspected as a key regulator of bone mass, and common polymorphic variations of this gene have been investigated, by association studies, for their relationship with BMD and fragility fracture in the general population. The two most investigated variants were the missense single nucleotide polymorphism (SNP) c.2047G>A, the Val667Met in exon 9 (rs4988321), and the missense SNP c.4037C>T, Ala1330Val in exon 18 (rs3736228). Both c.2047A and c.4037T alleles were associated with reduced lumbar bone mineral content, vertebral bone area, and stature in Caucasian men, but not in women [9], accounting for up to 15% of variance for these traits. In the same year, a study on young Korean men failed to find any association between *LRP5* polymorphism and peak bone mass and BMD at any site [10]. In a case-control study on middle-aged men (mean age 50 years) with idiopathic osteoporosis, both the rare alleles of these two polymorphisms and their haplotype have been associated with a threefold high risk of low BMD [11]. In 2006 the Rotterdam Study confirmed the association between the 1330Val allele and a reduced lumbar spine area and a higher risk of fracture at the femur, humerus, and pelvis in elderly men, but not in women [12]. The same study evidenced an interaction between the 1330Val allele and a missense SNP Ile1062Val in the *LRP6* gene (rs2302685), showing that 1330Val and 1062Val alleles have a synergic effect on fracture risk [12]. In 2008 a Bayesian meta-analysis on 10 association studies, including a total of 16,705 individual (of whom the great majority were women (8444) aged 18–81 years) indicated that 1330Val variant has a modest association with BMD and authors concluded that this aspect may limit its clinical use [13]. More recently, a prospective, multicenter, and large-scale study on 37,534 individuals from 18 participating teams in Europe and North America by the GENOMOS study group confirmed that genetic variations of the *LRP5* gene are associated with both BMD and fracture risk, very consistently across analyzed populations but with a modest clinical effect [14]. Conversely, the Ile1062Val SNP of *LRP6* did not show a significant association with BMD [14].

2.2.2 Vitamin D Receptor (*VDR*) Gene

Bioactive form of vitamin D is fundamental for the acquisition of bone mass pick and for the maintenance of bone homeostasis. It acts through its binding to the vitamin D receptor (VDR). Mutations of the *VDR* gene cause the syndrome of vitamin-resistant rickets a recessive Mendelian condition, characterized by severe rickets, hypocalcemia, and hypophosphatemia, which is resistant to vitamin D supplementation. Due to the importance of vitamin D in bone metabolism, *VDR* has been the first candidate gene whose polymorphic variants have been analyzed in association studies for osteoporosis in 1994, showing that common allelic variants of *VDR* can be used to predict differences in BMD, accounting for up to 75% of the total genetic effect on BMD in healthy individuals [15]. Association studies between *VDR* and osteoporosis have been principally focused on two polymorphisms in intron 8 (*BsmI* and *ApaI*), one silent polymorphism in exon 9 (*TaqI*), a polymorphism affecting exon 2 and creating an alternative start codon and responsible for two different isoforms of VDR protein which differ in length by three amino acids (*FokI*), and a functional polymorphism in the promoter region at the binding site for the transcription factor Cdx-2. *BsmI*, *ApaI*, and *TaqI* are in linkage disequilibrium, and maybe they are also in linkage disequilibrium with other sequence variations in the 3′ untranslated region (UTR) of the *VDR* gene that could affect mRNA stability and, thus, VDR protein expression. Numerous association studies have been published, presenting conflicting and/or inconclusive data, maybe due to inadequate population sampling, ethnicity, gender, age, confounding factors, gene-gene interactions, and gene-environment interactions; a linkage disequilibrium between *VDR* polymorphisms and other bone metabolism genes cannot be excluded. Today, results of association studies on large populations seem to strongly reduce the role of *VDR* polymorphisms in the risk of osteoporosis and fragility fractures. The GENOMOS study (26,242 participants; 18,405 women) evaluated association between *Cdx-2*, *FokI*, *BsmI*, *ApaI*, and *TaqI* polymorphisms, and DXA-measured femoral neck and lumbar spine BMD, and fractures concluding that *FokI*, *BsmI*, *ApaI*, and *TaqI* are not associated with BMD or with fractures, and only *Cdx-2* showed a very modest effect on the risk of vertebral fractures [16].

A haplotype meta-analysis by Thakkinstian et al. [17] evidenced that *VDR* single polymorphisms were not significantly associated to osteoporosis, while specific *BsmI/ApaI/TaqI* haplotypes were significantly associated to the clinical condition. Data from this study seem to indicate a gain in power when considering *VDR* haplotypes rather than polymorphisms separately, demonstrating the importance of haplotype studies rather than single polymorphism studies for the *VDR* gene.

In addition, some studies suggested a possible interaction between calcium and vitamin D intake and *VDR* polymorphisms in the regulation of BMD [6, 18], with the possibility that effect of *VDR* genotypes on BMD would be visible only in the presence of a low calcium intake [19] or a vitamin D deficiency. Conversely, the association between *VDR* genotypes and bone mass would be hidden by high calcium and/or vitamin D intake.

2.2.3 Estrogen Receptor Alpha (*ERα*) Gene

Estrogens are very important for the correct bone metabolism, for the skeletal growth, and for the maintenance of bone mass. Indeed, severe depletion of estrogens at menopause results in a rapid loss of bone mass, and it is one major cause of higher incidence of osteoporosis and fragility fractures in women than in men. Estrogens exert their action on bone cells through their specific steroid receptors (ERs). An inactivating mutation of the estrogen receptor alpha (*ERα* or *ESR1*) gene was identified in men affected by severe juvenile osteoporosis. This fact prompted *ERα* as an important candidate gene for osteoporosis. *ERα* and, very less frequently, estrogen receptor beta (*ERβ* or *ESR2*) genes have been widely studied about the association of their polymorphisms with osteoporosis and fragility fractures at the wrist, hip, and spine. In the last two decades, a large number of studies investigated about an association between *ERα* polymorphisms and bone mass, mostly focusing on two SNPs in the intron 1 of the gene, recognized, respectively, by the *XbaI* and *PvuII* restriction enzymes, and on a variable TA repeat in the promoter region. *PvuII* maps within consensus recognition sites for AP4 and Myb transcription factors and influences Myb-associated transcription in vitro [20]. Both *XbaI* and *PvuII* have shown to influence report gene transcription in vitro [21]. These data suggest a direct functional effect of *XbaI* and *PvuII* on *ERα* expression, but it is also possible a linkage disequilibrium with other functional polymorphic variations within *ERα* gene and/or contiguous genes.

Association studies between *ERα* polymorphisms and BMD showed inconsistent and controversial results. A meta-analysis by Ioannidis et al. [22], including more than 5000 women from 22 different studies (of which 11 including Caucasian women and 11 including Asian women), evidenced an association between *XbaI* genotypes and both BMD and fractures, with the XX genotype (*XbaI*) resulting associated with higher femur and spine BMD values (+1 to 2%) and with a reduced risk of fractures.

In 2004, the GENOMOS study group performed a large-scale association study between *XbaI*, *PvuII*, and TA repeat polymorphisms of *ERα* (both as single polymorphism and as haplotypes) and both BMD and occurrence of fragility fractures in 18,917 unrelated individuals from eight European centers [23]. None of the three polymorphisms or haplotypes showed any statistically significant effect on BMD. Conversely women with the homozygote XX genotype of *XbaI* had a reduced incidence of 19% for all fractures and of 35% for vertebral fractures. No significant effects on fracture risk were seen for *PvuII* and TA repeats. The study seems to indicate *XbaI* as a risk marker for fracture, independently by BMD values [23].

Very few studies investigated the role of polymorphic variants of *ERβ* in determining BMD and fracture risk, principally focused on a CA repeat in the intron 5 of the gene. The Framingham study analyzed the association of this genetic variation and four other intronic polymorphisms with BMD in 723 men and 795 women [24]. The CA repeat genotypes resulted associated with femoral BMD but not with the spine BMD, both in women and in men. Two other SNPs, *rs1256031* and *rs1256059* (respectively, in the intron 11 and the intron 15 of *ERβ*), showed an association with femoral BMD in men, and *rs1256031*, in particular, accounted for up to 4.0% difference in mean femoral BMD. The haplotype C-23CA-T (*rs1256031*, CA repeat, *rs1256059*) was significantly associated with reduced femoral BMD in women, with BMD value differences ranging from 3.0 to 4.3%. In the same year, the CA repeat was investigated for its association with BMD in 226 healthy postmenopausal women (60–98 years), evidencing that women with less than 25 CA repeats had significantly higher BMD at the total skeleton, lumbar spine, and femoral neck with respect to women bearing more than 25 CA repeats [25].

Two years later a large population-based cohort study analyzed the association of *ERβ* polymorphisms with risk of vertebral and incident fragility fracture in postmenopausal women, alone or in association with polymorphisms of *ERα* and insulin-like growth factor I (*IGF1*) genes, showing a synergic effect of genotypes interaction on fracture risk, and, thus, reinforcing the idea of the polygenic and complex nature of osteoporosis [26].

2.2.4 Aromatase Gene (*CYP19*)

The *CYP19* gene encodes for aromatase, the enzyme responsible for estrogen synthesis by catalyzing the aromatization of C19 androgens to C18 estrogens. Inactivating mutations of *CYP19* cause aromatase deficiency, and they have been associated to clinical conditions affecting also bone growth and mineralization. Common polymorphisms of *CYP19* have been, in vitro, associated with enzymatic activity. A study by Masi et al. first reported an association between a tetranucleotide (TTTA) repeat polymorphism in intron 4 of the *CYP19* gene and BMD in postmenopausal Italian women [27]. The association of these polymorphisms with BMD was also studied in Italian elderly men but without evidencing a statistical significance [28]. The association between TTTA repeat and BMD was not confirmed in Finnish early postmenopausal women [29]. Another study reported an association between a common SNP in the 5′ untranslated region (UTR) of *CYP19* (rs1062033) and BMD in Spanish late postmenopausal women [30]. More recently, six polymorphisms (rs4646, rs10046, rs3784307, rs1062033, rs936306, and rs190258), located throughout the entire *CYP19* gene (including also the 5′ and 3′ UTRs), were associated with bone mass in 286 Spanish postmenopausal women [31]. The rs10046 SNP in the 3′UTR resulted associated with BMD; the postmenopausal decrease in bone mass appeared to be slower in women with the AA genotype, than in those with AG or GG genotypes. This polymorphism is in strongly linkage disequilibrium with the TTTA repeat and the rs4646 SNP in the 3′UTR, and they are all three associated with BMD. Two SNPs, located in exon I.6 and promoter I.6 of *CYP19*, were analyzed in a cohort of 256 Spanish postmenopausal women [32], and rs4775936 was associated with lumbar spine BMD, with the homozygote AA genotype exhibiting a significantly higher lumbar spine BMD if compared with GG or GA women.

Association of *CYP19* functional polymorphisms with BMD and/or fracture was also confirmed by other studies on different populations [33–37].

2.2.5 Collagen Type I Alpha I (*COLIA1*) Gene

Collagen type 1 is the most represented protein of bone extracellular matrix (about 80% of total proteins in bone tissue). Alterations of collagen synthesis, properties, and relative quantity of its two chains affect mechanical features of bone tissue and increase susceptibility to fragility fractures. Inactivating mutations of the gene encoding the alpha I chain of type I collagen (*COLIA1*) are responsible for *osteogenesis imperfecta*, a hereditary Mendelian disorder characterized by severe osteoporosis and skeletal fracture in early life. Therefore, *COLIA1* is one of the principal candidate genes for fragility fractures in osteoporosis. A common polymorphism in the intron 1 of the *COL1A1* gene, (Sp1 polymorphism, rs1800012) alters the binding site for the Sp1 transcription factor, affecting *COL1A1* transcription and resulting in an alteration of the normal equilibrium between α_1 and α_2 chains (2:1). In particular, the s allele has an increased affinity for Sp1, resulting in a higher amount of α_1 with respect to α_2 chain; the Ss genotype is responsible for a collagen chain ratio of 2.3 (respect to the normal 2, typical of the SS genotype) [38]. Association studies evaluated the effect of Sp1 polymorphism on BMD and fragility fractures, showing a mild association with BMD values but a stronger relationship to osteoporotic fractures, particularly at the spine [38–41]. In particular, a higher prevalence of fragility fracture was found among ss and Ss genotypes with respect to the SS genotype [38–41], with an increase in fracture risk of about 68% for each copy of the s allele and independently by a significant reduction of BMD value [38].

The GENOMOS study evaluated *COLIA1* Sp1 alleles as a predictor of BMD and fracture in 20,786 unrelated individuals from several European countries and found only a modest association between the ss genotype and reduced BMD; no reduction of BMD was observed in Ss individuals [42]. Moreover, the s allele could predispose to incident vertebral fractures in women, but not in men, and the association with vertebral fracture has a 40% increase of risk for each copy of the s allele carried [42], independently by BMD.

A study by Uitterlinden et al. [43] investigated the interaction of polymorphisms of *VDR* and *COLI1A* genes in susceptibility to fractures in 1004 postmenopausal women. The "baT" (*BsmI-ApaI-TaqI*) *VDR* risk haplotype was evaluated in association with ss and Ss *COLI1A* risk genotypes, showing a significant interaction ($p = 0.03$) between *VDR* and *COLIA1* genotype effects. In subjects bearing the SS genotype, the fracture risk was not *VDR* genotype-dependent. Conversely, in subjects carrying ss or Ss genotypes, the contemporaneous presence of the baT haplotype was associated with a higher risk of fracture of 4.4 and 2.1, respectively [43].

Moreover, an additive effect of the *COLIA1* Sp1 polymorphism with 10565insGGA polymorphism of the sclerostin (*SOST* gene) was evidenced in an elderly male and female Caucasian healthy population [44].

Data from these two studies further confirmed the polygenic nature of osteoporosis and fracture risk.

2.2.6 Transforming Growth Factor Beta (*TGF-β1*)

Transforming growth factor beta (TGF-β1) is largely expressed by osteoclasts, and it has shown to control bone resorption and formation by directly acting on both osteoblasts and osteoclasts [45]. Therefore, polymorphic variants of *TGF-β1* gene have been extensively studied in relation to osteoporosis. A C/T transition in exon 1 which causes a proline-leucine substitution at position 10 has been associated with higher level of circulating TGF-β1 protein, and the C allele was associated with higher BMD values and lower occurrence of fragility fractures in two Japanese populations [46]. A rare polymorphism in intron 4 (713-8delC variant) was associated with very low BMD, severe osteoporosis, and fracture risk in women with osteoporosis and with low bone mass and increased bone turnover in both osteoporotic and normal women [47]. The same research group evaluated, in 2003, the association between 8 polymorphisms of the *TGF-β1* gene and osteoporosis in a case-control study of 96 osteoporotic patients with vertebral fractures vs 330 normal individuals, evidencing that the TT genotype of the 816-20 T>C variant in the intron 5 was less common in fractured osteoporotic patients than in healthy controls and that it was associated with higher lumbar spine and hip bone mass [48].

The GENOMOS study investigated associations between five *TGF-β1* polymorphisms [G–1639A (G–800A, rs1800468), C–1348T (C–509T, rs1800469), T29C (Leu10Pro, rs1982073), G74C (Arg25Pro, rs1800471), and C788T (Thr263Ile, rs1800472)] and BMD and fractures in 28,924 male and female individuals from 10 different European research studies [49]. Only weak associations between the C–1348T SNP and lumbar spine BMD in men and between the C788T SNP and risk of incident vertebral fractures were reported [49], presumably indicating that polymorphic variations of the *TGF-β1* gene do not play a major role in regulating BMD or susceptibility to fragility fractures.

Recently, a meta-analysis integrated all the eligible studies, including a total of 8 studies involving 1851 cases and 2247 controls, and it investigate whether T869C and T29C polymorphisms of the *TGF-β1* gene were correlated with postmenopausal osteoporosis [50]. A significant association between T29C or T869C polymorphisms and osteoporosis risk was observed only in Asian, but not in Caucasian, population [50].

2.2.7 Other Genes

Polymorphisms of other genes, involved in the regulation of bone metabolism and turnover, have been, although more rarely, investigated about their association with BMD and fractures. They include sclerostin (*SOST*), bone morphogenetic protein 2 (*BMP2*), bone morphogenetic protein 4 (*BMP4*), osteoprotegerin (*OPG*, *TNFRSF11B*), receptor activator of nuclear factor kappa-B (*RANK*; *TNFRSF11A*), RANK ligand (RANKL; TNFSF11), and runt-related transcription factor 2 (*RUNX2*; *CBFA1*).

Principal results from their association and/or linkage studies are depicted in Table 2.1.

Table 2.1 Other candidate genes in osteoporosis association and/or linkage studies

Gene	Role on bone tissue	Analyzed polymorphisms	Analyzed population	Association of each polymorphism with BMD, osteoporosis, and/or fracture	References
SOST (sclerostin)	SOST is a secreted osteoclast-derived BMP antagonist that represses BMP-induced osteoblast differentiation and/or function	rs1230399 (−9247 T/C)	1243 Chinese subjects with low BMD	1. Significant genotypic/allelic associations with the spine, femoral neck, trochanter, and total hip BMD 2. The T allele increases the risk of osteoporosis	[51]
SOST (sclerostin)		rs1513670 rs1107748	1012 Chinese healthy women	1. Significant association between rs1513670 and total hip BMD 2. Significant association between rs1107748 and osteoporotic fracture	[52]
SOST (sclerostin)		rs10534024 rs9902563	1383 Danish men	Significant association of rs9902563 with femoral neck BMD	[53]
SOST (sclerostin)		rs1234612 rs1513670 rs1634330 rs1708635 rs2023794 rs7220711 rs74252774 rs851057 rs851058 rs865429	Original study: 703 healthy postmenopausal Chinese women Update study: 1379 healthy postmenopausal Chinese women including 703 from the previous study	The original study failed to identify any significant association between SOST SNPs or haplotypes and BMD In the update study: the CC genotype of rs2023794 and the TT genotype of rs74252774 were associated with higher BMD values at lumbar spine (but not at hip), than other genotypes	[54] [55]
SOST (sclerostin)		C4102G C10356T 10565insGGA G11988A C17965G A18292G T42722C A58874G A75707G	1939 Dutch white elderly men and women	1. The 3-bp insertion of 10565insGGA was associated with decreased BMD at the femoral neck, in women 2. The G allele of A75707G was associated with increased BMD at the femoral neck, in men	[44]

(continued)

Table 2.1 (continued)

Gene	Role on bone tissue	Analyzed polymorphisms	Analyzed population	Association of each polymorphism with BMD, osteoporosis, and/or fracture	References
BMP2 (bone morphogenetic protein 2)	BMP2 acts in osteoblast differentiation	Ser37Ala Arg190Ser	Caucasian elderly women and men from the Rotterdam study	No association with BMD, bone loss, hip structural analysis, and incident fractures	[56]
BMP2 (bone morphogenetic protein 2)		Ser37Ala (rs2273073) rs235710 rs235767 rs235754	1059 young Swedish women (over 25 years) 1044 elderly Swedish women (over 75 years)	1. No association with BMD and fracture 2. rs235754 was associated with the ultrasound parameters speed of sound and stiffness	[57]
BMP2 (bone morphogenetic protein 2)		Ser37Ala Ala94Ser Arg189Ser	1. Osteoporosis families from Iceland 2. A cohort of Danish postmenopausal women with persistently low BMD 3. A group of Danish postmenopausal osteoporotic fracture patients	Ser37Ala showed a strong association with osteoporosis	[58]
BMP4 (bone morphogenetic protein 4)	BMP4 is a potent osteotropic factors, acting on osteoblasts and promoting bone formation in vivo and in vitro	rs1957860 rs2855528 rs2761885 rs2855532 rs2071047 rs17563	1232 postmenopausal women (mean age 75 years)	1. rs17563 was associated with total and intertrochanteric hip BMD; BMD was 32% lower in the CC genotype 2. No association with fractures 3. The G-C-T haplotype (rs1957860-rs2855532-rs17563) was associated with high bone mass	[59]

TNFRSF11B (OPG; osteoprotegerin)	Osteoprotegerin is a soluble receptor for RANKL and therefore a competitive inhibitor of osteoclast differentiation and activity	A163G T245G T950C G1181C A6890C	1. 217 osteoporotic women and 51 osteoporotic men 2. 255 healthy women and 72 healthy men	1. The G allele of A163G was more common in individuals with spine fractures 2. The G allele of T245G was more common in osteoporotic patients 3. The CC genotype of G1181C was less common among patients with spine fractures	[60]
TNFRSF11B (OPG; osteoprotegerin)		G209A T245G C889T T950C	103 osteoporotic postmenopausal women	1. Statistically significant association of genotypes with BMD at the lumbar spine was observed for G209A and T245G 2. The heterozygote GATG haplotype (G209A and T245G) was associated with lower BMD with respect to the homozygote wild-type GGTT haplotype	[61]
TNFRSF11B (OPG; osteoprotegerin)		Lys3Asn	205 Chinese postmenopausal women	1. The homozygote Asn genotype was associated with a significantly higher BMD at the lumbar spine with respect to the other two genotypes 2. The homozygote Lys genotype had a 2.7 times greater risk for osteopenia/osteoporosis than the homozygote Asn genotype	[62]
TNFRSF11B (OPG; osteoprotegerin)		4752_4753delCT G1181C C1217T G1284A C4501T A6893G A6950C T8738A	60 osteoporotic postmenopausal women	Individuals with the homozygote GG genotype (G1181C) had a significantly lower lumbar spine BMD than subjects with the heterozygote GC genotype	[63]

(continued)

Table 2.1 (continued)

Gene	Role on bone tissue	Analyzed polymorphisms	Analyzed population	Association of each polymorphism with BMD, osteoporosis, and/or fracture	References
TNFRSF11B (OPG; osteoprotegerin)		A163G T950C G1181C	126 postmenopausal Maltese women	1. The TT genotype (T950C) was more frequently associated with low BMD 2. The A-T-G haplotype, from the three polymorphisms, was found to be more frequent in individuals with low BMD	[64]
TNFRSF11B (OPG; osteoprotegerin)		T245G G1181C	478 postmenopausal women	1. Lumbar spine BMD was associated with polymorphisms T245G and G1181C, as well as with CT haplotype 2. Femoral neck BMD showed an association with T245G polymorphism	[65]
TNFRSF11B (OPG; osteoprotegerin)		g.21775C>T g. 23367T>C	336 osteoporotic postmenopausal Chinese women	The TT genotype (g.23367T>C) was associated with lower BMD at the spine, but not at the neck hip or total hip	[66]
TNFRSF11B (OPG; osteoprotegerin)		g.18861A>G g.25548C>T	1. 338 osteoporotic postmenopausal Chinese women 2. 367 healthy postmenopausal Chinese women	The AA genotype (g.18861A>G) was significantly higher in women with osteoporosis	[67]
TNFRSF11B (OPG; osteoprotegerin)		g.27450A>T	1. 441 osteoporotic postmenopausal Chinese women 2. 445 healthy postmenopausal Chinese women	The AA genotype was significantly higher in women with osteoporosis	[68]
TNFRSF11B (OPG; osteoprotegerin)		A163G T245G G1181C	327 postmenopausal Slovak women	The G allele (T245G) was more frequent in subjects with vertebral, non-vertebral, and total fractures	[69]

TNFRSF11A (RANK)	RANK is the receptor for the RANK ligand and is involved in the regulation of osteoclast differentiation and activity	25 polymorphisms (of which 7 were newly identified in the study)	560 postmenopausal Korean women	34863G>A and 35928insdelC polymorphisms were significantly associated with lumbar spine BMD	[70]
TNFRSF11A (RANK)		C421T C575T	1. 100 osteoporotic postmenopausal Turkish women 2. 78 healthy postmenopausal Turkish women	No association with osteoporosis, BMD value, or fracture, both as single polymorphisms and haplotypes	[71]
TNFRSF11A (RANK)		rs996215 rs4603673 rs7239261 rs4500848 rs6567270 rs1805034 rs4303637 rs4941131 rs964662	1026 postmenopausal women	rs7239261 was significantly associated with femoral neck BMD	[72]
TNFSF11 (RANKL; RANK ligand)	RANKL binds to RANK on the surface of osteoclasts and their precursors and leads to their differentiation and survival	rs9594738 rs9525641 rs2277439 rs232485 rs287545 rs2200287 rs953316	1026 postmenopausal women	1. rs2277439 and rs2324851 were significantly associated with femoral neck BMD 2. The haplotype TGACGT (rs9525641-rs2277439-rs2324851-rs2875459-rs2200287-rs953316) was a genetic risk factor for lower femoral neck BMD 3. The haplotype TAGCGT was a genetic protective factor for lumbar spine BMD	[72]
TNFSF11 (RANKL; RANK ligand)		−290C>T −643C>T −693G>C −1594G>A	115 postmenopausal Slovenian women	The CC genotype (−290C>T) was associated with lower BMD than the TT genotype	[73]

(continued)

Table 2.1 (continued)

Gene	Role on bone tissue	Analyzed polymorphisms	Analyzed population	Association of each polymorphism with BMD, osteoporosis, and/or fracture	References
RUNX2 (runt-related transcription factor 2)	RUNX2 is a transcription factor essential to osteoblast differentiation, bone remodeling, and fracture healing	11Ala/17Ala repeat 11GCA>GCG (Ala11Ala)	495 osteoporotic women	1. The A allele (11GCA>GCG) was associated with higher BMD at the lumbar spine, femoral neck, whole body, ultradistal (UD), and mid-forearm sites 2. The A allele (11GCA>GCG) was significantly protective against Colles' fracture in elderly women, but not spine and hip fracture	[74]
RUNX2 (runt-related transcription factor 2)		−330 G>T −1025 T>C	821 postmenopausal Spanish women	The TC genotype (−1025 T>C) was associated with higher mean of femoral neck BMD values with respect to the TT genotype	[75]
RUNX2 (runt-related transcription factor 2)		Complete sequence of *RUNX2* exons and intron-exon junctions	729 postmenopausal Korean women	The homozygote CC genotype of −1025 T>C was associated with reduced lumbar spine BMD and reduced BMDs at proximal femur sites (trochanter and total femur)	[76]
RUNX2 (runt-related transcription factor 2)		−1025 T>C +198 G>A	689 postmenopausal and 87 pre-perimenopausal Spanish women	TC and CC genotypes −1025 T>C were associated with higher femoral neck BMD with respect to the TT genotype	[77]
RUNX2 (runt-related transcription factor 2)		rs7771980	907 healthy postmenopausal Korean women	TC and CC genotypes were associated with a lower vertebral fracture risk with respect to the TT genotype	[78]

2.3 Novel Approaches to the Genetics of Osteoporosis: Genome-Wide Association Studies (GWAS)

Because of the polygenic nature of osteoporosis, in which few genes exert major effects on bone metabolism and homeostasis, while a large number of genes have only minor effects, classical single gene association and/or linkage studies present numerous limitations, such as inconclusive or controversial results, false-positive and/or false-negative associations, reduced sensibility in identifying genotype-phenotype associations, and inability to identify novel candidate genes and their genetic variants. The recent development of next generation sequencing (NGS) technique has allowed to design gene chips for the simultaneous analysis of hundreds genes and their polymorphic variants. Genome-wide association studies (GWAS) have opened new horizons for the discovery of genetic loci and variants associated with osteoporosis and fracture risk, and the application of this novel approach, in the last years, has obtained success in identifying replicated genetic loci associated with osteoporosis.

The first GWAS in osteoporosis was performed in 2007 and analyzed 100,000 SNPs in 1141 individuals from the Framingham Osteoporosis Study to examine genetic associations with bone quantitative traits: BMD (including the femoral neck, trochanter, and lumbar spine), calcaneal ultrasound, and geometric indices of the hip [79]. Of the 40 top SNPs with the highest number of significantly associations with BMD traits, a variable percentage of 30–50% of them maps within genetic loci or near genes that have not previously been studied for osteoporosis. The others were polymorphisms located within known osteoporosis candidate genes, such as rs1884052 and rs3778099 in *ERα*, rs4988300 in *LRP5*, rs2189480 in *VDR*, rs2075555 in *COLIA1* and rs10519297, and rs2008691 in *CYP19*.

One year later, two major GWAS analyzed the association of over 300,000 SNPs with BMD and fractures [80, 81]. The first study [80] evidenced an association between BMD and two SNPs, rs4355801 on chromosome 8 near to the *TNFRSF11B* gene, and rs3736228, on chromosome 11 in the *LRP5* gene. The second study [81] identified five genomic regions significantly associated with BMD, both in the discovery set population and in the replication set populations. Three of these regions map close to or within genes known to be important in bone homeostasis: *TNFSF11*, *TNFRSF11B*, and *ERα*.

In 2009, a large-scale meta-analysis of five GWAS of femoral neck and lumbar spine BMD, including 19,195 individuals of Northern European descent, allowed to identify 20 genetic loci reaching the genome-wide significance (GWS; $p < 5 \times 10^{-8}$). Seven of them confirmed to be known bone-related loci/genes, 1p36 (*ZBTB40*), 6q25 (*ERα*), 8q24 (*TNFRSF11B*), 11q13.4 (*LRP5*), 12q13 (*SP7*), 13q14 (*TNFSF11*), and 18q21 (*TNFRSF11A*), while 13 mapped to new regions, not yet investigated as candidate genes for osteoporosis: 1p31.3 (*GPR177*), 2p21 (*SPTBN1*), 3p22 (*CTNNB1*), 4q21.1 (*MEPE*), 5q14 (*MEF2C*), 7p14 (*STARD3NL*), 7q21.3 (*FLJ42280*), 11p11.2 (*LRP4*, *ARHGAP1*, *F2*), 11p14.1 (*DCDC5*), 11p15 (*SOX6*), 16q24 (*FOXL1*), 17q21 (*HDAC5*), and 17q12 (*CRHR1*) [82].

Two years later, a larger meta-analysis of 17 GWAS of the femoral neck and lumbar spine BMD was performed on 32,961 subjects of European and East Asian ancestry and validated for marker replication of BMD association on 50,933 independent subjects and for association with risk of low-trauma fracture in 31,016 fractured individuals (cases) and 102,444 non-fractured controls [83]. The study identified 56 loci (32 novels) associated with BMD with a positive GWS; 14 of them resulted also associated with fracture risk. Numerous of these loci mapped near or within *TNFRSF11B*, *TNFRSF11A*, and *TNFSF11* genes or near or within genes involved in the Wnt signaling pathways, in the mesenchymal stem cell differentiation and in the endochondral ossification.

GWAS highlighted the highly polygenic and complex nature of osteoporosis and fracture susceptibility and the difficulty to predict the risk of osteoporosis on genetic bases. Anyway, since the first GWAS on osteoporosis was performed in 1997, numerous and great advances have been made in the discovery and validation of genes and loci involved in the predisposition to osteoporosis. GWAS allowed, to date, the identification of more than 60 loci associated with BMD, osteoporosis, and fragility fractures, including novel loci, whose functional analysis has demonstrated that they have a clear effect on bone metabolism and, presumably, also on osteoporosis pathophysiology.

The association of GWAS results with functional studies revealed very useful to identify novel molecular targets for anti-fracture drugs and, thus, allowed the design of novel target therapies for osteoporosis.

References

1. Ralston SH. Genetic determinants of susceptibility to osteoporosis. Curr Opin Pharmacol. 2003;3:286–90.
2. Guéguen R, Jouanny P, Guillemin F, Kuntz C, Pourel J, Siest G. Segregation analysis and variance components analysis of bone mineral density in healthy families. J Bone Miner Res. 1995;10(12):2017–22.
3. Krall EA, Dawson-Hughes B. Heritable and life-style determinants of bone mineral density. J Bone Miner Res. 1993;8(1):1–9.
4. Arden NK, Baker J, Hogg C, Baan K, Spector TD. The heritability of bone mineral density, ultrasound of the calcaneus and hip axis length: a study of postmenopausal twins. J Bone Miner Res. 1996;11(4):530–4.
5. Garnero P, Arden NK, Griffiths G, Delmas PD, Spector TD. Genetic influence on bone turnover in postmenopausal twins. J Clin Endocrinol Metab. 1996;81(1):140–6.
6. Eisman JA. Genetics of osteoporosis. Endocr Rev. 1999;20:788–4.
7. MacGregor A, Snieder H, Spector TD. Genetic factors and osteoporotic fractures in elderly people. Twin data support genetic contribution to risk of fracture. BMJ. 2000;320(7250):1669–70.
8. Yavropoulou MP, Yovos JG. The role of the Wnt signaling pathway in osteoblast commitment and differentiation. Hormones. 2007;6(4):279–94.
9. Ferrari SL, Deutsch S, Choudhury U, Chevalley T, Bonjour JP, Dermitzakis ET, Rizzoli R, Antonarakis SE. Polymorphisms in the low-density lipoprotein receptor-related protein 5 (LRP5) gene are associated with variation in vertebral bone mass, vertebral bone size, and stature in whites. Am J Hum Genet. 2004;74(5):866–75.
10. Koh JM, Jung MH, Hong JS, Park HJ, Chang JS, Shin HD, Kim SY, Kim GS. Association between bone mineral density and LDL receptor-related protein 5 gene polymorphisms in young Korean men. J Korean Med Sci. 2004;19(3):407–12.

11. Ferrari SL, Deutsch S, Baudoin C, Cohen-Solal M, Ostertag A, Antonarakis SE, Rizzoli R, de Vernejoul MC. LRP5 gene polymorphisms and idiopathic osteoporosis in men. Bone. 2005;37(6):770–5.
12. van Meurs JB, Rivadeneira F, Jhamai M, et al. Common genetic variation of the low-density lipoprotein receptor-related protein 5 and 6 genes determined fracture risk in elderly white men. J Bone Miner Res. 2006;21(1):141–50.
13. Tran BNH, Nguyen ND, Eisman JA, Nguyen TV. Association between LRP5 polymorphism and bone mineral density: a Bayesian meta-analysis. BMC Med Genet. 2008;9:55.
14. van Meurs JBJ, Trikalinos TA, Ralston SH, et al. Large-scale analysis of association between LRP5 and LRP6 variants and osteoporosis. JAMA. 2008;299(11):1277–90.
15. Morrison NA, Qi JC, Tokita A, Kelly PJ, Crofts L, Nguyen TV, Sambrook PN, Eisman JA. Prediction of bone density from vitamin D receptor alleles. Nature. 1994;367(6460):284–7.
16. Uitterlinden AG, Ralston SH, Brandi ML, Carey AH, Grinberg D, Langdahl BL, Lips P, Lorenc R, et al. The association between common vitamin D receptor gene variations and osteoporosis: a participant-level meta-analysis. Ann Intern Med. 2006;145(4):255–64.
17. Thakkinstian A, D'Este C, Attia J. Haplotype analysis of VDR gene polymorphisms: a meta-analysis. Osteoporos Int. 2004;15(9):729–34.
18. Ferrari S, Rizzoli R, Chevalley T, et al. Vitamin-D-receptor-gene polymorphisms and change in lumbar-spine bone mineral density. Lancet. 1995;345(8947):423–4.
19. Ferrari S. Genetics, nutrition and bone health. In: Holick M, Dawson-Hughes E, editors. Nutrition and bone health. Totowa: The Humana press Inc; 2004. p. 19–41.
20. Herrington DM, Howard TD, Brosnihan KB, McDonnell DP, Li X, Hawkins GA, et al. Common estrogen receptor polymorphism augments effects of hormone replacement therapy on E-selectin but not C-reactive protein. Circulation. 2002;105:1879–82.
21. Maruyama H, Toji H, Harrington CR, Sasaki K, Izumi Y, Ohnuma T, et al. Lack of an association of estrogen receptor α gene polymorphisms and transcriptional activity with Alzheimer disease. Arch Neurol. 2000;57:236–40.
22. Ioannidis JP, Stravrou I, Trikalinos TA, Zois C, Brandi ML, Gennari L, et al. Association of polymorphisms of the estrogen receptor α gene with bone mineral density and fracture risk in women: a meta-analysis. J Bone Miner Res. 2002;17:2048–60.
23. Ioannidis JP, Ralston SH, Bennett ST, Brandi ML, Grinberg D, Karassa FB, et al. Differential genetic effects of ESR1 gene polymorphisms on osteoporosis outcomes. JAMA. 2004;292(17):2105–14.
24. Shearman AM, Karasik D, Gruenthal KM, Demissie S, Cupples LA, Housman DE, et al. Estrogen receptor beta polymorphisms are associated with bone mass in women and men: the Framingham Study. J Bone Miner Res. 2004;19(5):773–81.
25. Scariano JK, Simplicio SG, Montoya GD, Garry PJ, Baumgartner RN. Estrogen receptor beta dinucleotide (CA) repeat polymorphism is significantly associated with bone mineral density in postmenopausal women. Calcif Tissue Int. 2004;74(6):501–8.
26. Rivadeneira F, van Meurs JB, Kant J, Zillikens MC, Stolk L, Beck TJ, et al. Estrogen receptor beta (ESR2) polymorphisms in interaction with estrogen receptor alpha (ESR1) and insulin-like growth factor I (IGF1) variants influence the risk of fracture in postmenopausal women. J Bone Miner Res. 2006;21(9):1443–56.
27. Masi L, Becherini L, Gennari L, Amedei A, Colli E, Falchetti A, et al. Polymorphism of the aromatase gene in postmenopausal Italian women: distribution and correlation with bone mass and fracture risk. J Clin Endocrinol Metab. 2001;86:2263–9.
28. Gennari L, Masi L, Merlotti D, Picariello L, Falchetti A, Tanini A, et al. A polymorphic CYP19 TTTA repeat influences aromatase activity and estrogen levels in elderly men: effects on bone metabolism. J Clin Endocrinol Metab. 2004;89(6):2803–10.
29. Salmen T, Heikkinen AM, Mahonen A, Kröger H, Komulainen M, Pallonen H, et al. Relation of aromatase gene polymorphism and hormone replacement therapy to serum estradiol levels, bone mineral density, and fracture risk in early postmenopausal women. Ann Med. 2003;35(4):282–8.

30. Zarrabeitia MT, Hernández JL, Valero C, Zarrabeitia AL, García-Unzueta M, Amado JA, et al. A common polymorphism in the 5′-untranslated region of the aromatase gene influences bone mass and fracture risk. Eur J Endocrinol. 2004;150(5):699–704.
31. Riancho JA, Zarrabeitia MT, Valero C, Sañudo C, Hernández JL, Amado JA, et al. Aromatase gene and osteoporosis: relationship of ten polymorphic loci with bone mineral density. Bone. 2005;36(5):917–25.
32. Enjuanes A, Garcia-Giralt N, Supervía A, Nogués X, Ruiz-Gaspà S, Bustamante M, et al. A new SNP in a negative regulatory region of the CYP19A1 gene is associated with lumbar spine BMD in postmenopausal women. Bone. 2006;38(5):738–43.
33. Lorentzon M, Swanson C, Eriksson AL, Mellström D, Ohlsson C. Polymorphisms in the aromatase gene predict areal BMD as a result of affected cortical bone size: the GOOD study. J Bone Miner Res. 2006;21(2):332–9.
34. Mullin BH, Carter KW, Lewis JR, Ingley E, Wilson SG, Prince RL. Significant association between common polymorphisms in the aromatase gene CYP19A1 and bone mineral density in postmenopausal women. Calcif Tissue Int. 2011;89(6):464–71.
35. Koudu Y, Onouchi T, Hosoi T, Horiuchi T. Association of CYP19 gene polymorphism with vertebral fractures in Japanese postmenopausal women. Biochem Genet. 2012;50(5-6):389–96.
36. Markatseli AE, Lazaros L, Markoula S, Kostoulas H, Sakaloglou P, Tigas S, et al. Association of the (TTTA)n repeat polymorphism of CYP19 gene with bone mineral density in Greek peri- and postmenopausal women. Clin Endocrinol. 2014;81(1):38–44.
37. Casas-Avila L, Valdés-Flores M, Miranda-Duarte A, Ponce de León-Suárez V, Castro-Hernández C, Rubio-Lightbourn J, et al. Association of a (TTTA)n microsatellite and a TCT del/ins polymorphisms in the aromatase gene (CYP19) with hip fracture risk in Mexican postmenopausal women. Gynecol Endocrinol. 2015;31(12):987–91.
38. Mann V, Hobson EE, Li B, Stewart TL, Grant SF, Robins SP, et al. A COL1A1 Sp1 binding site polymorphism predisposes to osteoporotic fracture by affecting bone density and quality. J Clin Invest. 2001;107(7):899–907.
39. Uitterlinden AG, Burger H, Huang Q, Yue F, McGuigan FE, Grant SF, et al. Relation of alleles of the collagen type I alpha1 gene to bone density and the risk of osteoporotic fractures in postmenopausal women. N Engl J Med. 1998;338(15):1016–21.
40. Mann V, Ralston SH. Meta-analysis of COL1A1 Sp1 polymorphism in relation to bone mineral density and osteoporotic fracture. Bone. 2003;32(6):711–7.
41. Efstathiadou Z, Tsatsoulis A, Ioannidis JP. Association of collagen I alpha 1 Sp1 polymorphism with the risk of prevalent fractures: a meta-analysis. J Bone Miner Res. 2001;16(9):1586–92.
42. Ralston SH, Uitterlinden AG, Brandi ML, Balcells S, Langdahl BL, Lips P, et al. Large-scale evidence for the effect of the COLIA1 Sp1 polymorphism on osteoporosis outcomes: the GENOMOS study. PLoS Med. 2006;3(4):e90.
43. Uitterlinden AG, Weel AE, Burger H, Fang Y, van Duijn CM, Hofman A, et al. Interaction between the vitamin D receptor gene and collagen type I alpha1 gene in susceptibility for fracture. J Bone Miner Res. 2001;16(2):379–85.
44. Uitterlinden AG, Arp PP, Paeper BW, Charmley P, Proll S, Rivadeneira F, et al. Polymorphisms in the sclerosteosis/van Buchem disease gene (SOST) region are associated with bone-mineral density in elderly whites. Am J Hum Genet. 2004;75(6):1032–45.
45. Massagué J, Chen YG. Controlling TGF-β signalling. Genes Dev. 2000;14:627–44.
46. Yamada Y, Miyauchi A, Goto J, Takagi Y, Okuizumi H, Kanematsu M, et al. Association of a polymorphism of the transforming growth factor-beta1 gene with genetic susceptibility to osteoporosis in postmenopausal Japanese women. J Bone Miner Res. 1998;13(10):1569–76.
47. Langdahl BL, Knudsen JY, Jensen HK, Gregersen N, Eriksen EF. A sequence variation: 713-8delC in the transforming growth factor-beta 1 gene has higher prevalence in osteoporotic women than in normal women and is associated with very low bone mass in osteoporotic women and increased bone turnover in both osteoporotic and normal women. Bone. 1997;20(3):289–94.
48. Langdahl BL, Carstens M, Stenkjaer L, Eriksen EF. Polymorphisms in the transforming growth factor beta 1 gene and osteoporosis. Bone. 2003;32(3):297–310.

49. Langdahl BL, Uitterlinden AG, Ralston SH, Trikalinos TA, Balcells S, Brandi ML, et al. Large-scale analysis of association between polymorphisms in the transforming growth factor beta 1 gene (TGFB1) and osteoporosis: the GENOMOS study. Bone. 2008;42(5):969–81.
50. Sun J, Zhang C, Xu L, Yang M, Yang H. The transforming growth factor-β1 (TGF-β1) gene polymorphisms (TGF-β1 T869C and TGF-β1 T29C) and susceptibility to postmenopausal osteoporosis: a meta-analysis. Medicine. 2015;94(4):e461.
51. Huang QY, Li GH, Kung AW. The -9247 T/C polymorphism in the SOST upstream regulatory region that potentially affects C/EBP alpha and FOXA1 binding is associated with osteoporosis. Bone. 2009;45(2):289–94.
52. Valero C, Zarrabeitia MT, Hernández JL, Pineda B, Cano A, García-Pérez MA, Riancho JA. Relationship of sclerostin and secreted frizzled protein polymorphisms with bone mineral density: an association study with replication in postmenopausal women. Menopause. 2011;18(7):802–7.
53. Piters E, de Freitas F, Nielsen TL, Andersen M, Brixen K, Van Hul W. Association study of polymorphisms in the SOST gene region and parameters of bone strength and body composition in both young and elderly men: data from the Odense Androgen Study. Calcif Tissue Int. 2012;90(1):30–9.
54. He J, Zhang H, Wang C, Zhang Z, Yue H, Hu W, et al. Associations of serum sclerostin and polymorphisms in the SOST gene with bone mineral density and markers of bone metabolism in postmenopausal Chinese women. J Clin Endocrinol Metab. 2014;99(4):E665–73.
55. Zhang H, He JW, Wang C, Zhang Z, Yue H, Hu WW, et al. Associations of polymorphisms in the SOST gene and bone mineral density in postmenopausal Chinese Women. Osteoporos Int. 2014;25(12):2797–803.
56. Medici M, van Meurs JB, Rivadeneira F, Zhao H, Arp PP, Hofman A, Pols HA, Uitterlinden AG. BMP-2 gene polymorphisms and osteoporosis: the Rotterdam Study. J Bone Miner Res. 2006;21(6):845–54.
57. McGuigan FE, Larzenius E, Callreus M, Gerdhem P, Luthman H, Akesson K. Variation in the BMP2 gene: bone mineral density and ultrasound in young adult and elderly women. Calcif Tissue Int. 2007;81(4):254–62.
58. Styrkarsdottir U, Cazier JB, Kong A, Rolfsson O, Larsen H, Bjarnadottir E, et al. Linkage of osteoporosis to chromosome 20p12 and association to BMP2. PLoS Biol. 2003;1(3):E69.
59. Ramesh Babu L, Wilson SG, Dick IM, Islam FM, Devine A, Prince RL. Bone mass effects of a BMP4 gene polymorphism in postmenopausal women. Bone. 2005;36(3):555–61.
60. Langdahl BL, Carstens M, Stenkjaer L, Eriksen EF. Polymorphisms in the osteoprotegerin gene are associated with osteoporotic fractures. J Bone Miner Res. 2002;17(7):1245–55.
61. Arko B, Prezelj J, Komel R, Kocijancic A, Hudler P, Marc J. Sequence variations in the osteoprotegerin gene promoter in patients with postmenopausal osteoporosis. J Clin Endocrinol Metab. 2002;87(9):4080–4.
62. Zhao HY, Liu JM, Ning G, Zhao YJ, Zhang LZ, Sun LH, et al. The influence of Lys3Asn polymorphism in the osteoprotegerin gene on bone mineral density in Chinese postmenopausal women. Osteoporos Int. 2005;16(12):1519–24.
63. Arko B, Prezelj J, Kocijancic A, Komel R, Marc J. Association of the osteoprotegerin gene polymorphisms with bone mineral density in postmenopausal women. Maturitas. 2005;51(3):270–9.
64. Vidal C, Brincat M, Xuereb Anastasi A. TNFRSF11B gene variants and bone mineral density in postmenopausal women in Malta. Maturitas. 2006;53(4):386–95.
65. Mencej-Bedrač S, Preželj J, Marc J. TNFRSF11B gene polymorphisms 1181G > C and 245T > G as well as haplotype CT influence bone mineral density in postmenopausal women. Maturitas. 2011;69(3):263–7.
66. Zhang F, He C, Chen G, Li F, Gao H. Association analyses of osteoprotegerin gene polymorphisms with bone mineral density in Chinese postmenopausal women. Med Oncol. 2013;30(1):389.
67. Yu F, Huang X, Miao J, Guo L, Tao D. Association between osteoprotegerin genetic variants and osteoporosis in Chinese postmenopausal women. Endocr J. 2013;60(12):1303–7.

68. Lin H, Zhang G, Chen X, Wu X, Wu C, Ca H, et al. The relationship between the g.27450A>T genetic variant of OPG gene and osteoporosis in Chinese postmenopausal women. Int Immunopharmacol. 2014;21(2):464–7.
69. Boroňová I, Bernasovská J, Mačeková S, Petrejčíková E, Tomková Z, Kľoc J, et al. TNFRSF11B gene polymorphisms, bone mineral density, and fractures in Slovak postmenopausal women. J Appl Genet. 2015;56(1):57–63.
70. Koh JM, Park BL, Kim DJ, Kim GS, Cheong HS, Kim TH, et al. Identification of novel RANK polymorphisms and their putative association with low BMD among postmenopausal women. Osteoporos Int. 2007;18(3):323–31.
71. Işleten B, Durmaz B, Durmaz B, Onay H, Ozkınay F, Durmaz A, et al. The association of RANK gene C421T and C575T polymorphisms with bone mineral density in postmenopausal Turkish women. Arch Gynecol Obstet. 2013;288(4):917–23.
72. Tu P, Duan P, Zhang RS, Xu DB, Wang Y, Wu HP, et al. Polymorphisms in genes in the RANKL/RANK/OPG pathway are associated with bone mineral density at different skeletal sites in post-menopausal women. Osteoporos Int. 2015;26(1):179–85.
73. Mencej S, Prezelj J, Kocijancic A, Ostanek B, Marc J. Association of TNFSF11 gene promoter polymorphisms with bone mineral density in postmenopausal women. Maturitas. 2006;55(3):219–26.
74. Vaughan T, Pasco JA, Kotowicz MA, Nicholson GC, Morrison NA. Alleles of RUNX2/CBFA1 gene are associated with differences in bone mineral density and risk of fracture. J Bone Miner Res. 2002;17(8):1527–34.
75. Bustamante M, Nogués X, Agueda L, Jurado S, Wesselius A, Cáceres E, et al. Promoter 2 -1025 T/C polymorphism in the RUNX2 gene is associated with femoral neck bmd in Spanish postmenopausal women. Calcif Tissue Int. 2007;81(4):327–32.
76. Lee HJ, Koh JM, Hwang JY, Choi KY, Lee SH, Park EK, et al. Association of a RUNX2 promoter polymorphism with bone mineral density in postmenopausal Korean women. Calcif Tissue Int. 2009;84(6):439–45.
77. Pineda B, Hermenegildo C, Laporta P, Tarín JJ, Cano A, García-Pérez MÁ. Common polymorphisms rather than rare genetic variants of the Runx2 gene are associated with femoral neck BMD in Spanish women. J Bone Miner Metab. 2010;28(6):696–705.
78. Kim KC, Chun H, Lai C, Parnell LD, Jang Y, Lee J, et al. The association between genetic variants of RUNX2, ADIPOQ and vertebral fracture in Korean postmenopausal women. J Bone Miner Metab. 2015;33(2):173–9.
79. Kiel DP, Demissie S, Dupuis J, Lunetta KL, Murabito JM, Karasik D. Genome-wide association with bone mass and geometry in the Framingham Heart Study. BMC Med Genet. 2007;8(Suppl 1):S14.
80. Richards JB, Rivadeneira F, Inouye M, Pastinen TM, Soranzo N, Wilson SG, et al. Bone mineral density, osteoporosis, and osteoporotic fractures: a genome-wide association study. Lancet. 2008;371(9623):1505–12.
81. Styrkarsdottir U, Halldorsson BV, Gretarsdottir S, Gudbjartsson DF, Walters GB, Ingvarsson T, et al. Multiple genetic loci for bone mineral density and fractures. N Engl J Med. 2008;358(22):2355–65.
82. Rivadeneira F, Styrkársdottir U, Estrada K, Halldórsson BV, Hsu YH, Richards JB, et al. Twenty bone-mineral-density loci identified by large-scale meta-analysis of genome-wide association studies. Nat Genet. 2009;41(11):1199–206.
83. Estrada K, Styrkarsdottir U, Evangelou E, Hsu YH, Duncan EL, Ntzani EE, et al. Genome-wide meta-analysis identifies 56 bone mineral density loci and reveals 14 loci associated with risk of fracture. Nat Genet. 2012;44(5):491–501.

Osteoporosis Diagnosis

3

Claudio Marcocci and Federica Saponaro

Osteoporosis is a systemic disease characterized by decreased bone strength and an increased risk of fracture. Bone strength progressively declines with aging, and therefore osteoporosis is considered an inevitable process and is not approached as a relevant clinical problem. However, several intervening factors may accelerate this involutional process. One of the major reasons is that osteoporosis is asymptomatic until a fracture occurs, and therefore both the physician and the patients fail to appreciate its importance. As a matter of fact, many patients with osteoporosis and/or at increased risk of fracture are still underdiagnosed and undertreated.

Patients with known or suspected osteoporosis should undergo a through medical history and physical examination to discover risk factors that may have influenced bone accrual and peak bone mass and increased bone fragility (Table 3.1).

3.1 Clinical Evaluation

Individuals with known or suspected osteoporosis should be evaluated for several risk factors (modifiable or not), which can help estimate the individual peak bone mass and bone loss. At the initial visit, administering specific questionnaires could also be useful, but an accurate anamnesis and physical examination can be sufficient.

Questions about the following issues should be asked to help making the correct diagnosis and choose the management of patients with osteoporosis. The most important osteoporosis risk factors are summarized in Table 3.1.

C. Marcocci (✉) · F. Saponaro
Department of Clinical and Experimental Medicine,
University of Pisa, Endocrine Unit 2, University Hospital of Pisa, Pisa, Italy
e-mail: claudio.marcocci@med.unipi.it

A. Lenzi, S. Migliaccio (eds.), *Multidisciplinary Approach to Osteoporosis*,
https://doi.org/10.1007/978-3-319-75110-8_3

Table 3.1 Major risk factors of osteoporosis

• Genetic factor
• Environmental factors
–Alcohol abuse
–Cigarette smoking
–Physical inactivity and immobilization
–Low body weight and diet
–Limited exposure to sunlight
• Reproductive history and puberty
• Personal history of fractures and falls
• Drug therapy
• Comorbidities

3.1.1 Genetic Factors

Up to 80% of peak bone mass, depending on the skeletal site, is genetically determined: relevant factors are gender, race, and family history. A maternal history of hip fracture is particularly significant in increasing the fracture risk, but information about other fragility fractures and low BMD in first-degree and other relatives should also be collected [1]. The pathogenesis of osteoporosis is multifactorial, and only a few genes influencing bone mass have been identified (see Chap. 3). Moreover, some genetic diseases associated with osteoporosis, like "osteogenesis imperfecta," particularly late-onset variants, may present with vertebral fractures. Clue for the diagnosis is the family history or specific signs (blue sclerae, lax skin, hypermobile joints, deafness, and cardiac diseases).

3.1.2 Environmental Factors

3.1.2.1 Alcohol

Alcohol abuse (>14 g/day ethanol for women and >28 g/day ethanol for men) is associated with decreased BMD and increased fracture risk, the possible causal relationship being a direct suppression of osteoblasts by alcohol. Moderate to heavy alcohol consumption was also shown to be associated with changes in bone geometry, density, and microarchitecture, which affect bone quality [2]. On the other hand, some studies showed a favorable effect of small daily quantities of alcohol on the bone [3].

3.1.2.2 Cigarette Smoking

Smoking is another risk factor for bone loss. A higher the prevalence of osteoporosis is higher in smokers than in non-smokers, an increased risk of osteoporotic fractures has been shown in the former [4]. Recent studies have shown that smoking leads to a reduced bone resistance to mechanical stress because of deleterious microarchitectural changes in trabecular bone. Finally, cigarette smoking decreases estrogen levels and has influence on body weight [5].

3.1.2.3 Physical Inactivity and Immobilization

Gravity stimulates bone formation, and weight-bearing physical activity has a positive effect on bone mass, but it is difficult to document that exercise can increase bone density in adults. It is well known that athletes have high bone mass, but excessive exercise may also cause bone loss (marathon runners). On the other hand, periods of prolonged bed rest and immobilization due to neurological diseases led to rapid bone loss that can be reversible only in young patients.

3.1.2.4 Low Body Weight and Diet

Nutritional history should be evaluated, since thin habitus is a risk factor for low BMD and fractures. Caloric insufficiency during adolescence is associated with low peak bone mass and loss of weight at any age with bone loss. Inadequate calcium intake in the adolescence adversely affects peak bone mass and may contribute to age-related bone loss, particularly when accompanied by vitamin D deficiency. Conversely diets rich in sodium and animal proteins are associated with hypercalciuria and bone loss [6].

3.1.2.5 Limited Exposure to Ultraviolet Light

Ultraviolet light stimulates vitamin D production in the skin, mostly through sun exposure. Vitamin D insufficiency is rather common and is associated with decreased calcium absorption, subsequent secondary hyperparathyroidism, and bone loss. Long-standing severe vitamin D deficiency may result in osteomalacia.

3.1.3 Reproductive History and Puberty

The age of puberty affects bone mass both in males and females. Indeed, individuals with late pubertal development do not reach the adequate peak bone mass. In women, every condition characterized by a reduction in estrogen levels can be associated with bone loss: irregular menses, history of infertility, and prolonged uses of progesterone contraception [7]. Early menopause (before 45 years) is invariably associated with an increased risk of fractures, but particular attention should be paid to exclude concomitant secondary causes also in this setting. In men history of infertility, loss of libido, and sexual dysfunctions may suggest the presence of hypogonadism and suboptimal exposure of the bone to testosterone. Anorexia nervosa is a good example of a disease that can deeply influence pubertal development and the peak bone mass in both sexes, with a complex pathogenesis due to a combination of endocrine dysfunctions and nutritional deficit [8].

3.1.4 Personal History of Fractures and Falls

This aspect should be carefully investigated, particularly in elderly individuals. Of particular importance is to investigate the circumstances in which a fracture occurred, in order to identify the true "low-trauma, fragility fractures," namely, those related to a bone trauma, which should not cause a fracture in a healthy bone (i.e., a fall for the standing position). The hip, spine, and forearm are typically osteoporotic. In the position statement from the National Bone Health Alliance Working Group published in 2014, there was a consensus that the diagnosis of osteoporosis could be established in individuals who experienced a low-trauma hip fracture even without a BMD measurement and in those with osteopenia and a low-trauma clinical vertebral, proximal humerus, or pelvis fractures [9]. The position statement also indicated that a low-trauma distal forearm fracture in a patient with osteopenia at the lumbar spine or hip should be sufficient for the diagnosis of osteoporosis. Vertebral fractures directly reflect bone fragility and predict future new fractures. However, the large majority of spine fractures are not clinically evident, and imaging study can help to identify even old fractures: the incidental finding of a nontraumatic vertebral fracture on a radiograph (morphometric vertebral fracture) may also be considered as diagnostic of osteoporosis [10]. Fractures other than the spine, hip, or forearm should also be evaluated, since virtually all fractures are the results of bone strength and force applied on that bone and therefore could reflect bone fragility and osteoporosis [11].

Information of falls should also be collected, since most fractures are cause by falls. Fall prevention should also be included in an appropriate strategy of fracture prevention. A recent consensus statement recommends asking the patient the following question: “In the past month, have you had any fall including a slip or trip in which you lost your balance and landed on the floor or ground or lower level?” [12]. Indeed, fractures related to falls can be considered a major health problem: one third of people over 65 years falls once each year, and 5% of falls eventually leads to fractures, with subsequent increased mortality, morbidity, and costs for the community. Recent studies have shown the efficacy of physical exercise training as a program of fall prevention in elderly osteoporotic patients [13].

3.1.5 Drug Therapy

Osteoporosis is an adverse effect of many pharmacologic agents, like glucocorticoids, proton pump inhibitors, selective serotonin receptor inhibitors, thiazolidinediones, anticonvulsants, medroxyprogesterone acetate, aromatase inhibitors, heparin, calcineurin inhibitors, androgen deprivation therapy, and some chemotherapies. Glucocorticoid therapy is the most common cause of secondary osteoporosis and is associated with an increased rate of fractures, morbidity, and mortality. Glucocorticoids induce a rapid bone loss, and the fracture risks are already evident within 6 months of therapy, and several studies have shown that bone loss and fracture risk increase with the dose and duration of therapy [14]. The negative effects on bone are multifactorial, and not all of them can be explained by the reduction of BMD. They include direct effects like inhibition of osteoblast function, increased osteoblast and osteocyte apoptosis, and stimulation of the osteoclast, resulting in bone remodeling defects, bone loss, and a fracture risk [15]. Moreover, indirect effects (hypogonadism, kidney calcium loss, low levels of vitamin D) play a role [14]. Antiepileptic drugs, like phenobarbital and phenytoin, interfere with vitamin D metabolism and can cause osteomalacia, secondary hyperparathyroidism, and osteoporosis. Some anticoagulant drugs are known to interfere with bone density: long-term administration of unfractionated heparin is associated with an increased fracture risk, whereas no data are available on low molecular weight heparin; chronic use of warfarin, which interferes with γ-carboxylation of bone proteins, is associated with an increased risk of fractures [16]. Cyclosporin therapy in transplanted patients is associated with a 10–34% increase in clinical fractures particularly in the first year of treatment [17]. Finally, excessive administration of thyroxin can cause bone loss, particularly in postmenopausal women.

3.1.6 Comorbidities

Several diseases are known to have a deleterious effect on bone and may cause bone loss. Malabsorption syndromes like coeliac disease, peptic ulcer, gastrointestinal inflammatory diseases, chronic liver diseases, and chronic obstructive pulmonary disease can have negative effects on the bone by a combination of factors: excessive cytokine production, nutritional deficiency, decreased physical inactivity, and chronic drug use. The direct effects of cytokines on osteoblast and osteoclast activity and the use corticosteroid therapy can explain why rheumatologic diseases are associated with low BMD and increased fracture risk. Finally, some endocrine disorders cause osteoporosis: primary hyperparathyroidism, thyrotoxicosis, Cushing's syndrome, Addison syndrome, hypogonadism, and type 1 diabetes mellitus. Type 2 diabetes even if usually associated with normal or even increased BMD is also associated with an increased fracture rate [18], which seems to be mediated by the negative effect of advanced glycation end products on bone quality [19].

3.1.7 Physical Examination

Medical history should always be completed with an accurate physical examination. A high loss >4 cm compared with young age or >2 cm from the last visit may suggest a prior vertebral fracture. Thoracic kyphosis, even if it is not diagnostic, can be indicative of the presence of vertebral fractures. Finally, frailty and fall risk should be evaluated by inspection of muscle mass and direct strength testing and gait and stability when the patient is standing.

3.1.8 Algorithms

Fracture risk assessment has been evaluated for many years by BMD, on the basis of the inverse relationship between BMD and fractures. Despite high specificity, this method has low sensitivity since many fractures occur in individuals with osteopenia and several clinical risk factors for fractures are independent from BMD. For this reason, some algorithms based on clinical parameters with and without BMD values have been proposed and now accepted by international guidelines. FRAX is a World Health Organization-sponsored algorithm introduced in 2008 and endorsed by the US National Osteoporosis Foundation (NOF) and other national and international guidelines for osteoporosis management [20]. It is based on well-validated and weighted clinical risk factors for fracture and can predict hip, spine, humerus, and forearm fractures in males and women aged between 40 and 90 years. It was elaborated on data collected in large prospective studies and subsequently validated in a cohort of more than 230,000 patients.

The 2015 position statement from the National Bone Health Alliance Working Group for clinical diagnosis of osteoporosis agreed that a probability of hip fracture ≥3% or of major osteoporotic fracture ≥20% calculated with FRAX could be considered as an appropriate treatment intervention threshold, as suggested in US NOF Clinician's Guidelines, and could also be used as cutoff for the diagnosis of osteoporosis [9]. There is still an on-going debate in literature regarding the real utility of FRAX and the need of further improvement to the algorithm. Some strengths and limits of FRAX have been recognized. FRAX is free and easily accessible to clinicians and is particularly useful to identify old women with high fracture risk, still untreated. Moreover, it can help in reducing overtreatment in young postmenopausal women, with low BMD and low fracture risk. One possible limit of FRAX is that vertebral fractures have the same value of other fractures in the algorithm, leading to a possible underestimation of fracture risk. Another limit is the age cutoff: the NOF suggests that FRAX should be used for a target age between 50 and 90 years, excluding risk assessment in young people. Moreover, epidemiologic data on which FRAX is based upon were proven in Caucasian women, and few data were available in man and other races. Another limitation of the algorithm is that it does not take into account the dose and duration of glucocorticoid drug therapy. It should be underlined that in the large majority of studies that evaluated osteoporosis treatment efficacy, eligibility criteria were based on BMD and not on FRAX. In conclusion, FRAX algorithm is a valuable and well-recognized tool in the evaluation of fracture risk in osteoporotic patients, but the final decision and treatment threshold should also take into account the clinician experience and judgment.

Other algorithms different from FRAX have been created: in the UK, the National Institute for Health and Care Excellence (NICE) recognizes both FRAX and Qfracture that includes also alcohol, smoking, and falls in the risk assessment [21]. In Italy, an algorithm called DeFRA (an algorithm derived from FRAX and based on fracture risk in Italian population) has been proposed, which includes the same continuous variable of FRAX (age, BMI, BMD) but a more detailed evaluation of other clinical factors (site and number of previous fractures, vertebral BMD in addition to hip BMD, other comorbidities) and more accurate informations on dichotomous variables (smoking, corticosteroid dose, alcohol units) [22].

3.2 Laboratory Testing

No specific biochemical abnormalities are present in patients with involutional osteoporosis. However, biochemical testing may be of help in several instances: (1) uncover metabolic bone diseases which may be associated with clinical features and bone imaging (BMD and X-ray) similar to those typical of osteoporosis, (2) identify secondary causes of osteoporosis and choice of therapy, and (4) evaluate adherence to therapy.

Secondary causes are found in about 60% of men and 50% of premenopausal women with osteoporosis. Thus an underlying disorder should be searched in all men and premenopausal women with low bone mass. In postmenopausal women secondary causes of osteoporosis are less frequent (20–30% of cases). How extensive the search for secondary causes of osteoporosis should be based on medical history and clinical examination.

The most common causes of secondary osteoporosis are reported in Table 3.2. Most of these conditions may be clinically unapparent and may be discovered only by laboratory testing. The initial evaluation should include the first level tests that, if normal, would exclude other metabolic bone diseases or secondary cause of osteoporosis in about 90% of cases (Table 3.3). An increase of erythrocyte sedimentation rate associated with anemia and an abnormal electrophoretic pattern may suggest the diagnosis of multiple myeloma, which can be confirmed by the finding of elevated light chains at immunoelectrophoretic of serum or urine. A high 24-h urinary calcium excretion (>250 mg in women and >300 in men) in the presence of normal serum calcium may rise the suspicion of idiopathic hypercalciuria, a disorder found in approximately 10% of the general population. Conversely a low 24-h urinary calcium vitamin D deficiency of a malabsorptive state can be suspected. An isolated increase of alkaline phosphatase (especially the bone isoform) with normal levels of other liver enzymes is highly indicative of Paget's disease.

In selected cases, addition tests (Table 3.3, second level) are justified and should be selected on the basis of medical history and clinical examination. For instance, serum PTH should be assayed for the differential diagnosis of hypercalcemia. Serum cortisol should be measured in all cases of unexplained osteoporosis, particularly men, to rule out Cushing's disease. Anti-transglutaminase antibodies

Table 3.2 Most common secondary causes of low bone mass or osteoporosis

Male hypogonadism
Vitamin D deficiency
Malabsorption (especially celiac disease)
Primary hyperparathyroidism
Thyrotoxicosis
Multiple myeloma
Chronic liver diseases
Chronic obstructive pulmonary diseases
Rheumatoid arthritis
Idiopathic hypercalciuria
Solid organ transplantation
Alcohol abuse
Cigarette smoking
Physical inactivity and immobilization
Osteogenesis imperfecta
Anorexia nervosa
Drugs (glucocorticoids, antiepileptic drugs, excessive thyroxin and hydrocortisone replacement therapy)

Table 3.3 Laboratory tests to exclude/identify secondary causes of osteoporosis

First level
• Erythrocyte sedimentation rate
• Full blood count
• Albumin-corrected serum calcium
• Serum phosphate
• Serum alkaline phosphatase
• Protein electrophoresis
• Serum creatinine
• Serum testosterone in males[1] (preferably together with sex-hormone binging protein)
• 24/h urinary calcium[2]
Second level
• Ionized calcium
• TSH
• PTH
• 25OHD
• Morning cortisol after administration overnight of 1 mg dexamethasone
• Anti-transglutaminase antibodies (IgA)
• Tryptase

[1]Preferably together with sex-hormone binging globulin measuremnet, to calculate the free-androgen index

[2]Calcium supplement, if taken by the patient, should be stopped for 2 weeks before urine collection

should be measured in addition to serum 25OHD when urinary calcium excretion is low or in premenopausal women with low bone mass or postmenopausal women with osteoporosis. Once the diagnostic workup is completed, it is prudent to measure serum 25OHD to determine the vitamin D status and, if deficient, guide supplementation in order to reach adequate value.

Several markers of bone turnover (BTM) are currently available, reflecting the process of bone resorption and bone formation [23]. The most widely used are serum C-telopeptide of type 1 collagen (CTX) and urinary deoxypyridinoline for resorption and serum alkaline phosphatase (bone isoform) and procollagen type 1 aminoterminal propeptide (P1NP) for formation. Measurement of BTM has limited, if any, diagnostic value. In adults, an increase of BMT may suggest an accelerated bone loss or other bone disorders (osteomalacia, Paget's disease, bone metastases). Measurement of BTM may provide information that is complementary to BMD measurement. Indeed, high levels of bone resorption markers predict fracture independent of BMD [24] and may suggest pharmacologic therapy even if BMD is not sufficiently low. High levels of bone resorption markers may also predict a benefit of antiresorptive therapy, whereas low levels may suggest continued monitoring. The most valuable use of bone markers is to monitor therapy and check whether patient's adherence to pharmacologic therapy is adequate. Indeed, measurement of either bone resorption or bone formations marks at baseline and 3 months after the institution of therapy. Indeed, if a significant decrease is detected, the treatment can continue. Conversely, if no decrease is found, it will be important to reassess the patient to identify problems with the treatment [25]. In addition, BTM measurement may be used for assessing the response to therapy. Indeed, compared to BMD, a shorter time (3–6 months) is needed in each patient to evaluate the efficacy of both antiresorptive and anabolic therapies.

3.3 Bone Imaging

The main role of bone imaging in osteoporosis is the detection of vertebral fractures (VF). As a matter of fact, identification of VF is clinically relevant both in terms of further fracture risk, independent of other risk factors, and to select patients for anti-osteoporosis therapy.

Osteoporosis does not cause pain in the absence of fractures, but VF may also be asymptomatic, particularly in patients taking glucocorticoids. Back pain due VF has some typical features. It usually follows a fall or when some strain is applied to the back, such as lifting a suitcase or working in the garden. Loss of height and the finding of kyphosis at clinical examination, even in an asymptomatic patient, may suggest the presence of VF.

Indication for VF assessment therefore includes the presence of symptoms or signs suggestive of vertebral fractures and, in the absence of symptoms, other indications, which include previous fragility fractures and glucocorticoid treatment for more than 3 months using a daily dose of >5 mg daily of prednisone or equivalents (Table 3.3). Finally the search for VF is appropriate in all women aged >70 years and men between 70 and 79 years if T score is <−1.5 and in postmenopausal women and men with specific risk factors.

Spine images can be obtained using plain radiographs of the thoracic and lumbar spine in anteroposterior and, especially, lateral positions or by DXA, using the vertebral fracture assessment (VFA) software program provided with some densitometry devices. The advantage of FVA is the low radiation exposure (3 vs 600 μSv for a lateral lumbar spine X-ray) [26]. When VF are initially detected with VFA in patients in whom conditions other than osteoporosis are suspected, conventional X-ray of the spine should be performed and second-line imaging techniques (CT or MRI) be considered.

Table 3.4 Indication for vertebral fracture testing

• Suggestive symptoms (i.e., back pain that worsen with standing) and signs (i.e., kyphosis)
• Asymptomatic cases:
–All women aged >70 years and men between 70 and 79 years if T score is <−1.5
–Postmenopausal women and men aged 50 years or older with specific risk factors:
Previous fragility fractures
A high loss >4 cm compared with young age or >2 cm from the last visit
Marked reduction of BMD values (T score < −3)
Glucocorticoid therapy with >5 mg daily of prednisone or equivalents for >3 months
Comorbidities associated with increased risk of vertebral fractures *per se*

3.3.1 Conventional X-ray of the Spine

Lateral radiograph alone is often taken, but the anteroposterior images may help to identify the level of vertebral deformity and exclude other causes (i.e., absence of pedicles suggests malignancy).

Three types of vertebral deformities may be detected: wedge, end plate (biconcave if both plates are involved), and crush [27]. The method most commonly used to evaluate VF is based on the semiquantitative method devised by Genant [28]. This method is based on a visual inspection of the lateral spine images, and three deformity grades are defined: (1) mild or grade 1 (approximately 20–25% reduction in the anterior, middle (compared with the posterior height), and/or posterior height and a 10–20% reduction in area), (2) moderate or grade 2 (25–40% reduction in any height and a 20–40% reduction in area), and (3) severe or grade 3 (>40% reduction in any height and area) (Fig. 3.1).

Some vertebral deformities mimic fractures, as in Scheuermann's disease, a self-limiting skeletal disorder of children in which vertebrae grow unevenly resulting in a wedge shape of the vertebrae, causing kyphosis. Malignancy can also cause vertebral deformity, but in this case, erosion of the pedicle, a feature not found in osteoporotic vertebral deformity, is typically present. Paget's disease may affect the spine: the vertebral body may be enlarged, and the bone appears sclerotic with a

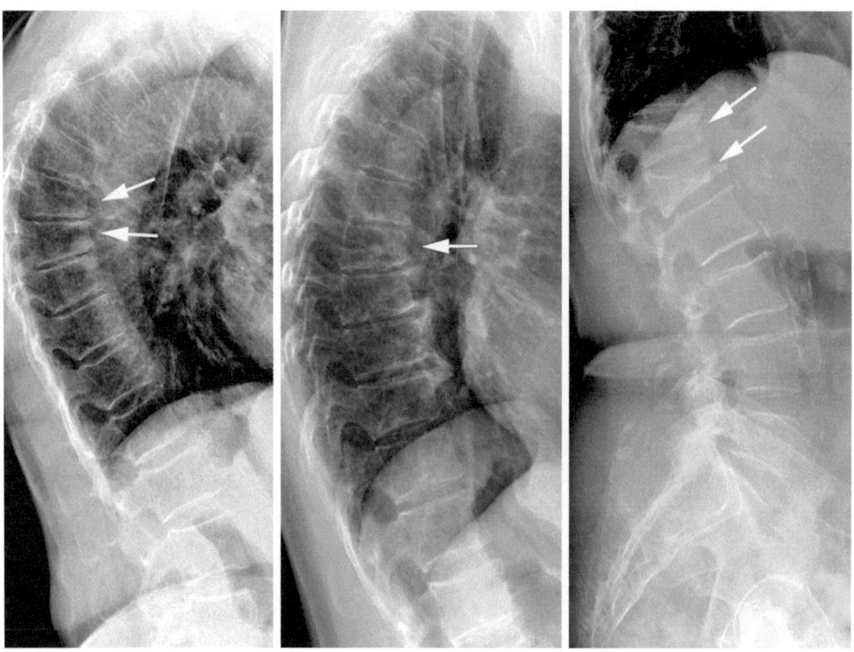

Fig. 3.1 Lateral X-rays of the spine showing a mild (left), moderate (middle), and severe (right) vertebral deformities (with the courtesy of Dr. Daniele Diacinti, University of Rome "La Sapienza," Rome, Italy)

disorganized texture appearance. Osteomalacia may cause vertebral deformities, often involving adjacent vertebrae, with atypical ground-glass appearance. Vertebral plates are deformed with a biconcave appearance (cod-fish appearance).

Vertebral morphometry is a quantitative method of diagnosis of VF based on the measure of anterior, middle, and posterior vertebral heights. It should always follow a qualitative analysis of the spine X-ray. It is performed by a six-point approach, corresponding to the four corners of the vertebral body and the midpoints of the end plate, by which the anterior, middle, and posterior heights are measured from T4 to L5. Several approaches have been proposed to quantify the shape of a vertebral body, based upon the anterior-posterior ratio, middle-posterior ratio, and posterior-posterior adjacent ratio. The algorithm developed by Eastell et al. defines a vertebral fracture if any of the ratio falls 3 SD below the sex- and vertebra-specific mean ratio in normal [29]. A more complex algorithm has been proposed by McCloskey et al. based on the reduction in the ratios, as in Eastell's algorithm, as well as a reduction in the ratios calculated with the "predicted posterior height" [30].

As mentioned before vertebral morphometry can be also performed on images obtained from DXA (VFA) (see chapter "New technologies for skeletal evaluation).

References

1. Bonjour JP, Chevalley T. Pubertal timing, bone acquisition, and risk of fracture throughout life. Endocr Rev. 2014;35(5):820–47. https://doi.org/10.1210/er.2014-1007.
2. Gaddini GW, Turner RT, Grant KA, Iwaniec UT. Alcohol: a simple nutrient with complex actions on bone in the adult skeleton. Alcohol Clin Exp Res. 2016;40(4):657–71. https://doi.org/10.1111/acer.13000.
3. Kanis JA, Johansson H, Johnell O, Oden A, De Laet C, Eisman JA, Pols H, Tenenhouse A. Alcohol intake as a risk factor for fracture. Osteoporos Int. 2005;16(7):737–42. https://doi.org/10.1007/s00198-004-1734-y.
4. Bijelic R, Milicevic S, Balaban J. Risk factors for osteoporosis in postmenopausal women. Med Arch. 2017;71(1):25–8. https://doi.org/10.5455/medarh.2017.71.25-28.
5. Brook JS, Balka EB, Zhang C. The smoking patterns of women in their forties: their relationship to later osteoporosis. Psychol Rep. 2012;110(2):351–62. https://doi.org/10.2466/13.18.PR0.110.2.351-362.
6. Pietschmann F, Breslau NA, Pak CY. Reduced vertebral bone density in hypercalciuric nephrolithiasis. J Bone Miner Res. 1992;7(12):1383–8. https://doi.org/10.1002/jbmr.5650071205.
7. Kaunitz AM, Arias R, McClung M. Bone density recovery after depot medroxyprogesterone acetate injectable contraception use. Contraception. 2008;77(2):67–76. https://doi.org/10.1016/j.contraception.2007.10.005.
8. Thornton D, Gordon CM. Restrictive eating disorders and skeletal health in adolescent girls and young women. Calcif Tissue Int. 2017;100(5):449–60. https://doi.org/10.1007/s00223-016-0164-0.
9. Siris ES, Adler R, Bilezikian J, Bolognese M, Dawson-Hughes B, Favus MJ, Harris ST, Jan de Beur SM, Khosla S, Lane NE, Lindsay R, Nana AD, Orwoll ES, Saag K, Silverman S, Watts NB. The clinical diagnosis of osteoporosis: a position statement from the National Bone Health Alliance Working Group. Osteoporos Int. 2014;25(5):1439–43. https://doi.org/10.1007/s00198-014-2655-z.
10. Melton LJ, Atkinson EJ, Cooper C, O'Fallon WM, Riggs BL. Vertebral fractures predict subsequent fractures. Osteoporos Int. 1999;10(3):214–21.

11. Mackey DC, Lui LY, Cawthon PM, Bauer DC, Nevitt MC, Cauley JA, Hillier TA, Lewis CE, Barrett-Connor E, Cummings SR, Study of Osteoporotic F, Osteoporotic Fractures in Men Study Research G. High-trauma fractures and low bone mineral density in older women and men. JAMA. 2007;298(20):2381–8. https://doi.org/10.1001/jama.298.20.2381.
12. Gillespie LD, Robertson MC, Gillespie WJ, Sherrington C, Gates S, Clemson LM, Lamb SE. Interventions for preventing falls in older people living in the community. Cochrane Database Syst Rev. 2012;9:CD007146. https://doi.org/10.1002/14651858.CD007146.pub3.
13. Smulders E, Weerdesteyn V, Groen BE, Duysens J, Eijsbouts A, Laan R, van Lankveld W. Efficacy of a short multidisciplinary falls prevention program for elderly persons with osteoporosis and a fall history: a randomized controlled trial. Arch Phys Med Rehabil. 2010;91(11):1705–11. https://doi.org/10.1016/j.apmr.2010.08.004.
14. Compston J. Clinical question: what is the best approach to managing glucocorticoid-induced osteoporosis? Clin Endocrinol. 2011;74(5):547–50. https://doi.org/10.1111/j.1365-2265.2011.03994.x.
15. Paggiosi MA, Peel NF, Eastell R. The impact of glucocorticoid therapy on trabecular bone score in older women. Osteoporos Int. 2015;26(6):1773–80. https://doi.org/10.1007/s00198-015-3078-1.
16. Panday K, Gona A, Humphrey MB. Medication-induced osteoporosis: screening and treatment strategies. Ther Adv Musculoskelet Dis. 2014;6(5):185–202. https://doi.org/10.1177/1759720X14546350.
17. Tufano A, Coppola A, Contaldi P, Franchini M, Minno GD. Oral anticoagulant drugs and the risk of osteoporosis: new anticoagulants better than old? Semin Thromb Hemost. 2015; 41(4):382–8. https://doi.org/10.1055/s-0034-1543999.
18. Vestergaard P. Discrepancies in bone mineral density and fracture risk in patients with type 1 and type 2 diabetes--a meta-analysis. Osteoporos Int. 2007;18(4):427–44. https://doi.org/10.1007/s00198-006-0253-4.
19. Yamagishi S, Maeda S, Matsui T, Ueda S, Fukami K, Okuda S. Role of advanced glycation end products (AGEs) and oxidative stress in vascular complications in diabetes. Biochim Biophys Acta. 2012;1820(5):663–71. https://doi.org/10.1016/j.bbagen.2011.03.014.
20. Kanis JA, Hans D, Cooper C, Baim S, Bilezikian JP, Binkley N, Cauley JA, Compston JE, Dawson-Hughes B, El-Hajj Fuleihan G, Johansson H, Leslie WD, Lewiecki EM, Luckey M, Oden A, Papapoulos SE, Poiana C, Rizzoli R, Wahl DA, McCloskey EV, Task Force of the FI. Interpretation and use of FRAX in clinical practice. Osteoporos Int. 2011;22(9):2395–411. https://doi.org/10.1007/s00198-011-1713-z.
21. Compston J. Osteoporosis: advances in risk assessment and management. Clin Med. 2016;16(Suppl 6):s121–4. https://doi.org/10.7861/clinmedicine.16-6-s121.
22. Adami S, Bianchi G, Brandi ML, Di Munno O, Frediani B, Gatti D, Giannini S, Girasole G, Minisola G, Minisola S, Nuti R, Pedrazzoni M, Rossini M, Varenna M. Validation and further development of the WHO 10-year fracture risk assessment tool in Italian postmenopausal women: project rationale and description. Clin Exp Rheumatol. 2010;28(4):561–70.
23. Naylor K, Eastell R. Bone turnover markers: use in osteoporosis. Nat Rev Rheumatol. 2012;8(7):379–89. https://doi.org/10.1038/nrrheum.2012.86.
24. Garnero P, Shih WJ, Gineyts E, Karpf DB, Delmas PD. Comparison of new biochemical markers of bone turnover in late postmenopausal osteoporotic women in response to alendronate treatment. J Clin Endocrinol Metab. 1994;79(6):1693–700. https://doi.org/10.1210/jcem.79.6.7989477.
25. Diez-Perez A, Naylor KE, Abrahamsen B, Agnusdei D, Brandi ML, Cooper C, Dennison E, Eriksen EF, Gold DT, Guanabens N, Hadji P, Hiligsmann M, Horne R, Josse R, Kanis JA, Obermayer-Pietsch B, Prieto-Alhambra D, Reginster JY, Rizzoli R, Silverman S, Zillikens MC, Eastell R, Adherence Working Group of the International Osteoporosis F, the European Calcified Tissue S. International Osteoporosis Foundation and European Calcified Tissue Society Working Group. Recommendations for the screening of adherence to oral bisphosphonates. Osteoporos Int. 2017;28(3):767–74. https://doi.org/10.1007/s00198-017-3906-6.

26. Lewiecki EM, Laster AJ. Clinical review: clinical applications of vertebral fracture assessment by dual-energy X-ray absorptiometry. J Clin Endocrinol Metab. 2006;91(11):4215–22. https://doi.org/10.1210/jc.2006-1178.
27. Jiang G, Eastell R, Barrington NA, Ferrar L. Comparison of methods for the visual identification of prevalent vertebral fracture in osteoporosis. Osteoporos Int. 2004;15(11):887–96. https://doi.org/10.1007/s00198-004-1626-1.
28. Genant HK, Wu CY, van Kuijk C, Nevitt MC. Vertebral fracture assessment using a semiquantitative technique. J Bone Miner Res. 1993;8(9):1137–48. https://doi.org/10.1002/jbmr.5650080915.
29. Eastell R, Cedel SL, Wahner HW, Riggs BL, Melton LJ. Classification of vertebral fractures. J Bone Miner Res. 1991;6(3):207–15. https://doi.org/10.1002/jbmr.5650060302.
30. McCloskey EV, Spector TD, Eyres KS, Fern ED, O'Rourke N, Vasikaran S, Kanis JA. The assessment of vertebral deformity: a method for use in population studies and clinical trials. Osteoporos Int. 1993;3(3):138–47.

Functional Evaluation of the Subjects with Skeletal Alterations

4

Giovanni Iolascon, Alessandro de Sire, Marco Paoletta, Antimo Moretti, and Francesca Gimigliano

4.1 Introduction

Health and well being of an individual are directly related to the functional status of the various systems of the human body. The World Health Organization (WHO) defines health as "a state of complete physical, mental and social well-being and not merely the absence of disease or infirmity" [1]. In 2001, a new classification system based on this bio-psychosocial model [2], the "International Classification of Functioning, Disability and Health" (ICF), was proposed to provide a unified and international common language and framework for the description of functioning, disability and health [3]. In the term "functioning" WHO includes all body functions and structures, personal activities and social participation. In this framework, "functioning" and "disability" become the centre of health-care provision. Therefore any health-care intervention should be intended to restore impaired body structures and functions, to overcome activity limitations and participation restrictions, and to prevent new alterations and disabilities from developing, especially in case of a chronic disease [4].

The most common diseases affecting the musculoskeletal system are osteoarthritis and osteoporosis. In this chapter we will only deal with the functional evaluation of osteoporotic patients.

In the past, osteoporosis used to be defined as a silent disease and it was identified only after the occurrence of a fragility fracture. Nowadays the appropriate management of osteoporotic patients requires an accurate functional evaluation even before the appearance of a fragility fracture. The cornerstone of this management is to identify the prodromal symptoms and signs of a fragility fracture and of its risk factors.

G. Iolascon (✉) · A. de Sire · M. Paoletta · A. Moretti
Department of Medical and Surgical Specialties and Dentistry,
University of Campania "Luigi Vanvitelli", Naples, Italy

F. Gimigliano
Department of Mental and Physical Health and Preventive Medicine,
University of Campania "Luigi Vanvitelli", Naples, Italy

A. Lenzi, S. Migliaccio (eds.), *Multidisciplinary Approach to Osteoporosis*,
https://doi.org/10.1007/978-3-319-75110-8_4

4.2 Functional Evaluation

The functional evaluation of osteoporotic patients is a part of the physical examination aimed to identify systemic alterations that induce an increased risk of fracturing or are consequences of fragility fractures. For example, the inspection allows the identification of postural alterations, such as increased kyphosis of the thoracic spine, protruded abdomen or loss of body height that might be ascribed to the presence of one or more vertebral deformities. Measurement of height is probably one of the easiest ways to identify patients with vertebral deformities due to osteoporosis. A height reduction of 4 cm or more is a reliable sign of a vertebral fracture. After sustaining this kind of fracture, patients frequently refer that their clothes are longer or do not fit as they used to. For an objective evaluation of the severity of the kyphosis, the wall-occiput distance (WOD) can be measured quantifying the distance from the bony prominence of the seventh cervical vertebra (occiput) to the wall, while standing against the wall [5, 6]. The measurement of WOD is one of the most useful maneuver for the clinical assessment of kyphosis. It has been proved that a WOD >4 cm can detect the presence of a prevalent thoracic vertebral fracture with a sensitivity of 41% and specificity of 92% [7]. Another measurement to take is the Rib-Pelvis Distance (RPD) (see Fig. 4.1) that can localize vertebral fractures at the lumbar spine level, a distance of <2 fingerbreadths (about 3.5 cm) has a high sensitivity (87%) for detecting a lumbar vertebral fracture with a specificity of 47% [8].

It is worthwhile to remember that patients with multiple vertebral fractures, with a significant kyphosis, might have severe respiratory consequences such as chronic obstructive pulmonary disease and pneumonia both increasing their mortality risk [9].

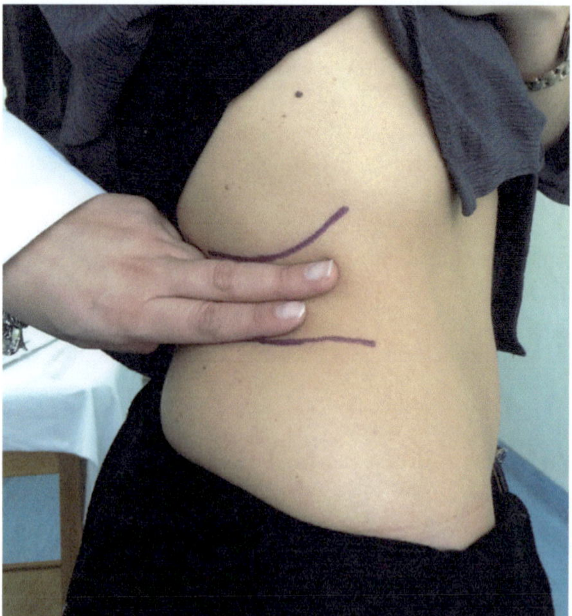

Fig. 4.1 The rib-pelvis distance

During the functional evaluation it is mandatory to investigate the following parameters: range of motion (ROM), muscle assessment (mass, strength, and power), balance, and disability. An accurate investigation of pain and quality of life is also necessary to complete the framework.

4.2.1 Range of Motion

The ROM is defined as the extent of passive or active joint mobility, measured in degrees. It can vary according to age, gender, functioning, body habitus, and genetics. Passive ROM should be performed through all planes of motion (sagittal, coronal and transverse), by the examiner when the patient is in a relaxed position. We define the ROM as active when the patient performs the same movements by himself. An impaired joint should be always compared with the contralateral one, whenever it is possible. The flexibility of the trunk is the most difficult to be assessed as no measurement tools can be used and it is necessary to rely on functional tests. One of these is the Schober test: while the patient is in a standing position, the examiner marks two points along the proximal and distal ends of the lumbar spine and this distance is taken when the trunk is in a flexed, neutral, and extended position. An alternative is the Modified Schober Test that propose to mark a point located 5 cm below and 10 cm above the lumbosacral junction for a total of 15 cm distance, if when flexing the distance between the two marks do not reach 20 cm it means that there is a limitation in lumbar flexion (see Fig. 4.2).

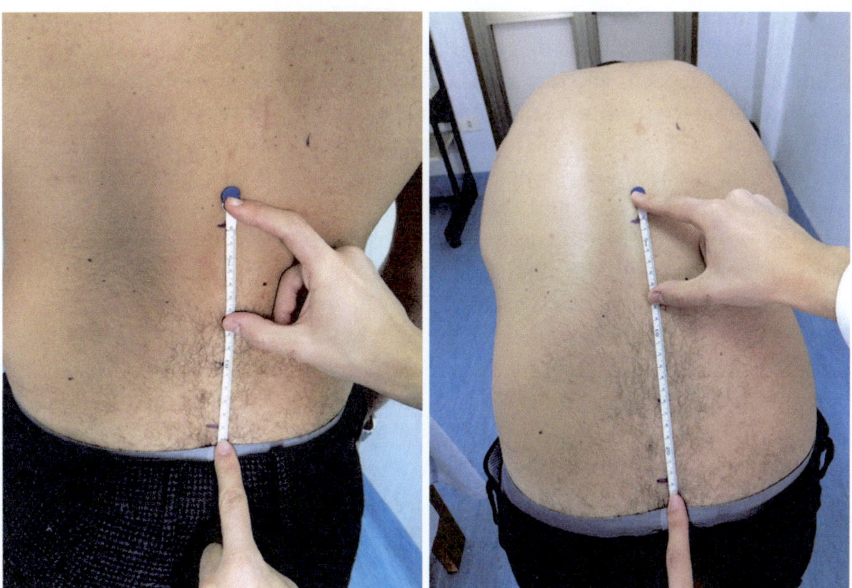

Fig. 4.2 Modified Schober test

These tests seem to be more reliable than others, such as the measurement of the distance of the fingers to the floor or the inclinometer technique of Loebl. These tests can result positive in case of vertebral fragility fractures [10].

4.2.2 Muscle Assessment

An accurate assessment of muscle functioning in osteoporotic patients should include the evaluation of muscle mass, muscle strength, and muscle power. The last one is an important predictor of physical functioning. Alterations in muscle functioning are important reasons for the loss of independence [11].

In the past, age-related muscle alterations were identified only with the loss of muscle mass, the so called "sarcopenia"; the term was coined to describe the loss of lean mass and derived from the Greek "sarcos" referring to flesh and "penia," a lack of. Recently it has been proposed to introduce the term "dynapenia" in addition to "sarcopenia" when specifically referring to the loss of muscle function [12, 13]. More recently it was introduced the term "osteosarcopenia" to better identify those people affected both by a loss of muscle mass and a reduction of BMD, as they are supposed to be strictly related as they share common physio-pathological pathways [14].

In order to better explain muscle assessment we divided the topic in three different paragraphs: muscle mass, muscle strength, and muscle power and physical performance.

4.2.2.1 Muscle Mass Assessment

Considering that the clinical evaluation by anthropomorphic measurements is scarcely correlated with the diagnosis of sarcopenia (as changes in body composition like fat deposits and loss of skin elasticity might be possible confounders), it is preferable to perform an instrumental evaluation of muscle mass. Computed Tomography (CT) and Magnetic Resonance Imaging are considered as the gold standard for an accurate estimate of muscle mass and body composition. The high costs of both techniques and the high radiation exposure of the CT limit their use to research. Dual-energy X-ray absorptiometry (DXA), using a lower dose of radiation with the similar accuracy to discriminate fat, BMD and lean tissues, is a valid alternative. The Total Body examination with DXA can be considered the gold standard in the measurement of the loss of muscle mass as it can define the appendicular lean mass (ALM). According to the Foundation of the National Institutes of Health (FNIH), a reduced muscle mass is defined by gender-specific cut-offs: ratio ALM to body mass index <0.512 for women and <0.789 for men [15]. When a DXA evaluation cannot be available, the Bioelectrical Impedance Analysis (BIA) might represent an easy and inexpensive alternative tool.

4.2.2.2 Muscle Strength Assessment

Muscle strength is defined as the maximum amount of force a muscle can generate during its contraction [16]. Size and innervation of muscle fibers are responsible of the strength.

It is important to measure muscle strength of both upper and lower limbs. Handgrip strength is well correlated to physical performance and it is also strongly related with lower extremity muscle power, and with the level of disability in activities of daily living (ADL) [17]. Upper limb muscle strength can be calculated with the Hand Grip Strength Test (HGS), through the hand-held Jamar dynamometer, considering the maximum value (in kilograms) of three consecutive measurements of the upper dominant limb (with a pause of 1 min after each measurement). The cut-off to define hand grip muscle weakness is <16 kg [15]. Lower limbs muscular strength can be measured isokinetically with an isokinetec device or isometrically with the Knee Extension Strength Test (KES). The KES is performed by a hand-held dynamometer and the mean value (in kilograms) of three consecutive measurements (with a pause of 1 min after each measurement) is assumed for each patient [18]. A ratio of KES and body weight (BW) (KES/BW) inferior to 0.31 defines lower limb muscle weakness.

4.2.2.3 Muscle Power and Physical Performance Assessment

Muscle power represents the maximum rate of work undertaken by a muscle per unit of time. It plays a key role in functional independence; in particular, the peak muscle power seems to be associated with physical performance more than strength in older people [19] Common activities such as walking, climbing stairs, and standing from a seated position require sufficient leg muscle power [20]. Physical performance is defined as the ability to perform a physical task consisting in aerobic and anaerobic capacity, balance, coordination, flexibility; it results from several factors, such as age, sex, hereditary factors, nutrition, and training [21].

Muscle power can be assessed using evaluation tools, such as the sit to stand test, that investigate the ability and the time to stand up from a sitting position. Patients are first asked to stand from a sitting position for five times, as fast as possible, without using their arms. The test is performed twice with an interval of 1 min and it is considered the time of the best performance. "Normal" times for community dwelling older adults are: 11.4 s at 60–69 years, 12.6 s at 70–79, and 14.8 s over 80 years old [22].

Buatois et al. demonstrated that subjects requiring more than 15 s to complete the task showed a risk of recurrent falls twice higher than those performing in <15 s [23]. The sit-to-stand test is easy as it can be performed everywhere and by everybody just using a chair and a stopwatch and its results are directly related with the level of independence in elderly people [24].

Another test generally used to assess leg muscle power is the Stair Climb Power Test, consisting in recording the time necessary to climb a 10-stair flight of stairs, with the use of the handrail if needed; the average time of two trials is considered.

The test is easy to perform as it can be completed in <1 min and requires only a scale and a stopwatch [25].

One of the most widely used assessment tools for physical performance is the Short Physical Performance Battery (SPPB), including three sub-items: balance, gait, and sit to stand test. For the evaluation of balance we ask subjects to stand in three different positions (with feet in side-by-side, in a semi-tandem, and in tandem positions) for 10 s; the score goes from 0 (unable to hold any of the three positions) to 4 (able to hold all the three positions for 10 s). Gait speed is assessed asking subjects to walk for 4 m at a normal pace; a score of 0 is given when the patients cannot perform the test, while 4 means that the task is completed in <4.1 s. Furthermore, the sit to stand test assesses the lower limb strength with participants instructed to sit in and fully rise from a chair five times as quickly as possible, without using arms for supporting. The score goes from 0 when the task is not completed to 4 when it is done in <11.1 s [26].

The overall score of SPPB ranges therefore from 0 to 12. The test can be administered in about 10 min and uniformly performed in each context by all researchers and clinicians. It has an excellent degree of reliability [27] and it is a good predictor of the functional status in older people, where a low score is associated with a higher risk of disability and hospitalization [28, 29].

Another very common and quick test is the 6-minute walk test (6MWT), performed asking the patient to walk as far as possible on a flat indoor course for 6 min. This test can measure muscle tolerance and endurance as well.

4.2.3 Balance Assessment

The aims of balance assessments is to identify the presence of any balance impairment and its possible cause in order to predict the risk of falling [30].

Fall is probably the most important risk factor for fragility fractures. The history of falls, including the number, the circumstances and other risk factors have to be consistently investigated [31]. Risk factors of falls can be broadly classified into intrinsic and extrinsic. The intrinsic risk factors include all the age-related physiological changes (such as visual impairments and/or senile gait), cognitive impairments (delirium, anxiety, depression, reduced attention and psychomotor restlessness), several medical conditions (all the diseases affecting the sensory and neuromuscular system contributing to postural stability) and drugs (the risk of falling is significantly increased when a person is on more than four medications, irrespective of the type of drug). Extrinsic risk factors account for the 33–50% of overall falls. Environmental factors include narrow steps or unmarked floor rises, slippery surfaces, low light or excessive glare, and ill-fitting footwear. Activity-related risk factors are associated to the person's need for or inappropriate use of assistive devices and the so called "furniture cruising" [32]. The acronym DAME (D: drugs and alcohol; A: age-related physiological changes; M: medical problems; E: environment) can be used to recall all the necessary information to investigate during the anamnesis [33].

A commonly used test for predicting risk of falls is the Timed Up and Go test (TUG); it measures the time necessary to stand up from a chair, walk for 3 m, turn around, come back, and sit again; normal values for elderly range from 7 to 10 s [34]. The TUG is considered the simplest and most reliable test for balance assessment [30].

The Berg Balance Scale (BBS) is a complex assessment tool, constituted by 14 items, used to assess balance and risk of falls in older community-dwelling adults [35].

It can be completed in 10–20 min and it measures the ability of the patient to maintain balance while standing or when performing different movements. Each item is scored from 0 (inability to complete the task) to 4 (ability to complete it independently). Therefore the global score ranges from 0 to 56. Scores from 0 to 20 reflect the presence of a balance impairment, 21–40 an acceptable balance, and 41–56 a good balance. The BBS involves minimal equipment (chair, stopwatch, ruler, step) and space and requires no specialized training.

Another example of a complex scale is the Performance Oriented Mobility Assessment (POMA) or Tinetti test, a standardized assessment tool for both balance and gait. With POMA, balance is assessed while the patient is sitting, arising, standing, and turning; the right and left feet are separately evaluated for both step length and clearance, and then compared for symmetry and continuity. Additionally, any path deviation and trunk instability are searched. A score of 22 or less, out of a maximum score of 28, indicates that the patient is at high risk of falling [36].

Another simple and easy to perform test to assess balance is the Unipedal Stance Test (UST). It consists in measuring the length of time a patient is able to stand on one foot first with eyes open and then closed. Hurvitz et al. report that a UST lower than 30 s in an older ambulatory outpatient population is associated with a history of falling, while a UST higher than 30 s is associated with a low risk of falling [37]. The test was demonstrated to be age-specific but not gender-related [38].

Furthermore, the Functional Reach (FR) test could measure anterior and posterior instability [39]; the patient is asked to slide a peg mounted on a horizontal bar, settled on a tripod, as far as possible without loosing his/her balance, while standing and with the other hand on the umbilicus. The test includes 3 trials and the mean distance is entered in the analysis.

4.2.4 Disability Assessment

The most used disability assessment tools are the Barthel Index (BI) and the Functional Independence Measure (FIM).

The BI or its modified version (Modified Barthel Index, MBI) assesses the ability of an individual to care for him/herself during different ADL. The BI maximum score is 20, while the MBI is 100; in both cases 0 refers to the complete dependence and the maximum score to complete autonomy.

The FIM was designed to provide a consistent data collection tool for comparison of rehabilitation outcomes across the continuum of healthcare. It consists of

18 items assessing the patient's degree of disability and burden of care, of these 13 items define the disability in motor functions and the others the disability in cognitive functions [40]. Each item is rated on a 7-point scale, with 1 = total assistance (<25% independence) and 7 = complete independence (100% independence). The total score is useful to determine the degree of help the patient needs to accomplish basic daily tasks. The degree of dependency ranges from no help needed to complete dependence on a caregiver. The FIM should be performed at admission to rehabilitation and at discharge [41].

Other two disability scales are the ADL and instrumental activities of daily living (IADL) that measure respectively the autonomy of the patient in performing several activities without or with the use of different tools.

The term ADL is used in healthcare to refer to people's daily self care activities. This concept was originally proposed in the 1950s by Sidney Katz [42]. ADL include self-care tasks, such as: bathing/showering, bowel and bladder management, dressing/undressing, eating (or swallowing), feeding, functional mobility such as transfers and bed mobility, sexual activities, toilet hygiene, and the care of personal devices such as hearing aids, orthotics, and splints.

The IADL scale was developed to assess more complex activities necessary for functioning in community settings (e.g., shopping, cooking, managing finances). The capacity to handle these complex functions normally is lost earlier than the basic ADL [43].

4.3 Pain Assessment

From Aristotle, through Descartes, to arrive to the early nineteenth century evolutionists, pain has been described as a mechanism to protect the body, and therefore as useful. A modern and widely accepted definition of pain was formulated by the IASP (International Association for the Study of Pain) that defined it "an unpleasant sensory and emotional experience which we primarily associate with tissue damage or describe in terms of such damage, or both". Recently Kandel defined pain as "not the direct expression of a sensory event but rather the product of elaborate processing by the brain of a variety of neural signals". Nociception is the most common starting mechanism of pain; it can be elicited by the stimulation of nociceptors and transmitted by myelin (Aδ) and non-myelin (C) sensitive nerve fibers [44].

Osteoporotic bone does not activate the pain pathway present in the bone tissue; therefore the disease remains asymptomatic until the fracture occurs [45]. On the other hand, vertebral fractures are the main cause both of acute and chronic pain in osteoporotic patients. Acute pain is generally a consequence of a sudden vertebral collapse and it generally increases in the standing position and decreases during rest. Pain can be aroused pushing on the spinous processes and it might bring to different degrees of functional limitation till immobility.

A comprehensive assessment of pain is required to characterize and quantify its impact on a patient's health status and well being, with special attention to its onset, location, intensity, characteristics and its effects on patient's functioning and ADL. Pain should be assessed both qualitatively and quantitatively.

Qualitatively, pain can be described as burning, clamping, electric-like, compressive, prickly, pincer etc. Moreover, it is important to define the site and irradiation of pain and the condition that cause or relieve it like movements, posture, bedsores etc.

Quantitatively, we can perform an objective measurement of pain using a pressure algometer, an instrument for measuring sensitivity to pressure or to pain (Fig. 4.3).

More often pain assessment is done subjectively, using mono-dimensional or multidimensional scales. Unidimensional scales measure only the intensity pain, whereas multidimensional ones can assess, apart from its intensity, the extent to which pain impacts on other components, such as affective, cognitive and behavioural parameters.

The Visual Analogic Scale (VAS) and the Numerical Rating Scale (NRS) are the most widely known and used mono-dimensional scales for the measurement of pain. VAS is based on an analogic measure of pain asking to the patient to point the intensity of pain on a 10 cm line. The lower and the upper limits correspond to the absence of pain and the worst imaginable pain respectively [46]. NRS is a segmented version of VAS, where patients express on a 0–10 scale the intensity of their pain. NRS is easier to use than VAS, because it is simpler to be understood and

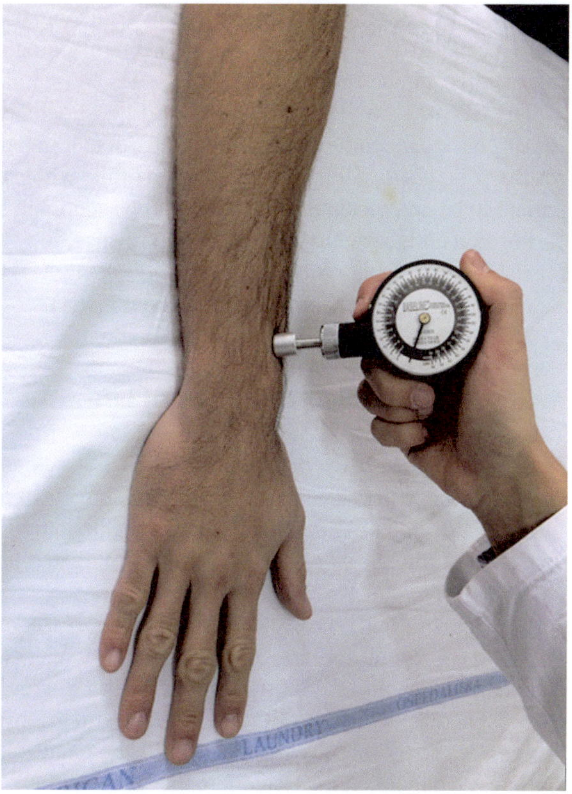

Fig. 4.3 Algometer

executed by patients. Other mono-dimensional scale is the Verbal Categorical Rating Scale (VRS); which consists of a list of adjectives describing increasing pain intensities (no pain, mild pain, moderate pain, and severe or intense pain) [47].

Multidimensional scales measure several dimensions of pain, such as quality, intensity, interference with functioning and the effects on the quality of life. They are more complete and useful than mono-dimensional ones. Good examples of multidimensional scales are: the McGill Pain Questionnaire (MPQ) and its short form (SF-MPQ); the Brief Pain Inventory (BPI); and Spine Pain Index (SPI).

The MPQ is formed of two parts: the Pain Rating Index and the Present Pain Intensity. The questionnaire can be completed in 20 min plus 2–5 min to score it [48]. Its short form, the SF-MPQ is composed of the same two parts, but takes about 2–5 min to be executed and only 1 min to be scored [49].

The BPI [50] assesses pain severity and its interference with functioning, using a 0–10 NRS for each item. The Pain Intensity Score is the results of the average of the item "worst pain", "least pain, "average pain", over the last 24 h and finally the "present pain". The Pain Interference Score estimates patient's limits due to pain using a numeric scale from 1 to 10, going to "no interference" to "interferes completely". The seven domains investigated are: general activity, walking, normal work, interpersonal relations, mood, sleep and enjoyment of life [51]. The score is obtained by an arithmetic average of the interference item's rating. The questionnaire also gives the possibility to indicate the location of pain on a body chart and to describe it as stabbing, tingling, oppressive, pulsing, burning. The percentage of the relief achieved as a consequence of a pharmacological or non-pharmacological intervention can be easily calculated.

The SPI is a simple self-administered questionnaire that investigates the influence of back pain on functioning and in particular in the execution of ADL. It analyses the patient's disability due to the pain of the whole column requiring <5 min for patient to be completed and about 20 s to be scored [52].

For non collaborating patients there are specific pain assessment scales such as the Pain Assessment in Advanced Dementia (PAINAD) and the Non-Communicative Patient's Pain Assessment Instrument (NOPPAIN).

4.4 Health-Related Quality of Life

Health-Related Quality of Life (HRQoL) is "a concept representing individual responses to the physical, mental and social effects of illness on daily living, which influence the extent to which personal satisfaction with life circumstances can be achieved…it includes perceptions of well-being and basic level of satisfaction and a general sense of self-worth" [53].

Osteoporosis and fragility fractures might have a considerable impact on HRQoL.

There are several scales available for its assessment that can be roughly classified as generic (such as The Short Form 36 Health Survey, SF36, European Quality of Life–5 Dimensions index, EQ-5D index, and the EuroQol-Visual Analogue Scale scores, EQ VAS) and disease specific (as the Quality of Life Questionnaire of the European Foundation for Osteoporosis, QUALEFFO).

The SF36 is one of the most used instruments to assess quality of life in different diseases. It comprises 36 items, with six possible answers, from "none" to "very severe" according to an ordinal scale, investigating eight domains (physical functioning, social functioning, physical role functioning, emotional role functioning, mental well-being, vitality, bodily pain, and general health perceptions). Two summary scores are calculated: the physical (PCS) and mental (MCS) components. Shorter versions of this questionnaire are the SF-12 and SF-8 [54].

Another generic scale is the EQ-5D, a self-administered and short questionnaire [55]. It consists of two main parts: the first including five dimensions, EQ-5D index [56], the second part is a VAS, which has as end points "the best imaginable health states" and "the worst imaginable health state" indicated on a scale from 100 to 0 respectively.

As for the HRQoL measuring instruments specifically built for osteoporotic women, the most used is the QUALEFFO, a self-administered questionnaire for patients with vertebral fractures, developed by European Foundation for Osteoporosis. It includes five domains: pain, physical activity, social, general, and mental.

References

1. World Health Organization. Preamble to the Constitution of the World Health Organization as adopted by the International Health Conference, New York, 19–22 June, 1946; signed on 22 July 1946 by the representatives of 61 States (official records of the World Health Organization, no. 2, p. 100) and entered into force on 7 April 1948.
2. Engel GL. The need for a new medical model: a challenge for biomedicine. Science. 1977; 196(4286):129–36.
3. World Health Organization. International classification of functioning disability, and health: ICF. Geneva: WHO; 2001.
4. Cieza A, Stucki G. Content comparison of health-related quality of life (HRQOL) instruments based on the international classification of functioning, disability and health (ICF). Qual Life Res. 2005;14(5):1225–37.
5. Antonelli-Incalzi R, Pedone C, Cesari M, Di Iorio A, Bandinelli S, Ferrucci L. Relationship between the occiput-wall distance and physical performance in the elderly: a cross sectional study. Aging Clin Exp Res. 2007;19:207–12.
6. Balzini L, Vannucchi L, Benvenuti F, Benucci M, Monni M, Cappozzo A, et al. Clinical characteristics of flexed posture in elderly women. J Am Geriatr Soc. 2003;51:1419–26.
7. Siminoski K, Warshawski RS, Jen H, Lee KC. The accuracy of clinical kyphosis examination for detection of thoracic vertebral fractures: comparison of direct and indirect kyphosis measures. J Musculoskelet Neuronal Interact. 2011;11(3):249–56.
8. Siminoski K, Warshawski RS, Jen H, Lee KC. Accuracy of physical examination using the rib-pelvis distance for detection of lumbar vertebral fractures. Am J Med. 2003;115(3):233–6.
9. Kado DM, Browner WS, Palermo L, et al. Vertebral fractures and mortality in older women: a prospective study. Study of Osteoporotic Fractures Research Group. Arch Intern Med. 1999; 159:1215–20.
10. Cifu DX. Braddom's physical medicine and rehabilitation. 5th ed; 2016. ISBN: 978-0-323-28046-4.
11. Hars M, Biver E, Chevalley T, Herrmann F, Rizzoli R, Ferrari S, Trombetti A. Low lean mass predicts incident fractures independently from FRAX: a prospective cohort study of recent retirees. J Bone Miner Res. 2016;31(11):2048–56. https://doi.org/10.1002/jbmr.2878. Epub 2016 Jun 27.

12. Clark BC, Manini TM. Sarcopenia ≠ Dynapenia. J Gerontol A Biol Sci Med Sci. 2008; 63(8):829–34.
13. Clark BC, Manini TM. Functional consequences of sarcopenia and dynapenia in the elderly. Curr Opin Clin Nutr Metab Care. 2010;13(3):271–6.
14. Huo YR, Suriyaarachchi P, Gomez F, Curcio CL, Boersma D, Muir SW, Montero-Odasso M, Gunawardene P, Demontiero O, Duque G. Phenotype of osteosarcopenia in older individuals with a history of falling. J Am Med Dir Assoc. 2015;16(4):290–5.
15. Studenski SA, Peters KW, Alley DE, Cawthon PM, McLean RR, Harris TB, Ferrucci L, Guralnik JM, Fragala MS, Kenny AM, Kiel DP, Kritchevsky SB, Shardell MD, Dam TT, Vassileva MT. The FNIH sarcopenia project: rationale, study description, conference recommendations, and final estimates. J Gerontol A Biol Sci Med Sci. 2014;69(5):547–58.
16. Cooper C, Fielding R, Visser M, van Loon LJ, Rolland Y, Orwoll E, Reid K, Boonen S, Dere W, Epstein S, Mitlak B, Tsouderos Y, Sayer AA, Rizzoli R, Reginster JY, Kanis JA. Tools in assessment of sarcopenia. Calcif Tissue Int. 2013;93(3):201–10.
17. Cruz-Jentoft AJ, Baeyens JP, Bauer JM, Boirie Y, Cederholm T, Landi F, Martin FC, Michel JP, Rolland Y, Schneider SM, Topinková E, Vandewoude M, Zamboni M, European Working Group on Sarcopenia in Older People. Sarcopenia: European consensus on definition and diagnosis: report of the European Working Group on Sarcopenia in Older People. Age Ageing. 2010;39(4):412–23.
18. Andrews AW, Thomas MW, Bohannon RW. Normative values for isometric muscle force measurements obtained with hand-held dynamometers. Phys Ther. 1996;76(3):248–59.
19. Bassey EJ, Fiatarone MA, O'Neill EF, Kelley M, Lipsitz LA, Evans WJ. Leg extensor power and functional performance in very old men and women. Clin Sci. 1992;82:321–7.
20. Foldvari M, Clark M, Laviolette LC, Bernstein MA, Kaliton D, Castaneda C, Pu CT, Hausdorff JM, Fielding RA, Singh MA. Association of muscle power with functional status in community-dwelling elderly women. J Gerontol A Biol Sci Med Sci. 2000;55(4):M192–9.
21. Tsianos GI, Evangelou E, Boot A, Zillikens MC, van Meurs JB, Uitterlinden AG, Ioannidis JP. Associations of polymorphisms of eight muscle- or metabolism-related genes with performance in Mount Olympus marathon runners. J Appl Physiol. 2010;108:567–74.
22. Bohannon RW. Reference values for the five-repetition sit-to-stand test: a descriptive meta-analysis of data from elders. Percept Mot Skills. 2006;103(1):215–22.
23. Buatois S, Perret-Guillaume C, Gueguen R, Miget P, Vançon G, Perrin P, Benetos A. A simple clinical scale to stratify risk of recurrent falls in community-dwelling adults aged 65 years and older. Phys Ther. 2010;90(4):550–60.
24. Corrigan D, Bohannon RW. Relationship between knee extension force and stand-up performance in community-dwelling elderly women. Arch Phys Med Rehabil. 2001;82(12):1666–72.
25. Bean JF, Kiely DK, LaRose S, Alian J, Frontera WR. Is stair climb power a clinically relevant measure of leg power impairments in at-risk older adults? Arch Phys Med Rehabil. 2007;88(5):604–9.
26. Guralnik JM, Ferrucci L, Pieper CF, Leveille SG, Markides KS, Ostir GV, Studenski S, Berkman LF, Wallace RB. Lower extremity function and subsequent disability: consistency across studies, predictive models, and value of gait speed alone compared with the short physical performance battery. J Gerontol A Biol Sci Med Sci. 2000;55(4):M221–31.
27. Ostir GV, Volpato S, Fried LP, Chaves P, Guralnik JM. Reliability and sensitivity to change assessed for a summary measure of lower body function: results from the Women's health and aging study. J Clin Epidemiol. 2002;55:916–21.
28. Ahmed T, Vafaei A, Auais M, Guralnik J, Zunzunegui MV. Gender roles and physical function in older adults: cross-sectional analysis of the international mobility in aging study (IMIAS). PLoS One. 2016;11(6):e0156828.
29. Keeler E, Guralnik JM, Tian H, Wallace RB, Reuben DB. The impact of functional status on life expectancy in older persons. J Gerontol A Biol Sci Med Sci. 2010;65(7):727–33.
30. Mancini M, Horak FB. The relevance of clinical balance assessment tools to differentiate balance deficits. Eur J Phys Rehabil Med. 2010;46(2):239–48.
31. Iolascon G, Gravina P, Luciano F, Palladino C, Gimigliano F. Characteristics and circumstances of falls in hip fractures. Aging Clin Exp Res. 2013;25(Suppl 1):S133–5.

32. World Health Organization. Global report on falls prevention in older age. Geneva: WHO; 2007.
33. Close JCT. Falls in older people: risk factors, assessment and intervention. IBMS BoneKey. 2009;6(10):368–84.
34. Podsiadlo D, Richardson S. The timed "Up & Go": a test of basic functional mobility for frail elderly persons. J Am Geriatr Soc. 1991;39(2):142–8.
35. Berg KO, Wood-Dauphinee SL, Williams JI, Maki B. Measuring balance in the elderly: validation of an instrument. Can J Public Health. 1992;83(Suppl 2):S7–11.
36. Tinetti ME. Performance-oriented assessment of mobility problems in elderly patients. J Am Geriatr Soc. 1986;34:119–26.
37. Hurvitz EA, Richardson JK, Werner RA, Ruhl AM, Dixon MR. Unipedal stance testing as an indicator of fall risk among older outpatients. Arch Phys Med Rehabil. 2000;81(5):587–91.
38. Springer BA, Marin R, Cyhan T, Roberts H, Gill NW. Normative values for the unipedal stance test with eyes open and closed. J Geriatr Phys Ther. 2007;30(1):8–15.
39. Duncan PW, Weiner DK, Chandler J, Studenski S. Functional reach: a new clinical measure of balance. J Gerontol. 1990;45(6):M192–7.
40. Horn SD, DeJong G, Smout R, Gassaway J, James R, Conroy B. Stroke rehabilitation patients, practice, and outcomes: is earlier and more aggressive therapy better? Arch Phys Med Rehabil. 2005;86(12 Suppl 2):S101–14.
41. Linacre JM, Heinemann AW, Wright BD, Granger CV, Hamilton BB. The structure and stability of the functional independence measure. Arch Phys Med Rehabil. 1994;75(2):127–32.
42. Noelker LS, Browdie R. Sidney Katz, MD: a new paradigm for chronic illness and long-term care. Gerontologist. 2014;54(1):13–20. https://doi.org/10.1093/geront/gnt086. Epub 2013 Aug 22.
43. Graf C. The Lawton instrumental activities of daily living (IADL) scale. Medsurg Nurs. 2009;18(5):315–6.
44. Martin CD, Jimenez-Andrade JM, Ghilardi JR, Mantyh PW. Organization of a unique net-like meshwork of CGRP+ sensory fibers in the mouse periosteum: implications for the generation and maintenance of bone fracture pain. Neurosci Lett. 2007;427(3):148–52.
45. Iolascon G, Gimigliano F, Moretti A, Bianco M, Cannaviello G, Gimigliano R. Dolore e osteoporosi. In: Saggini R, Buoso S, Pestelli G, editors. Dolore e riabilitazione; 2014. p. 187–202. ISBN: 9788877118134.
46. Williamson A, Hoggart B. Pain: a review of three commonly used pain rating scales. J Clin Nurs. 2005;14(7):798–804.
47. Breivik H, Borchgrevink PC, Allen SM, Rosseland LA, Romundstad L, Hals EK, Kvarstein G, Stubhaug A. Assessment of pain. Br J Anaesth. 2008;101(1):17–24.
48. Melzack R. The McGill pain questionnaire: major properties and scoring methods. Pain. 1975;1(3):277–99.
49. Melzack R. The short-form McGill pain questionnaire. Pain. 1987;30:191–7.
50. Daut RL, Cleeland CS, Flanery RC. Development of the Wisconsin brief pain questionnaire to assess pain in cancer and other diseases. Pain. 1983;17:197–21.
51. Cleeland CS, Ryan KM. Pain assessment: global use of the brief pain inventory. Ann Acad Med Singap. 1994;23(2):129–38.
52. Iolascon G, Gimigliano F, Gison A, et al. Validazione di un nuovo score di disabilita` da lombalgia: lo Spine Pain Index. Europa Medicophysica. 2003;39(suppl 1):600–3.
53. Bowling A. Measuring health: a review of quality of life measurement scales. 2nd ed. Buckingham: Open University Press; 1997.
54. Ware JE Jr, Sherbourne CD. The MOS 36-item short-form health survey (SF-36). I. Conceptual framework and item selection. Med Care. 1992;30(6):473–83.
55. Walters SJ, Brazier JE. Comparison of the minimally important difference for two health state utility measures: EQ-5D and SF-6D. Qual Life Res. 2005;14(6):1523–32.
56. Janssen MF, Birnie E, Haagsma JA, Bonsel GJ. Comparing the standard EQ–5D three level system with a five level version. Value Health. 2008;11:275–84.

Part I

Endocrinologicic and Metabolic Regulation

Skeletal Alterations and Parathyroid Function

5

Elisabetta Romagnoli and Vincenzo Carnevale

5.1 Introduction

Parathyroid hormone (PTH) action on bone is essential to regulate calcium and phosphorus metabolism as well as skeletal turnover.

The hormone is released from the chief cells of the parathyroid glands. The calcium-sensing receptor (CaSR) expressed in the parathyroid cell membrane is the most important regulator of PTH synthesis and secretion. It is able to register subtle variations of extracellular ionized calcium concentration and, consequently, tightly regulates PTH levels.

PTH plays its functions by binding to the PTH/PTH-related peptide (PTHrP) type 1 receptor (PTHR1), a G-protein-coupled receptor. This receptor is widely expressed on many types of cells, but it is mainly represented on bone and kidney, where PTH exerts its most important functions.

In recent years, accumulating evidences showed that the actions of PTH on bone are much more complex than previously known. In fact, PTH regulates bone turnover by stimulating both bone resorption and bone formation, being the hormone catabolic or anabolic on the skeleton depending on the dose and periodicity of its signal. These different responses are mediated by the complex effects of PTH on bone cells that are, until now, not completely understood [1–3].

E. Romagnoli (✉)
Department of Experimental Medicine, University of Rome "Sapienza", Rome, Italy
e-mail: elisabetta.romagnoli@uniroma1.it

V. Carnevale
Unit of Internal Medicine, "Casa Sollievo della Sofferenza" Hospital,
San Giovanni Rotondo, Italy

A. Lenzi, S. Migliaccio (eds.), *Multidisciplinary Approach to Osteoporosis*,
https://doi.org/10.1007/978-3-319-75110-8_5

5.2 Effect on Bone Resorption

Primary hyperparathyroidism (PHPT) is the most representative human disease in which the catabolic action of PTH on bone is mainly expressed. At the cellular level, this catabolic effect is achieved by the continuous exposure of bone cells to the PTH action. The hormone acts directly on osteoblasts and osteocytes, and, through its effects on these cells, it regulates the activity of osteoclasts, the bone resorbing cells. In turn, bone resorption is controlled by several cellular pathways, the most important of which being represented by the OPG-RANKL-RANK system. In recent years it has been demonstrated that PTH hormone regulates the expression of this pathway not only in the osteoblast lineage but also in the osteocytes, which probably most contribute to the resorpting signal for osteoclasts. Briefly, the increase of RANKL expression and the decrease of OPG expression in both osteoblasts and osteocytes lead to an increased RANKL/OPG ratio; this imbalance seems to be the main determinant of the enhanced osteoclastogenesis induced by PTH. Studies carried out in humans with PHPT seem to support this hypothesis also "in vivo": circulating levels of RANKL and the RANKL/OPG ratio are higher in PHPT patients compared to controls, and, after successful parathyroidectomy, the RANKL/OPG ratio shows a significant reduction [3–5].

5.3 Effect on Bone Formation

The discovery in recent years of the anabolic effect of PTH on bone has established a new potential role of the hormone as a promising therapy for osteoporosis. This action of PTH is evident when it is administered by intermittent injection. This modality leads to an increase in bone mass, contrary to what is observed with the continuous infusion of the hormone, causing a reduction of skeletal mass.

The stimulation of bone formation results from several mechanisms, among which the increased osteoblastogenesis, the decrease of osteoblasts apoptosis and the activation of dormant lining cells.

However, the most important mechanism increasing bone formation is the inhibition of the sclerostin action. This is a glycoprotein, secreted primarily by osteocytes, that antagonizes the osteoanabolic Wnt/β-catenin signalling pathway. So in this sense, PTH acts as an "inhibitor of the inhibitor".

According to "in vitro" studies, also in humans it has been demonstrated that patients with PHPT have lower serum sclerostin levels compared to normal subjects or patients who had undergone parathyroidectomy. Moreover, patients treated with PTH for postmenopausal osteoporosis show reduced serum sclerostin levels. The effect of PTH on the activity of Dickkopf1 (DKK1), another endogenous inhibitor of Wnt signalling, is less well known. In fact, results of "in vitro" studies are not consistent with those obtained in humans: while anabolic treatment with PTH reduces DKK1 mRNA levels in mice, serum levels of the protein are increased in both postmenopausal women treated with anabolic regimen and in patients with PHPT [3–5].

5.4 Primary Hyperparathyroidism

The classical picture of severe skeletal involvement of PHPT includes bone pain and pathologic fractures, subperiosteal erosions and resorption of the distal phalanges, salt-and-pepper appearance of the skull, brown tumours and bone cysts. Such a clinical presentation is now quite uncommon among patients with PHPT, at least in developed countries. Instead, the hallmark of PHPT is an increase of bone turnover rate, which is found also in patients with minimal clinical manifestations and without radiological signs of skeletal involvement [6]. The enhanced activation frequency of bone multicellular units and the corresponding decrease of quiescent surfaces in turn expand the remodelling space. According to histomorphometric studies, as a consequence of such an increase of skeletal turnover rate, the cortical bone would appear more affected than trabecular tissue. In cancellous tissue, at least with mild to moderate PTH excess, the increased turnover rate induces a more active bone formation by the osteoblasts, whereas the tangential erosion of the trabeculae by the osteoclasts would make them thinner but still well connected. The more pronounced involvement of cortical tissue could instead derive from its lower turnover rate, bone resorption prevailing over the less activated formation process or, alternatively, a higher activity of the osteoclasts at the cortico-medullary junction. The higher activation frequency also translates in a less densely mineralized tissue, due to the shortening of secondary mineralization (the recovery of bone mineral density—BMD—following parathyroidectomy partly depends on the higher mineralization of bone matrix), as well as in lower maturation of collagen crosslinks (also ameliorating after surgery).

The histological consequence of this mechanism is the preferential loss of cortical tissue and the relative preservation of the trabecular bone, as is observed in specimens obtained from the biopsy of the iliac crest. Patients with PHPT display thinner and porous cortices, while the microarchitecture of the cancellous bone is substantially unaffected, since the trabeculae have higher number, thickness and connectivity and lower separation than age-matched control subjects. The three-dimensional observation of biopsy blocks by microcomputed tomography (μCT) coincides with the two-dimensional appearance of histological sections [6]. In other words, the modest to moderate increase of PTH levels which usually characterizes the nowadays clinical presentation of PHPT appears to exert an anabolic action on the trabecular tissue, delaying some features of its ageing process.

Under a clinical point of view, the enhanced rate of turnover is reflected by a diffuse increase of the skeletal uptake of bone-seeking tracers, as well as by the augmented concentration of biochemical markers of bone formation and resorption in serum and urine [7]. Bone markers may be frankly elevated when the skeletal involvement is more pronounced but may also remain in the upper range of normal in milder forms of PHPT. Even in the latter cases, however, the significant decrease of both resorption and formation markers after surgery reflects their previous up-regulation due to PTH excess [8].

With the current clinical presentation of PHPT, the measurement of areal BMD (aBMD) by dual-energy X-ray absorptiometry (DXA) due to the wide availability, accuracy, precision and low radiation exposure of this technique has become part of the standard clinical evaluation of these patients [9]. The current guidelines on PHPT recommend aBMD assessment of the third distal radius, lumbar spine, total hip and femoral neck every 1–2 years. Furthermore, in postmenopausal women and men 50 years and older showing a *T*-score value ≤ -2.5 at these sites, parathyroidectomy is indicated [10]. Although the aBMD of the forearm is not routinely measured in many centres, about 5% of patients would fulfil criteria for surgery based only on the *T*-score of the distal radius [11]. In any case, the measurement of aBMD at multiple sites is wise in PHPT, because preferential bone loss occurs at the 1/3 distal radius (where cortical tissue prevails), whereas aBMD of the lumbar spine (having a higher proportion of trabecular tissue) is relatively preserved. Femoral sites, having about equal proportions of the trabecular and cortical bone, show intermediate decreases of aBMD. Such a typical picture of PHPT is almost opposite to what is seen in patients with postmenopausal osteoporosis, whose trabecular bone loss usually anticipates the decline of aBMD detected at sites prominently composed of cortical tissue. However, most cases of PHPT occur in postmenopausal women, so that different patterns of aBMD loss, reflecting the variable influence of the two conditions, may be found in individual patients [9, 12]. DXA aBMD assessment is also a precious tool to monitor patients' skeletal involvement over time. In fact, following parathyroidectomy, aBMD increases, mostly and more rapidly, at the lumbar spine and hip, whereas, if any, the recovery of aBMD is least and lowest at the distal radius. This has also been observed in a small sample of patients with normocalcemic PHPT. In PHPT patients who were not surgical candidates, a cornerstone longitudinal study showed a substantial stability of aBMD values over about 10 years of observation [13]. After longer follow-up periods, bone loss can be detected, particularly in patients younger than 50 years and at sites enriched in cortical tissue, such as distal radius and hip [14].

The DXA assessment of aBMD has invaluable clinical utility. However, although aBMD findings appear overall consistent with those of histomorphometric and μCT studies, they do not explain the increased risk of both vertebral and non-vertebral fractures of patients with PHPT. In particular, postmenopausal women with PHPT, independently of the severity of the disease, have a higher rate of morphometric vertebral fractures, even if aBMD appears preserved [15]. This apparent discrepancy probably relies to the fact that DXA may only provide an integrated estimate of areal density, but does not allow to distinguish between the trabecular and cortical compartments of the examined bone site. High-resolution peripheral quantitative computed tomography (HR-pQCT) is a newer non-invasive technique, hitherto only available in research units, which allows to separately measure the true volumetric density (vBMD) of cortical and trabecular compartments of the radius and the tibia. It also allows to appreciate aspects of bone microarchitecture and strength, which cannot be detected by the DXA technique. In patients with PHPT, through HR-pQCT, it has been shown that vBMD is decreased, besides the whole skeletal site, in both cortical and trabecular compartments. Cortices are thinner, and the trabeculae are fewer, thinner, more spaced and heterogeneously distributed. The alterations of the tibia (a weight-bearing site) are less pronounced than that of the radius, suggesting that gravity could partly mitigate the effects of PTH excess. The abnormalities of vBMD and microarchitecture are associated to altered biomechanical competence, and whole-bone and trabecular strength are decreased by 22% and 46%, respectively [16]. According to a longitudinal study, HR-pQCT-measured vBMD and microarchitecture of the radius and (even slightly more) of the tibia improve following parathyroidectomy.

Despite its speculative relevance, HR-pQCT remains an interesting research tool, still not widely available even in specialized bone units. Another measurement, obtained through the application of a software to DXA devices, the trabecular bone score (TBS), is rapidly gaining wide acceptance and diffusion. It is based on a grey-level textural analysis of the DXA scans of the lumbar spine and can be performed also by analysing previous measurements. TBS has been reported to provide an indirect estimate of trabecular microarchitecture. Its results correlate to the findings of μCT studies, and low values reflect worse bone structure. TBS values significantly correlate with HR-pQCT indices of total, cortical, trabecular vBMD, as well as with trabecular number and whole-bone stiffness of both the radius and the tibia [17]. Low TBS values are actually found also in many PHPT patients with normal aBMD of the lumbar spine. In adjunct, in a group of patients with PHPT, we found that their TBS values were lower than those of control subjects, although the respective aBMD values at the lumbar spine did not differ. Moreover, among PHPT patients, those with vertebral fractures had lower mean TBS values than patients without fractures, whereas TBS did not discriminate patients with and without non-vertebral fractures [18]. So, TBS seems capable to identify vertebral fracture risk better than aBMD measurement, in patients with PHPT as previously found in patients with postmenopausal osteoporosis. Finally, as shown in a small group of PHPT patients followed-up for about 2 years, TBS values may recover after parathyroidectomy more than aBMD values, while they do not significantly change in non-operated patients [19].

5.5 Hypoparathyroidism

Hypoparathyroidism is an endocrine disease characterized by the absent or inappropriately low serum levels of PTH. In recent years it has been demonstrated that chronic PTH deficiency may profoundly affects the bone; however, these skeletal effects are difficult to completely elucidate because of the influence of concomitant chronic vitamin D treatment that clearly interferes with bone metabolism [20].

In general, chronic PTH deficiency leads to a marked reduction of bone turnover; bone resorption and bone formation are either depressed, but over time the remodelling balance favours bone formation. The final result is an increase of bone mass which is evident in both cancellous and cortical compartments. The histomorphometry and μCT of iliac crest bone biopsies give the most comprehensive information about the effects of PTH deficiency on the skeleton. These techniques showed that the reduction of both bone resorption and bone formation was evident at all three envelopes of the bone (cancellous, endocortical and intracortical). Bone formation rate was reduced mostly because of both a decrease in mineralizing surface and mineral apposition rate. μCT confirmed that the higher cancellous bone volume was due to increased trabecular thickness, number and connectivity [20–22].

Non-invasive assessment of skeletal status by DXA consistently shows, across several studies, that BMD in patients with hypoparathyroidism was significantly above the average at lumbar spine and femoral sites. In some cohorts, BMD was also increased at the 1/3 distal and ultradistal radius. The increase in aBMD is probably due to the increased mineralization. However, TBS, that at least indirectly evaluates trabecular microarchitecture, was not changed in hypoparathyroid patients [22].

New insights in the evaluation of bone properties in hypoparathyroidism have been provided by the application of advanced imaging techniques, such as HR-pQCT of the radius and finite element analysis (FEA). These techniques allow to estimate skeletal microarchitecture and estimated bone strength. Trabecular and cortical vBMD, cortical area and cortical thickness were all increased in hypoparathyroidism; on the contrary, cortical porosity was reduced. However, ultimate stress and failure load were not different between hypoparathyroid patients and controls [23]. Changes in skeletal properties showed by the various imaging techniques may divergently affect the propensity to fragility fractures in these patients. However, data published so far concerning the risk of fractures are inconclusive and, sometimes, also divergent. It has been demonstrated that long-term overall fracture risk in patients with hypoparathyroidism was similar compared to controls; however, according to some authors, the risk of upper extremity fractures was increased, while, on the contrary, it was significantly reduced based on other studies. Similar divergent results have been reported also for vertebral fractures [24, 25].

5.6 Effects of Parathyroid Hormone Treatment in Hypoparathyroidism

The administration of hormone replacement therapy with PTH in patients with hypoparathyroidism may help to elucidate the effect of treatment on skeletal abnormalities.

Data of long-term administration of rhPTH 1-84 for up to 6 years have been recently published [26]. This study showed that BMD significantly increased at lumbar spine and femoral neck, while it progressively and significantly decreased at the distal 1/3 radius. Concomitantly, treatment induced an early stimulation of bone remodelling, reflected by a marked increase of both bone formation and bone resorption markers. After the first year, markers of bone turnover progressively declined but remained to levels always above baseline values. These findings are consistent with the different effects of PTH treatment at cortical or trabecular skeletal sites. Long-term administration in hypoparathyroidism leads to beneficial effect on the trabecular bone, increasing areal and volumetric BMD at the lumbar spine as well as TBS values. On the contrary, the effects on the cortical bone (mostly represented at the distal 1/3 radius) are consistent with an increase in cortical porosity and endosteal resorption. The analysis of iliac crest bone biopsies shows that long-term hormone replacement is associated with a decrease in trabecular thickness and an increase in both trabecular number and cortical porosity [27]. Moreover, administration of rhPTH 1-84 is associated with early but transient increase in trabecular bone strength, as demonstrated by the microfinite element (μFE) analysis that is generally accepted as a surrogate marker of bone strength [28]. However, how PTH-induced changes in skeletal properties observed in different studies might reflect a modification of fracture risk still remains to be elucidated. More long-term data about incidence of fractures in hypoparathyroid patients treated with replacement therapy clearly are needed.

References

1. Goltzman D. Physiologic actions of PTH (I). PTH action on the skeleton. In: Bilezikian JP, Marcus R, Levine MA, Marcocci C, Silverberg SJ, Potts Jr JT, editors. The parathyroids: basic and clinical concepts. 3rd ed. London: Academic Press-Elsevier; 2015. p. 139–52.
2. Divieti Pajevic P, Wein MN, Kronenberg HM. Parathyroid hormone actions on bone and kidney. In: Brandi ML, Brown EM, editors. Hypoparathyroidism. Milan: Springer-Verlag; 2015. p. 99–109.
3. Silva BC, Bilezikian JP. Parathyroid hormone: anabolic and catabolic actions on the skeleton. Curr Opin Pharmacol. 2015;22:41–50.
4. Silva BC, Kousteni S. Cellular actions of PTH. Osteoblasts, osteoclasts, and osteocytes. In: Bilezikian JP, Marcus R, Levine MA, Marcocci C, Silverberg SJ, Potts Jr JT, editors. The parathyroids: basic and clinical concepts. 3rd ed. London: Academic Press-Elsevier; 2015. p. 127–37.
5. Silva BC, Bilezikian JP. Anabolic and catabolic pathways of parathyroid hormone on the skeleton. In: Bilezikian JP, Marcus R, Levine MA, Marcocci C, Silverberg SJ, Potts Jr JT, editors. The parathyroids: basic and clinical concepts. 3rd ed. London: Academic Press-Elsevier; 2015. p. 233–44.
6. Dempster DW, Silverberg SJ, Shane E, Bilezikian JP. Bone histomorphometry and bone quality in primary hyperparathyroidism. In: Bilezikian JP, Marcus R, Levine MA, Marcocci C, Silverberg SJ, Potts Jr JT, editors. The parathyroids: basic and clinical concepts. 3rd ed. London: Academic Press-Elsevier; 2015. p. 429–45.
7. Scillitani A, Dicembrino F, Chiodini I, et al. Global skeletal uptake of ^{99m}Tc-methylene diphosphonate (GSU) in patients affected by endocrine diseases: comparison with biochemical markers of bone turnover. Osteoporos Int. 2002;13:829–34.
8. Carnevale V, Pacitti MT, Pileri M, et al. Short-term effects of surgery in post-menopausal patients with primary hyperparathyroidism and normal bone turnover. J Endocrinol Invest. 2001;24:575–9.
9. Silva BC, Cusano NE, Hans D, Lewiecki EM, Bilezikian JP. Skeletal imaging in primary hyperparathyroidism. In: Bilezikian JP, Marcus R, Levine MA, Marcocci C, Silverberg SJ, Potts Jr JT, editors. The parathyroids: basic and clinical concepts. 3rd ed. London: Academic Press-Elsevier; 2015. p. 447–54.
10. Bilezikian JP, Brandi ML, Eastell R, et al. Guidelines for the management of asymptomatic primary hyperparathyroidism: summary statement from the Fourth International Workshop. J Clin Endocrinol Metab. 2014;99:3561–9.
11. Castellano E, Attanasio R, Cesario F, Tassone F, Borretta G. Forearm DXA increases the rate of patients with asymptomatic primary hyperparathyroidism meeting surgical criteria. J Clin Endocrinol Metab. 2016;101:2728–32.

12. Silverberg SJ. Primary hyperparathyroidism. In: Rosen CJ, editor. Primer on the metabolic bone diseases and disorders of mineral metabolism. 8th ed. New York: John Wiley & Sons; 2013. p. 543–52.
13. Silverberg SJ, Shane E, Jacobs TP, Siris E, Bilezikian JP. A 10-year prospective study of primary hyperparathyroidism with or without surgery. N Engl J Med. 1999;341:1249–55.
14. Rubin MR, Bilezikian JP, McMahon DJ, et al. The natural history of primary hyperparathyroidism with or without surgery after 15 years. J Clin Endocrinol Metab. 2008;93:346–3470.
15. De Geronimo S, Romagnoli E, Diacinti D, D'Erasmo E, Minisola S. The risk of fractures in postmenopausal women with primary hyperparathyroidism. Eur J Endocrinol. 2006;155:415–20.
16. Stein EM, Silva BC, Boutroy S, et al. Primary hyperparathyroidism is associated with abnormal cortical and trabecular microstructure and reduced bone stiffness in postmenopausal women. J Bone Miner Res. 2013;28:1029–40.
17. Silva BC, Boutroy S, Zhang C, et al. Trabecular bone score (TBS)—a novel method to evaluate bone microarchitecture texture in patients with primary hyperparathyroidism. J Clin Endocrinol Metab. 2013;98:1963–70.
18. Romagnoli E, Cipriani C, Nofroni I, et al. "Trabecular bone score" (TBS): an indirect measure of bone microarchitecture in postmenopausal patients with primary hyperparathyroidism. Bone. 2013;53:154–9.
19. Eller-Vainicher C, Filopanti M, Palmieri S, et al. Bone quality, as measured by trabecular bone score, in patients with primary hyperparathyroidism. Eur J Endocrinol. 2013;169:155–62.
20. Bilezikian JP, Khan A, Potts JT Jr, et al. Hypoparathyroidism in the adult: epidemiology, diagnosis, pathophysiology, target-organ involvement, treatment, and challenges for future research. J Bone Miner Res. 2011;26:2317–37.
21. Dempster DW. Bone histomorphometry in hypoparathyroidism. In: Brandi ML, Brown EM, editors. Hypoparathyroidism. Milan: Springer-Verlag; 2015. p. 287–96.
22. Shoback DM, Bilezikian JP, Costa AG, et al. Presentation of hypoparathyroidism: etiologies and clinical features. J Clin Endocrinol Metab. 2016;101:2300–12.
23. Cusano NE, Nishiyama KK, Zhang C, et al. Noninvasive assessment of skeletal microstructure and estimated bone strength in hypoparathyroidism. J Bone Miner Res. 2016;31:308–16.
24. Mendonca ML, Pereira FA, Nogueira-Barbosa MH, et al. Increased vertebral morphometric fracture in patients with postsurgical hypoparathyroidism despite normal bone mineral density. BMC Endocr Disord. 2013;13:1–8.
25. Underbjerg L, Sikjaer T, Mosekilde L, Rejnmark L. Postsurgical hypoparathyroidism—risk of fractures, psychiatric diseases, cancer, cataract, and infections. J Bone Miner Res. 2014;29:2504–10.
26. Rubin MR, Cusano NE, Fan WW, et al. Therapy of hypoparathyroidism with PTH(1-84): a prospective six year investigation of efficacy and safety. J Clin Endocrinol Metab. 2016;101:2742–50.
27. Rubin MR, Dempster DW, Sliney J Jr, et al. PTH(1-84) administration reverses abnormal bone-remodeling dynamics and structure in hypoparathyroidism. J Bone Miner Res. 2011;26:2727–36.
28. Rubin MR, Zwahlen A, Dempster DW, et al. Effects of parathyroid hormone administration on bone strength in hypoparathyroidism. J Bone Miner Res. 2016;31:1–7.

GH/IGF-I and Bone

6

Stefano Frara, Filippo Maffezzoni, Mauro Doga, Anna Maria Formenti, Gherardo Mazziotti, and Andrea Giustina

6.1 Physiology

Growth hormone (GH) and insulin-like growth factor-I (IGF-I) are relevant regulators of bone homeostasis throughout human life, acting on both the trabecular and cortical bone [1]. The anabolic effects of these hormones are important to reach an adequate bone mass during puberty and early adulthood—a critical determinant for the future risk of osteoporosis—and for the maintenance of skeletal health during adult life [2–4]. The precise time of the attainment of peak bone mass is not clear-cut, but it is skeletal-site dependent, and the gonadal status plays a noteworthy role in regulating bone accretion [5].

Bone modeling occurs mostly during growth: this process is characterized by uncoupled bone formation and bone resorption [6, 7] and is regulated by mechanical forces in order to maintain bone shape and mass. During embryonic development, IGF-I is fundamental for growth, independently of GH action [8], while postnatally and till the end of puberty, GH and IGF-I play a critical role in determining longitudinal skeletal growth, bony maturation, and acquisition of bone mass [9], as demonstrated by short stature, skeletal deformities, and low bone mass in GH-deficiency (GHD) patients [10], which can be normalized by adequate GH replacement therapy [11, 12].

Longitudinal growth is determined by proliferation and differentiation of chondrocytes in the epiphyseal growth plate of long bones, leading to endochondral bone formation. Once chondrocyte proliferation, hypertrophy, and differentiation are

S. Frara · M. Doga · A. Giustina (✉)
Chair of Endocrinology, Università Vita-Salute San Raffaele, Milan, Italy

F. Maffezzoni · A. M. Formenti
ASST Spedali Civili, Brescia, Italy

G. Mazziotti
Endocrinology Unit, ASST Carlo Poma, Mantua, Italy

A. Lenzi, S. Migliaccio (eds.), *Multidisciplinary Approach to Osteoporosis*,
https://doi.org/10.1007/978-3-319-75110-8_6

completed, a new process starts: the newly formed cartilage is invaded by new blood vessels and then, modeled into bone trabeculae. This is called endochondral ossification and is influenced by genetic and hormonal factors, as well as by nutrition and the cellular environment [13, 14].

GH and IGF-I also act in the regulation of the coordinated process of bone resorption and bone formation occurring during bone remodeling in the microscopic basic multicellular units [6]: multinucleated osteoclasts are attracted to a specific site to resorb the bone; then, once resorption is completed, mononuclear osteoblasts are activated to fill the cavity with newly synthesized matrix. At the end of these events, a resting phase occurs. The skeleton is, therefore, an extremely dynamic tissue with a continuous remodeling process which regulates calcium homeostasis and removes potentially damaged bone [5].

The synthesis and release of GH from pituitary cells is under control of several signals, both from the central nervous system and the periphery: traditionally, GHRH promotes it, while somatostatin acts in an inhibitory fashion, and they are both regulated by a negative feedback mechanism. Moreover, IGF-I is secreted by the liver under GH control and inhibits GH secretion directly at the somatotroph level and, indirectly, by stimulating the release of somatostatin [15]. Serum GH levels decline with age, due to a decrease in GHRH production and an increased somatostatin tone. As a consequence, also, systemic IGF-I levels decline in elderly with a progressive loss of muscle mass and strength, a decline in physical performance, an increased body fat, and a reduced bone mineral density (BMD) [16, 17].

Most of GH circulates bound to a GH-binding protein, which is the extracellular domain of the GH receptor (GHR) [18, 19], and once the dimerization and phosphorylation of the internalized receptor are completed, the signal transduction process is started involving different proteins, such as the signal transducers and activators of transcription (STAT) [20]. The GHRs are highly expressed in several organs, in particular on surface cells of the liver, adipose tissue, heart, kidneys, intestine, cartilage, and skeletal muscles. Even if GH predominantly induces IGF-I synthesis by the liver, the physiology is more complex because IGF-I acts both as a circulating hormone and as a local growth factor. Actually, in this latter condition, IGF-I is synthesized, at least in part, in a GH-independent manner, and its production by different extrahepatic tissues is under the control of several peptides [21].

In the bone, GHRs are densely expressed by chondrocytes and osteoblasts [22–25], and in vitro studies showed that GH is able to stimulate the proliferation of cells of the osteoblastic lineage through both STAT and ERK-1 and ERK-2/mitogen-activated protein (MAPK) pathways [5]. Moreover, GH affects directly the fate of mesenchymal precursors opposing adipogenesis and favoring osteoblastogenesis and chondrogenesis [26]. Indirectly, it stimulates the expression of bone morphogenetic proteins, which play a major role for bone synthesis and for the differentiation of osteoblasts [27, 28].

In addition to these effects on their precursors, GH induces, directly or through IGF-I, the differentiated function of mature osteoblasts as well as the carboxylation of osteocalcin, a marker of osteoblastic activity [29]. Moreover, GH and IGF-I variably stimulate the production of the receptor activator of nuclear factor κB ligand (RANK-L) and its decoy receptor osteoprotegerin which are essential for all the cascade events of osteoclastogenesis [30–33].

Moreover, GH may act either directly to stimulate the replication of cells in the germinal layer of the epiphyseal plate or indirectly through its stimulatory effect on IGF-I secretion at the latter stages of maturation [34]. The growth plate is composed of three layers of chondrocytes in various stages of differentiation: the resting zone, where chondrocytes replicate at a slow rate and act to replenish the pool of proliferative chondrocytes; the proliferative zone, where chondrocytes replicate at high rate and the resulting daughter cells line up along the long axis of the bone; and the hypertrophic zone, where cells differentiate terminally into hypertrophic chondrocytes [35–37]. At the end of this process, the hypertrophic zone is invaded by blood vessels and bone cells in order to calcify it and form a new endochondral bone [38].

GH also influences bone metabolism indirectly through the modulation of parathyroid hormone (PTH) secretion and its circadian levels [39] (mediated in part by changes in serum phosphate levels) [40] and enhances the activity of renal 1α-hydroxylase while inhibiting 24-hydroxylase, with an increase in the synthesis of active 1,25-dihydroxyvitamin D_3 that contributes to an increased extracellular calcium-phosphate product and bone mineralization [41].

When synthesized by peripheral tissues, IGF-I secretion is under control of several hormones and growth factors. For example, in chondrocytes, its expression is regulated by GH, while in osteoblasts, it is controlled by PTH and other inducers of cAMP [34, 42]. Moreover, IGF-I mediates selected anabolic effects of PTH in both in vivo and in vitro bone cells [43, 44].

Conversely, estrogens and glucocorticoids act decreasing IGF-I transcription in osteoblasts [42, 45, 46], and some selected inhibitory effects of steroids on bone metabolism can be explained by the reduced IGF-I levels in osseous microenvironment [5]. Also growth factors with mitogenic properties such as platelet-derived growth factor (PDGF) and fibroblast growth factor (FGF) may have a role reducing IGF-I synthesis and release in osteoblast cells [47].

Thyroid hormones are important factors for the regulation of skeletal development and maturation, increasing bone remodeling. Triiodothyronine (T_3) stimulates IGF-I synthesis in osteoblasts [48], and, at the same time, IGF-I can mediate anabolic actions of T_3 on the bone [49].

IGF-I receptor (IGF-IR) expression in osteoblasts is regulated by PDGF, glucocorticoids, and 1,25-dihydroxyvitamin D_3 [50–52]. Once dimerized and autophosphorylated, IGF-IR is able to activate insulin receptor substrate (IRS)-1 and IRS-2 [53], which mediate the effects of IGF-I in osteoblasts, through the phosphatidylinositol-3 kinase (PI3K) and MAPK pathways [54–56].

In vitro studies showed similar biological actions for IGF-I and IGF-II, which are both expressed by osteoblasts, even though IGF-II exerts less efficacious effects than IGF-I [5]. IGF-I strongly stimulates the osteoblastic function and bone formation, enhancing the activity of mature osteoblast cells. In contrast, its effect on osteoblastic cell proliferation is modest as well as its direct action on the differentiation of undifferentiated stromal cells toward osteoblastic lineage [56]. Indirectly, IGF-I might favor osteoblastogenesis stabilizing β-catenin, a signaling molecule implicated in Wnt signaling pathway, which is fundamental for osteoblastogenesis [57, 58].

The action of IGF-I at the osteoclast level is not completely understood, even though osteoclasts express IGF-IRs and IGF-I has direct effects on their functions

[59]. In fact, IGF-I is able to induce RANK-L synthesis and, as a consequence, osteoclastogenesis [60]. This might explain the stimulatory effects on bone resorption, while the induction of osteoprotegerin by GH may counterbalance these actions, justifying the modest effect of IGF-I on bone mass in vivo [5].

Moreover, few studies have recently shown a role for IGF-I in chondrogenesis, inducing adipose-derived mesenchymal cell toward chondrogenic differentiation [61]. In vivo studies showed that *Igf-1* null mice present impaired chondrocyte maturation and shortened femoral length; however, only cortical bone is reduced, probably caused by a compensatory hypersecretion of GH or a decrease in trabecular bone resorption [62, 63]. They also exhibit decreased number of functional osteoclasts, confirming that IGF-I plays a part in normal osteoclastogenesis [64].

In contrast with the role of systemic IGF-I, some authors evidence a different role for locally produced hormones, suggesting that systemic IGF-I is necessary to maintain cortical bone structure, whereas skeletal IGF-I seems to play a predominant role in maintaining the trabecular bone [65].

Actually, only about 1% IGF-I is free in the circulation, while the majority is bound with specific proteins, called IGF-binding proteins (IGFBPs), which are a family of evolutionary conserved-related peptides with different affinity for IGF-I and IGF-II [66, 67]. Even if they usually sequester these growth factors, precluding their interactions with cell surface receptor, in selected conditions, IGFBPs may sometimes increase the effective concentrations of IGF-I in the cellular environment, resulting in enhanced IGF-I effects [68].

In cells of the osteoblastic lineage, the pattern of IGFBP expression depends on the stage of cell differentiation [69] and may be regulated by the autocrine and paracrine factors that are participating in the cellular environment [70]: IGFBP-2 and IGFBP-5 levels are highest in the proliferative phase, while IGFBP-3, IGFBP-4, and IGFBP-6 are elevated during terminal cell differentiation [71].

IGFBP expression is regulated in a complex manner [72]: for example, GH increases IGFBP-3, IGF-I stimulates the IGFBP-5 expression (which is inhibited by other growth factors with mitogenic activity), 1,25-dihydroxyvitamin D_3 augments osteoblast IGFBP-3 and IGFBP-4 production, and all the cAMP inducers amplify the synthesis of almost all IGFBPs [71, 73, 74].

The abundance of IGFBPs is regulated by matrix metalloproteases and serine proteases, secreted by osteoblasts as well [75]. Pregnancy-associated plasma protein-A (PAPP-A) is a metalloproteases expressed by bony cells that play a critical role in osteoblastic function by modulating IGF-I bioavailability [76], cleaving the inhibitory IGFBP-4 in an IGF-dependent manner [77].

IGFBP-1 role in skeletal cells has not been completely clarified; however, recent studies affirm that elevated values of this protein are strongly associated with high fracture risk, independently of IGF-I circulating levels [78]. In vitro, IGFBP-2 prevents the effects of IGF-I on osteoblast activity, and it has been demonstrated that IGFBP-2 serum levels are inversely related with BMD and bone turnover in the elderly [79].

IGFBP-3 is a major component of the circulating IGF complex; its concentrations are GH dependent [66, 67], and in vitro it can either inhibit or stimulate IGF activity by upregulating IGF-I delivery to cell surface receptors [80]. However, in vivo studies are less contradictory: overexpression of IGFBP-3 causes growth retardation and osteopenia [81]. This is the only IGFBP cleaved also by plasmin, so the bioavailability of IGF-I in the bone microenvironment can be regulated by activators and inhibitors of plasminogen [82].

IGFBP-4 [83] and IGFBP-5 [84] are usually inhibitors of IGF-I, but under certain experimental conditions, autonomously from IGF-I levels, they can stimulate bone cell formation depending on interactions with extracellular matrix proteins [85].

6.2 Clinical Consequences of GH Excess and Deficiency in Humans

6.2.1 Acromegaly

Acromegaly is an insidious disorder characterized by exaggerated circulating levels of GH and IGF-I, usually caused by a pituitary adenoma. Even though it is a rare disease, the diagnosis is challenging and, frequently, very delayed [86], being associated with reduced quality of life and an average 10-year reduction in life expectancy due to metabolic, cardiovascular, and cerebrovascular comorbidities [87].

The effects of GH and IGF-I hypersecretion on bone structure and metabolism have been long debated, after the first evidence that this hormonal excess may stimulate bone turnover [88]. In reality, initial studies failed to demonstrate a possible protective role of GH on the skeleton [89, 90], and acromegaly has been recently recognized as a possible cause of secondary osteoporosis, determining abnormalities in bone microstructure [91, 92] and predisposing patients to develop a specific bone metabolic disorder, also known as acromegalic osteopathy [93], with high bone turnover and increased risk of vertebral fractures [94].

Histomorphometric and clinical studies observed an increased bone turnover in close relationship with activity of disease in acromegaly patients [88]. Like in other forms of secondary osteoporosis, biochemical markers are a good tool for clinicians in order to evaluate the risk of skeletal fragility in acromegaly [95]: markers of bone formation (i.e., osteocalcin, bone isoenzyme of alkaline phosphatase, and procollagen type 1 *N*-propeptide, also known as P1NP) are direct or indirect products of active osteoblasts, while on the other hand, reference markers of bone resorption are released during osteoclast activity and include serum carboxy-terminal cross-linking telopeptide of type 1 collagen (CTX) and urinary *N*-telopeptide of type 1 collagen (NTX) [96]. Markers of bony resorption tended to be more increased in relation to markers of bone formation, so explaining, at least in part, bone loss induced by GH excess [97–99].

Hypovitaminosis D has been consistently reported in acromegaly patients, and this may be associated with its low bioavailability due to a GH excess-related effect on vitamin D-binding protein [100]. Furthermore, GH excess strongly influences PTH pulsatility, prolonging pulse half-duration and increasing pulse mass [101];

however, at the same time, parathyroid hormone secretion might be influenced by medical treatment with somatostatin analogs [102]. Patients with active acromegaly usually present calcium-phosphate metabolism abnormalities, including hyperphosphatemia (related to increased calcitriol-stimulated dietary absorption and a direct antiphosphaturic effect of IGF-I in the proximal renal tubule, but it could also represent a result of bone turnover) [103], high serum calcium levels, and hypercalciuria, caused by increased intestinal absorption and high bone turnover [103]. So, in this clinical setting, hypercalciuria may be considered, at least in part, as a marker of skeletal fragility [93].

Even though measurement of BMD at lumbar spine and hip by dual-energy X-ray absorptiometry (DXA) is the cornerstone for diagnosis of osteoporosis and prediction of fracture risk in clinical practice [104], the relief of osteoporosis cannot be easily performed in acromegaly patients. In fact, the DXA measurements of BMD may be affected by several pitfalls related to abnormalities of bone structures caused by GH excess: degenerative joint alterations, characterized by osteophyte formation and facet-joint hypertrophy that may lead to an overestimation of BMD [92, 95] or bone enlargement due to GH hypersecretion [93, 105].

In this clinical setting, the different effects of both somatotropic and peripheral hormones excess on cortical and trabecular bone are discordant: deleterious action on trabecular microarchitecture is associated with a tendency to an increased cortical bone density on periosteal ossification [5, 92]. Moreover, acromegaly patients show a compromised bone strength, macrostructure, microstructure, mineralization, microdamages, and alterations in collagen status, as confirmed in studies evaluating iliac crest biopsies that showed a reduced trabecular biomechanical competence in this clinical context [106]. Nevertheless, DXA scans do not distinguish between cortical and trabecular bone, leading to divergent results, which are largely influenced by the variable distribution of these compartments in different skeletal sites [107]. Actually, this peculiarity may justify different BMD values on lumbar spine and femoral neck, reflecting the different percentage of cortical and trabecular bone in these sites [95].

All these considerations explain at least in part why different studies show inconsistent patterns in BMD of acromegaly patients: they are reported to be normal, or even increased, while only few studies reported low BMD at the lumbar spine particularly in patients with concomitant hypogonadism, consistently with the hypothesis that loss of sex steroids may cause an increase in bone turnover with altered trabecular microarchitecture [99, 107, 108].

Many of the limitations of areal DXA estimation can be easily overcome by quantitative computed tomography (qCT) techniques. A few studies have already showed that qCT allows higher spatial resolution, improved delineation of bone architecture, and acquisition of near isotropic volumetric datasets [109]. They have also demonstrated that bone abnormalities were linked with duration of active acromegaly, hypogonadism, and coexistent diabetes mellitus [91, 92, 110].

In order to precociously identify deterioration of trabecular microstructure, a simpler and more practicable technique is now available: the trabecular bone score

(TBS). It is a gray-level textural metric extracted from the two-dimensional lumbar spine DXA image, and lower TBS values were reported in patients affected by acromegaly in respect with healthy subjects [111].

Even though in the past the first studies failed to demonstrate an increased fracture risk in osteoporosis [112], vertebral fractures are a very frequent complication of acromegaly osteopathy, but only a few are clinically recognized and quickly treated [94, 113]. In this clinical setting, the radiological and morphometric approach is the gold standard to evaluate the true prevalence and incidence of fractures, as already determined in population studies [114].

In 2005, the first study stating an increased prevalence of vertebral fractures in postmenopausal acromegaly women was published [115]. Since then, several cross-sectional [116–121] and prospective [113, 122] studies were completed, demonstrating that vertebral fractures—in particular at the thoracic spine, with a peculiar kyphosis [122]—may occur even after a few years after diagnosis of disease [113]. Prevalent fractures were associated with hypogonadism [116] and concomitant diabetes mellitus [123], and they correlate with the duration of active disease [113], but not with BMD, since it could be normal, slightly reduced, or even increased in this peculiar contest [115–117].

Moreover, in the prospective studies, patients with vertebral fractures—even when mild or single—were predisposed to develop incident deformities [124], consistently with the concept that these fractures are always a hallmark of skeletal fragility.

The role of overtreatment of coexistent hypopituitarism on skeletal health is still a matter of uncertainty [125, 126], and different questionnaires or the fracture risk assessment (FRAX) tool does not provide any help in identifying patients with increased vertebral fractures risk [121].

A recent study, evaluating the trabecular microstructure by cone-beam computed tomography analysis, confirms the hypothesis of a more severe deterioration in acromegaly patients with vertebral fractures as compared to non-fractured ones [92].

Albeit appropriate and effective management of acromegaly improves skeletal health [94], the fracture risk may remain augmented in those patients with preexistent fractures, hypogonadism, or significant reduction of BMD at the femoral neck during the follow-up period [113, 122], providing a need of anti-osteoporotic therapies in addition to treatment of acromegaly and, eventually, coexistent hypopituitarism [93].

Finally, it is important to underline the statements of revised guidelines on acromegaly that emphasized the concept that vertebral fractures may occur in all acromegaly patients, independently of BMD, and recommended performing thoracic and lumbar radiological evaluation in order to diagnose deformities [87]. Nevertheless, the therapeutic choice is still empiric, since no studies have tested the efficacy and safety of bone-active drugs [93] and it is unknown whether vertebral fractures may impact quality of life in this specific clinical setting [127–130].

6.2.2 GHD

Subjects with large nonfunctioning pituitary adenomas, patients who underwent neurosurgery for pituitary adenoma or craniopharyngioma, people who had pituitary or head irradiation and neck or brain tumors, or those who were affected by autoimmune hypophysitis, Sheehan syndrome, or cranial accidents frequently show GH deficiency [131].

GHD in adults is associated with increased fat mass, particularly distributed in the truncal region, reduced lean mass [132], osteopenia [133], adverse lipid profile [134, 135], glucose intolerance, insulin resistance [135, 136], impaired fibrinolysis, altered cardiac structure and function [137], reduced exercise capacity [138], and reduced quality of life [139].

As previously reported, GH and IGF-I play a key role in the control of longitudinal growth in addition to important stimulatory effects on bone remodeling and bone mass [1], whereas the progressive decline of GH secretion [15] is considered to be among the factors contributing to age-related and postmenopausal bone loss [140, 141].

GHD plays a negative role on the skeleton with a marked reduction in bone turnover [142], and this effect seems to be related to the age of the patients. In fact, young patients have been shown to have a greater impairment of BMD, as assessed by bidimensional radiological measurement, compared with the elderly [143–146]. Different bone turnover may explain such variable effects of GHD in two life periods [146]. In fact, it has been hypothesized that during adolescence and young adult life, when bone turnover is high and bone mass is being accrued, GHD would slow this acquisition determining osteopenia [147]. On the other hand, in patients who develop GH deficiency over 30 years, reduced BMD might be due to the lack of the important role of GH in bone metabolism [148].

In an investigational study of trabecular bone histomorphometry in 36 male adult patients with GHD, the analysis revealed decreased osteoid and mineralizing surfaces, decreased bone formation rate, and an increase in the eroded surface compared with the normal healthy bone [149], confirming the state of low bone turnover osteoporosis [1, 145, 150–154].

Although GHD deficiency was found to be the most important determinant of bone loss in hypopituitary patients [5], other pituitary hormone deficiencies as well as their replacement therapies may contribute to determining skeletal fragility in this clinical setting. In fact, hypogonadism, replacement therapy with levothyroxine (L-T4), and glucocorticoids in excess may influence BMD status in patients with multiple hormone deficiencies [155–157].

Wüster et al. observed a decrease in vertebral lumbar bone mass and in proximal femur measured with DXA in 73% of 122 hypopituitaric patients [158]; while Johansson and colleagues studied 17 GHD male patients showing that total, but not spinal, BMD, measured with DXA, was reduced [159]. Like in childhood onset GHD, there are no suggestive differences in Z-score of patients with both GHD and hypogonadism and those with GHD alone. Regarding a group of patients in which the GHD onset was around 30 years, a reduction in vertebral lumbar spine BMD was observed with both DXA and quantitative computed tomography (QCT), and older patients experience a lesser decrease in BMD compared to younger patients. Beshyah et al. compared lumbar spine BMD of 64 hypopituitary patients to control subjects and found it decreased in both male and female patients [160]. On the other hand, Degerblad et al. found a normal spine and hip BMD in adult-onset GHD male patients but a reduced total BMD in adult-onset GHD women both in the spine and hip [161].

A direct link between GHD and reduced bone mass in hypopituitarism is also supported by reports that GH replacement therapy with recombinant human GH (rhGH) can improve BMD and bone metabolism in these patients [162–164].

RhGH leads to an increase in bone turnover [165]. Moreover, GH replacement therapy increases serum and urinary calcium after 3–6 months, an effect caused by calcium mobilization from the skeleton, and increases intestinal and renal absorption of calcium due to an increased sensitivity to PTH [166–169]. It is noteworthy that the effect of rhGH on bone turnover is biphasic and dose dependent. In the first 6–12 months of treatment, rhGH has a predominant pro-resorptive effect, whereas the stimulation of bone formation becomes relevant and sustained after 12–18 months of treatment [1, 154, 165, 170–177]. This biphasic effect on bone turnover explains why a decline in BMD was reported in the first 6–12 months of treatment [161, 178–185], whereas a significant increase in BMD was observed only in longer-term studies [1, 162, 164, 186–193]. Indeed, the increase in BMD was described for up to 10 years follow-up in patients receiving continuous rhGH therapy [192, 194] and continued to increase even 18 months after rhGH discontinuation [195, 196].

RhGH increases bone mineral content to a greater extent than BMD because replacement therapy also increases bone area [171, 183]. This is supported by histomorphometric findings demonstrating an increase in periosteal bone formation during rhGH treatment [185].

Low bone turnover osteoporosis in adult patients with GHD leads to an increase in fracture risk, which may contribute to the increased risk of mortality observed in this clinical setting [1, 133].

The risk of non-vertebral fractures is about threefold increased in untreated GHD patients [197–199]. Fractures in GHD are frequently localized to the radius, suggesting a loss of cortical bone [197, 199], but GHD patients also have an increased incidence of vertebral fractures [200].

Previous studies suggested that GHD may be an independent risk factor for fractures in patients with anterior hypopituitarism without any significant effects of other pituitary hormone deficiencies. However, these data regarded mainly nonvertebral fractures and were based on a retrospective historical evaluation. In a cross-sectional study in GHD patients, Mazziotti et al. reported that hypogonadism was not associated with higher prevalence of fractures even in the presence of lower BMD as compared to eugonadic patients, and in both groups fractures were not correlated with BMD [155]. In another cross-sectional study by the same group [125], authors demonstrated that high replacement doses of glucocorticoid therapy may favor the occurrence of vertebral fractures in patients with untreated GHD. This finding was not observed in patients with treated GHD, suggesting that rhGH replacement therapy could protect the bone from the negative effects of glucocorticoid over-replacement.

Moreover, in GHD-treated patients with central hypothyroidism, overtreatment with L-T4 was associated with a high prevalence of radiological vertebral fractures, whereas when GHD was not treated, the prevalence of vertebral fractures was high regardless of L-T4 doses [126].

This different impact of other pituitary hormone deficiencies or hormonal replacement therapies on BMD and fractures is consistent with the finding that fractures do not correlate with BMD in GHD [155, 200]. This finding agrees with previous experiences who reported a poor predicted value of BMD for the risk of fractures in various forms of secondary osteoporosis, in which the fracture BMD threshold seems to be much lower than in postmenopausal osteoporosis.

Consistently with former cross-sectional studies [5], recent prospective studies reported a significant decrease in incident vertebral [11] and non-vertebral [12] fractures in adult GHD patients treated with rhGH, suggesting that skeletal integrity could be an emerging critical end point in the decision-making process to initiate GH replacement in hypopituitary patients with GHD [201].

Glucocorticoid-induced osteoporosis (GIO) is the most frequent secondary osteoporosis both in men and women [157]; it is usually caused by exogenous corticosteroid administration for the treatment of several autoimmune, pulmonary, and gastrointestinal disorders, but they are prescribed also in patients after organ transplantation or with cancer. Fracture risk increases precociously after starting treatment, and it is, at least in part, related to the dose and duration of glucocorticoid exposure [202]. Furthermore, even if it is much more uncommon, also, endogenous hypercortisolism may be a cause of GIO [203], and fragility fractures can be the presenting manifestation of Cushing's syndrome, either clinical or subclinical [204].

The pathophysiology of GIO is based on reduced bone formation, due to the actions of glucocorticoid excess on osteoblast differentiation and function [157], as well as on survival, metabolism, and function of osteocytes, causing high apoptosis rates and modifying the elastic modulus surrounding osteocytes lacunae [205].

All these negative effects account for a chronic impairment of bone quality and exaggerated loss of bone strength in relation to bone mass in this clinical setting [206]. However, during the first phases of steroid exposure, a significantly augmented bone resorption may occur, leading to the well-known early increase in fracture risk [157, 202].

Besides the direct action of these drugs on bone cells, they may also have indirect effects mediated by derangements in neuroendocrine signals, including the somatotropic axis. Glucocorticoids can both increase and inhibit the GH secretory response of somatotropes to GHRH and GH secretagogues (GHS) [207, 208]. Glucocorticoids may enhance the expression of GHRH and GHS receptors on pituitary cells: pretreatment with dexamethasone increases GH response to GHRH even after long-term exposure to the drug [15] and modulates GHRH receptor mRNA expression in the human pituitary [209]. At low concentrations, glucocorticoids increase GHRH content in hypothalamic cells, while at high levels a reduced neuronal content and release of GHRH together with an increase in hypothalamic production of somatostatin was reported both in in vitro [210] and in vivo studies. These observations have been described even when the glucocorticoid excess is mild, for example, in patients treated with inhaled steroids or those with subclinical endogenous hypercortisolism [211, 212].

Actually, the increase in somatostatin tone seems to be the most important mechanism involved in the pathogenesis of blunted GH secretion observed during chronic treatment with glucocorticoids [15], and somatostatin antibodies as well as other substances known to decrease somatostatin tone such as galanin, pyridostigmine, clonidine, or ghrelin may at least partially counteract these inhibitory effects [213–216]. Acute and chronic administration of glucocorticoids in healthy men induces a decrease in GH secretion throughout an augmented somatostatin tone [217–219], and, interestingly, GH inhibitory effects of hydrocortisone infusion were also demonstrated in acromegaly patients [220].

Furthermore, several studies reported a growth retardation at diagnosis in more than three-quarters of pediatric Cushing's syndrome patients due to the induced resistance of target tissues to IGF-I and other growth factors, together with a marked GH suppression [221, 222]. In this peculiar contest, an early appropriate treatment with GH appears to be indicated in the majority of patients, and it is able to considerably improve the final height [223]. Limited data are available regarding BMD, but a high prevalence of reduced values—in particular at the femoral neck [224]—associated with an increased fracture risk is commonly described [225–228]. It is noteworthy that the mild reduction in BMD in pediatric subjects is reversible after the cure of the primary disease and, eventually, the replacement of pituitary hormone deficiencies that could be present [229].

Finally, glucocorticoid excess may suppress the peripheral expression of GHRs impairing the GH-mediated synthesis of IGF-I and thus amplifying the effects of functional GHD on target tissues [230]. On the other hand, the peripheral metabolism of glucocorticoids by 11-β-hydroxysteroid dehydrogenase (11-βHSD) is modulated by GH, and activation of cortisone to cortisol in target tissues is amplified by GHD [231].

Although data are still few and not conclusive [232], some studies show that short-term rhGH treatment may significantly increase bone turnover markers, potentially leading to favorable chronic effects on bone remodeling [233], and it may positively contribute to reduce sarcopenia and the related protein wasting syndrome caused by glucocorticoid excess [234, 235].

Conclusions

Growth hormone and IGF-I play a major physiological role in the regulation of bone metabolism in adults. Interestingly, both a hyperactivity of the GH/IGF-I axis as in acromegaly and a hypoactivity of the axis are associated with an increased risk of fractures. Importantly, acromegaly and GHD osteopathy are characterized by opposite alterations in bone metabolism since GH excess is linked to a high bone turnover skeletal disease, whereas GHD causes low bone turnover. Prevention of vertebral fractures in status of altered GH secretion is a major clinical problem, and appropriate guidelines should be implemented, including DXA or X-ray morphometry.

References

1. Ohlsson C, Bengtsson BA, Isaksson OG, Andreassen TT, Slootweg MC. Growth hormone and bone. Endocr Rev. 1998;19:55–79.
2. Bangor JP, Theists G, Bushes B, Solomon D, Rizzoli R. Critical years and stages of puberty for spinal and femoral bone mass accumulation during adolescence. J Clin Endocrinol Metab. 1991;73:555–63.
3. Matkovic V, Jelic T, Wardlaw GM, Ilich JC, Goel PK, Wright JK, Andon MB, Smith KT, Heaney R. Timing of peak bone mass in Caucasian females and its implication for the prevention of osteoporosis: interference from a cross-sectional model. J Clin Invest. 1994; 93:799–808.
4. Theintz G, Buchs B, Rizzoli R, Slosman D, Clavein H, Sizonenko PC, Bonjour JP. Longitudinal monitoring of bone mass accumulation in healthy adolescents: evidence for a marked reduction after 16 years of age at the levels of lumbar spine and femoral neck in female subjects. J Clin Endocrinol Metab. 1992;75:1060–5.
5. Giustina A, Mazziotti G, Canalis E. Growth hormone, insulin-like growth factors and the skeleton. Endocr Rev. 2008;29:535–59.
6. Parfitt AM. The bone remodeling compartment: a circulatory function for bone lining cells. J Bone Miner Res. 2001;16:1583–5.
7. Canalis E. The fate of circulating osteoblasts. N Engl J Med. 2005;352:2014–6.
8. Woods KA, Camacho-Hubner C, Savage MO, Clark AJ. Intrauterine growth retardation and postnatal growth failure associated with deletion of the insulin-like growth factor I gene. N Engl J Med. 1996;335:1363–7.
9. Isaksson OG, Lindhal A, Nilsson A, Isgaard J. Mechanism of the stimulatory effect of growth hormone on longitudinal bone growth. Endocr Rev. 1987;8:426–38.
10. Guler HP, Zapf J, Scheiwiller E, Froesch ER. Recombinant human insulin-like growth factor I stimulates growth and has distinct effects on organ size in hypophysectomized rats. Proc Natl Acad Sci U S A. 1988;85:4889–93.
11. Mazziotti G, Doga M, Frara S, Maffezzoni P, Porcelli T, Cerri L, Maroldi R, Giustina A. Incidence of morphometric vertebral fractures in adult patients with growth hormone deficiency. Endocrine. 2016;52:103–10.
12. Mo D, Fleseriu M, Qi R, Jia N, Child CJ, Bouillon R, Hardin DS. Fracture risk in adult patients treated with growth hormone replacement therapy for growth hormone deficiency: a prospective cohort study. Lancet Diabetes Endocrinol. 2015;3:331–8.
13. Van der Eerden BC, Karperien M, Wit JM. Systemic and local regulation of the growth plate. Endocr Rev. 2003;24:782–801.
14. Nilsson O, Marino R, De Luca F, Philip M, Baron J. Endocrine regulation of the growth plate. Horm Res. 2005;64:157–65.
15. Giustina A, Veldhuis JD. Pathophysiology of the neuroregulation of growth hormone secretion in experimental animals and the human. Endocr Rev. 1998;19:717–97.
16. Savine R, Sonksen P. Growth hormone – hormone replacement for the somatopause? Horm Res. 2000;53:37–41.
17. Skelton DA, Grieg CA, Davies JM, Young A. Strength, power and related functional ability of healthy people aged 60–89 years. Age Ageing. 1994;23:371–7.
18. Clark RG, Mortensen DL, Carlsson LM, Spencer SA, McKay P, Mulkerrin M, Moore J, Cunningham BC. Recombinant human growth hormone (GH)-binding protein enhances the growth promoting activity of human GH in the rat. Endocrinology. 1996;137:4308–15.
19. Amit T, Youdim MB, Hochberg Z. Does serum growth hormone (GH) binding protein reflect human GH receptor function? J Clin Endocrinol Metab. 2000;85:927–32.
20. Fisker S. Physiology and pathophysiology of growth hormone-binding protein: methodological and clinical aspects. Growth Horm IGF Res. 2006;16:1–28.
21. Melmed S. Insulin-like growth factor I – a prototypic peripheral-paracrine hormone? Endocrinology. 1999;140:3879–80.

22. Barnard R, Haynes KM, Werther GA, Waters MJ. The ontogeny of growth hormone receptors in the rabbit tibia. Endocrinology. 1998;122:2562–9.
23. Werther GA, Haynes K, Edmonson S, Oakes S, Buchanan CJ, Herington AC, Waters MJ. Identification of growth hormone receptors on human growth plate chondrocytes. Acta Paediatr Suppl. 1993;82:50–3.
24. Kassem M, Mosekilde L, Eriksen EF, Kassem M, Mosekilde L, Eriksen EF. Growth hormone stimulates proliferation of normal human bone marrow stromal osteoblast precursor cells in vitro. Growth Regul. 1994;4:131–5.
25. Nilsson A, Swolin D, Enerback S, Ohlsson C. Expression of functional growth hormone receptors in cultured human osteoblast-like cells. J Clin Endocrinol Metab. 1995;80:3483–8.
26. Gevers EF, Loveridge N, Robinson IC. Bone marrow adipocytes: a neglected target tissue for growth hormone. Endocrinology. 2002;143:4065–73.
27. Canalis E, Economides AN, Gazzerro E. Bone morphogenetic proteins, their antagonists, and the skeleton. Endocr Rev. 2003;24:218–35.
28. Li H, Bartold PM, Zhang CZ, Clarkson RW, Young WG, Waters MJ. Growth hormone and insulin-like growth factor-1 induce bone morphogenetic proteins 2 and 4: a mediator role in bone and tooth formation. Endocrinology. 1998;139:3855–62.
29. Hubina E, Lakatos P, Kovacs L, Szabolcs I, Racz K, Toth M, Szucs N, Goth MI. Effects of 24 months of growth hormone (GH) treatment on serum carboxylated and undercarboxylated osteocalcin levels in GH-deficient adults. Calcif Tissue Int. 2004;74:55–9.
30. Simonet WS, Lacey DL, Dunstan CR, Kelley M, Chang MS, Luthy R, Nguyen HQ, Wooden S, Bennett L, Boone T, Shimamoto G, DeRose M, Elliott R, Colombero A, Tan HL, Trail G, Sullivan J, Davy E, Bucay N, Renshaw-Gegg L, Hughes TM, Hill D, Pattison W, Campbell P, Sander S, Van G, Tarpley J, Derby P, Lee R, Boyle WJ. Osteoprotegerin: a novel secreted protein involved in the regulation of bone density. Cell. 1997;89:309–19.
31. Rubin J, Ackert-Bicknell CL, Zhu L, Fan X, Murphy TC, Nanes MS, Marcus R, Holloway L, Beamer WG, Rosen CJ. IGF-I regulates osteoprotegerin (OPG) and receptor activator of nuclear factor-κB ligand in vitro and OPG in vivo. J Clin Endocrinol Metab. 2002;87:4273–9.
32. Ueland T, Bollerslev J, Flyvbjerg A, Hansen TB, Vahl N, Mosekilde L. Effects of 12 months of growth hormone (GH) treatment on cortical and trabecular bone content of insulin like growth factors (IGF) and osteoprotegerin in adults with acquired GH deficiency: a double-blind, randomized, placebo-controlled study. J Clin Endocrinol Metab. 2002;87:2760–3.
33. Mrak E, Villa I, Lanzi R, Losa M, Guidobono F, Rubinacci A. Growth hormone stimulates osteoprotegerin expression and secretion in human osteoblast-like cells. J Endocrinol. 2007; 192:639–45.
34. Ohlsson C, Nilsson A, Isaksson O, Lindahl A. Growth hormone induces multiplication of the slowly cycling germinal cells of the rat tibial growth plate. Proc Natl Acad Sci U S A. 1992;89:9826–30.
35. Lindahl A, Isgaard J, Nilsson A, Isaksson OG. Growth hormone potentiates colony formation of epiphyseal chondrocytes in suspension culture. Endocrinology. 1986;118:1843–8.
36. Lindahl A, Nilsson A, Isaksson OG. Effects of growth hormone and insulin-like growth factor-I on colony formation of rabbit epiphyseal chondrocytes at different stages of maturation. J Endocrinol. 1987;115:263–71.
37. Lindahl A, Isgaard J, Carlsson L, Isaksson OG. Differential effects of growth hormone and insulin-like growth factor I on colony formation of epiphyseal chondrocytes in suspension culture in rats of different ages. Endocrinology. 1987;121:1061–9.
38. Ohlsson C, Isaksson O, Lindahl A. Clonal analysis of rat tibia growth plate chondrocytes in suspension culture – differential effects of growth hormone and insulin-like growth factor I. Growth Regul. 1994;4:1–7.
39. Chiavistelli S, Giustina A, Mazziotti G. Parathyroid hormone pulsatility: physiological and clinical aspects. Bone Res. 2015;3:14049.
40. el-Hajj GF, Klerman EB, Brown EN, Choe Y, Brown EM, Czeisler CA. The parathyroid hormone circadian rhythm is truly endogenous – a general clinical research center study. J Clin Endocrinol Metab. 1997;82:281–6.

41. Wei S, Tanaka H, Kubo T, Ono T, Kanzaki S, Seino Y. Growth hormone increases serum 1,25-dihydroxyvitamin D levels and decreases 24,25-dihydroxyvitamin D levels in children with growth hormone deficiency. Eur J Endocrinol. 1997;136:45–51.
42. Ernst M, Heath JK, Rodan GA. Estradiol effects on proliferation, messenger ribonucleic acid for collagen and insulin-like growth factor-I, and parathyroid hormone stimulated adenylate cyclase activity in osteoblastic cells from calvariae and long bones. Endocrinology. 1989;125:825–33.
43. Canalis E, Centrella M, Burch W, McCarthy TL. Insulin-like growth factor I mediates selective anabolic effects of parathyroid hormone in bone cultures. J Clin Invest. 1989;83:60–5.
44. Bikle DD, Sakata T, Leary C, Elalieh H, Ginzinger D, Rosen CJ, Beamer W, Majumdar S, Halloran BP. Insulin-like growth factor I is required for the anabolic actions of parathyroid hormone on mouse bone. J Bone Miner Res. 2002;17:1570–8.
45. Ernst M, Rodan GA. Estradiol regulation of insulin-like growth factor-I expression in osteoblastic cells: evidence for transcriptional control. Mol Endocrinol. 1991;5:1081–9.
46. Delany AM, Durant D, Canalis E. Glucocorticoid suppression of IGF-I transcription in osteoblasts. Mol Endocrinol. 2001;15:1781–9.
47. Canalis E, Pash J, Gabbitas B, Rydziel S, Varghese S. Growth factors regulate the synthesis of insulin-like growth factor-I in bone cell cultures. Endocrinology. 1993;133:33–8.
48. Lakatos P, Caplice MD, Khanna V, Stern PH. Thyroid hormones increase insulin-like growth factor-I content in the medium of rat bone tissue. J Bone Miner Res. 1993;8:1475–81.
49. Huang BK, Golden LA, Tarjan G, Madison LD, Stern PH. Insulin-like growth factor I production is essential for anabolic effects of thyroid hormone in osteoblasts. J Bone Miner Res. 2000;15:188–97.
50. Bennett A, Chen T, Feldman D, Hintz RL, Rosenfeld RG. Characterization of insulin-like growth factor I receptors on cultured rat bone cells: regulation of receptor concentration by glucocorticoids. Endocrinology. 1984;115:1577–83.
51. Kurose H, Yamaoka K, Okada S, Nakajima S, Seino Y. 1,25-Dihydroxyvitamin D3 [1,25-(OH)2D3] increases insulin-like growth factor I (IGF-I) receptors in clonal osteoblastic cells. Study on interaction of IGF-I and 1,25-(OH)2D3. Endocrinology. 1990;126:2088–94.
52. Rubini M, Werner H, Gandini E, Roberts CT Jr, LeRoith D, Baserga R. Platelet-derived growth factor increases the activity of the promoter of the insulin-like growth factor-1 (IGF-1) receptor gene. Exp Cell Res. 1994;211:374–9.
53. Adams TE, Epa VC, Garrett TP, Ward CW. Structure and function of the type 1 insulin-like growth factor receptor. Cell Mol Life Sci. 2000;57:1050–93.
54. Giorgetti S, Ballotti R, Kowalski-Chauvel A, Tartare S, Van Obberghen E. The insulin and insulin-like growth factor-I receptor substrate IRS-1 associates with and activates phosphatidylinositol 3-kinase in vitro. J Biol Chem. 1993;268:7358–64.
55. Grey A, Chen Q, Xu X, Callon K, Cornish J. Parallel phosphatidylinositol-3 kinase and p42/44 mitogen-activated protein kinase signaling pathways subserve the mitogenic and antiapoptotic actions of insulin-like growth factor I in osteoblastic cells. Endocrinology. 2003;144:4886–93.
56. Xi G, Rosen CJ, Clemmons DR. IGF-I and IGFBP-2 stimulate AMPK activation and autophagy, which are required for osteoblast differentiation. Endocrinology. 2016;157:268–81.
57. Playford MP, Bicknell D, Bodmer WF, Macaulay VM. Insulin-like growth factor 1 regulates the location, stability, and transcriptional activity of β-catenin. Proc Natl Acad Sci U S A. 2000;97:12103–8.
58. Krishnan V, Bryant HU, MacDougald OA. Regulation of bone mass by Wnt signaling. J Clin Invest. 2006;116:1202–9.
59. Hou P, Sato T, Hofstetter W, Foged NT. Identification and characterization of the insulin-like growth factor I receptor in mature rabbit osteoclasts. J Bone Miner Res. 1997;12:534–40.
60. Mochizuki H, Hakeda Y, Wakatsuki N, Usui N, Akashi S, Sato T, Tanaka K, Kumegawa M. Insulin-like growth factor-I supports formation and activation of osteoclasts. Endocrinology. 1992;131:1075–80.

61. Zhou Q, Li B, Zhao J, Pan W, Xu J, Chen S. IGF-I induces adipose derived mesenchymal cell chondrogenic differentiation in vitro and enhances chondrogenesis in vivo. In Vitro Cell Dev Biol Anim. 2016;52:356–64.
62. Liu P, Baker J, Perkins AS, Robertson EJ, Efstratiadis A. Mice carrying null mutations of the genes encoding insulin-like growth factor I (Igf-1) and type 1 IGF receptor (Igf1r). Cell. 1993;75:59–72.
63. Bikle D, Majumdar S, Laib A, Powell-Braxton L, Rosen C, Beamer W, Nauman E, Leary C, Halloran B. The skeletal structure of insulin-like growth factor I-deficient mice. J Bone Miner Res. 2001;16:2320–9.
64. Wang Y, Nishida S, Elalieh HZ, Long RK, Halloran BP, Bikle DD. Role of IGF-I signaling in regulating osteoclastogenesis. J Bone Miner Res. 2006;21:1350–8.
65. Zhang M, Xuan S, Bouxsein ML, von Stechow D, Akeno N, Faugere MC, Malluche H, Zhao G, Rosen CJ, Efstratiadis A, Clemens TL. Osteoblast-specific knockout of the insulin-like growth factor (IGF) receptor gene reveals an essential role of IGF signaling in bone matrix mineralization. J Biol Chem. 2002;277:44005–12.
66. Jones JI, Clemmons DR. Insulin-like growth factors and their binding proteins: biological actions. Endocr Rev. 1995;16:3–34.
67. Hwa V, Oh Y, Rosenfeld RG. The insulin-like growth factor-binding protein (IGFBP) superfamily. Endocr Rev. 1999;20:761–87.
68. Jones JI, Gockerman A, Busby WH Jr, Camacho-Hubner C, Clemmons DR. Extracellular matrix contains insulin-like growth factor binding protein-5: potentiation of the effects of IGF-I. J Cell Biol. 1993;121:679–87.
69. Hassager C, Fitzpatrick LA, Spencer EM, Riggs BL, Conover CA. Basal and regulated secretion of insulin-like growth factor binding proteins in osteoblast-like cells is cell line specific. J Clin Endocrinol Metab. 1992;75:228–33.
70. Dong Y, Canalis E. Insulin-like growth factor (IGF) I and retinoic acid induce the synthesis of IGF-binding protein 5 in rat osteoblastic cells. Endocrinology. 1995;136:2000–6.
71. Birnbaum RS, Wiren KM. Changes in insulin-like growth factor-binding protein expression and secretion during the proliferation, differentiation, and mineralization of primary cultures of rat osteoblasts. Endocrinology. 1994;135:223–30.
72. McCarthy TL, Casinghino S, Centrella M, Canalis E. Complex pattern of insulin-like growth factor binding protein expression in primary rat osteoblast enriched cultures: regulation by prostaglandin E2, growth hormone, and the insulin-like growth factors. J Cell Physiol. 1994;160:163–75.
73. Canalis E, Gabbitas B. Skeletal growth factors regulate the synthesis of insulin-like growth factor binding protein-5 in bone cell cultures. J Biol Chem. 1995;270:10771–6.
74. Moriwake T, Tanaka H, Kanzaki S, Higuchi J, Seino Y. 1,25-Dihydroxyvitamin D3 stimulates the secretion of insulin-like growth factor binding protein 3 (IGFBP-3) by cultured human osteosarcoma cells. Endocrinology. 1992;130:1071–3.
75. Conover CA. Insulin-like growth factor binding protein proteolysis in bone cell models. Prog Growth Factor Res. 1995;6:301–9.
76. Boldt HB, Conover CA. Pregnancy-associated plasma protein-A (PAPP-A): a local regulator of IGF bioavailability through cleavage of IGFBPs. Growth Horm IGF Res. 2007;17:10–8.
77. Kanzaki S, Hilliker S, Baylink DJ, Mohan S. Evidence that human bone cells in culture produce insulin-like growth factor-binding protein-4 and -5 proteases. Endocrinology. 1994;134:383–92.
78. Lundin H, Sääf M, Strender LE, Nyren S, Johansson SE, Salminen H. High serum insulin-like growth factor-binding protein 1 (IGFBP-1) is associated with high fracture risk independent of insulin-like growth factor 1 (IGF-I). Calcif Tissue Int. 2016;99:333–9.
79. Amin S, Riggs BL, Atkinson EJ, Oberg AL, Melton LJ III, Khosla S. A potentially deleterious role of IGFBP-2 on bone density in aging men and women. J Bone Miner Res. 2004;19:1075–83.

80. Longobardi L, Torello M, Buckway C, O'Rear L, Horton WA, Hwa V, Roberts CT Jr, Chiarelli F, Rosenfeld RG, Spagnoli A. A novel insulin-like growth factor (IGF)-independent role for IGF binding protein-3 in mesenchymal chondroprogenitor cell apoptosis. Endocrinology. 2003;144:1695–702.
81. Silha JV, Mishra S, Rosen CJ, Beamer WG, Turner RT, Powell DR, Murphy LJ. Perturbations in bone formation and resorption in insulin-like growth factor binding protein-3 transgenic mice. J Bone Miner Res. 2003;18:1834–41.
82. Lalou C, Silve C, Rosato R, Segovia B, Binoux M. Interactions between insulin-like growth factor-I (IGF-I) and the system of plasminogen activators and their inhibitors in the control of IGF-binding protein-3 production and proteolysis in human osteosarcoma cells. Endocrinology. 1994;135:2318–26.
83. Zhang M, Faugere MC, Malluche H, Rosen CJ, Chernausek SD, Clemens TL. Paracrine overexpression of IGFBP-4 in osteoblasts of transgenic mice decreases bone turnover and causes global growth retardation. J Bone Miner Res. 2003;18:836–43.
84. Richman C, Baylink DJ, Lang K, Dony C, Mohan S. Recombinant human insulin-like growth factor-binding protein-5 stimulates bone formation parameters in vitro and in vivo. Endocrinology. 1999;140:4699–705.
85. Durant D, Pereira RM, Canalis E. Overexpression of insulin-like growth factor binding protein-5 decreases osteoblastic function in vitro. Bone. 2004;35:1256–62.
86. Frara S, Maffezzoni F, Mazziotti G, Giustina A. The modern criteria for medical management of acromegaly. Prog Mol Biol Transl Sci. 2016;138:63–83.
87. Melmed S, Casanueva FF, Klibanski A, Bronstein MD, Chanson P, Lamberts SW, Strasburger CJ, Wass JA, Giustina A. A consensus on the diagnosis and treatment of acromegaly complications. Pituitary. 2013;16:294–302.
88. Mazziotti G, Chiavistelli S, Giustina A. Pituitary diseases and bone. Endocrinol Metab Clin North Am. 2015;44:171–80.
89. Riggs L, Randall RV, Wanner HW, Jowsey J, Kelly PJ, Singh M. The nature of metabolic bone disorder in acromegaly. J Clin Endocrinol Metab. 1972;34:911–8.
90. Kayath MJ, Vieira JGH. Osteopenia occurs in a minority of patients with acromegaly and is predominant in the spine. Osteoporos Int. 1997;7:226–30.
91. Madeira M, Neto LV, de Paula Paranhos Neto F, Barbosa Lima IC, Carvalho de Mendonça LM, Gadelha MR, Fleiuss de Farias ML. Acromegaly has a negative influence on trabecular bone, but not on cortical bone, as assessed by high-resolution peripheral quantitative computed tomography. J Clin Endocrinol Metab. 2013;98:1734–41.
92. Maffezzoni F, Maddalo M, Frara S, Mezzone M, Zorza I, Baruffaldi F, Doglietto F, Mazziotti G, Maroldi R, Giustina A. High-resolution-cone beam tomography analysis of bone microarchitecture in patients with acromegaly and radiological vertebral fractures. Endocrine. 2016;54:532–42.
93. Mazziotti G, Maffezzoni F, Frara S, Giustina A. Acromegalic osteopathy. Pituitary. 2017;20:63–9. https://doi.org/10.1007/s11102-016-0758-6.
94. Mazziotti G, Biagioli E, Maffezzoni F, Spinello M, Serra V, Maroldi R, Floriani I, Giustina A. Bone turnover, bone mineral density, and fracture risk in acromegaly: a meta-analysis. J Clin Endocrinol Metab. 2015;100:384–94.
95. Claessen KM, Mazziotti G, Biermasz NR, Giustina A. Bone and joint disorders in acromegaly. Neuroendocrinology. 2016;103:86–95.
96. Vasikaran S, Eastell R, Bruyère O, Foldes AJ, Garnero P, Griesmacher A, McClung M, Morris HA, Silverman S, Trenti T, Wahl DA, Cooper C, Kanis JA. Markers of bone turnover for the prediction of fracture risk and monitoring of osteoporosis treatment: a need for international reference standards. Osteoporos Int. 2011;22:391–420.
97. Stěpán J, Marek J, Havránek T, Dolezal V, Pacovský V. Bone isoenzyme of serum phosphatase in acromegaly. Clin Chim Acta. 1979;93:355–63.
98. Scillitani A, Chiodini I, Carnevale V, Giannatempo GM, Frusciante V, Villella M, Pileri M, Guglielmi G, Di Giorgio A, Modoni S, Fusilli S, Di Cerbo A, Liuzzi A. Skeletal involvement in female acromegalic subjects: the effects of growth hormone excess in amenorrheal and menstruating patients. J Bone Miner Res. 1997;12:1729–36.

99. Ueland T, Bollerslev J, Godang K, Müller F, Frøland SS, Aukrust P. Increased serum osteoprotegerin in disorders characterized by persistent immune activation or glucocorticoid excess – possible role in bone homeostasis. Eur J Endocrinol. 2001;145:685–90.
100. Mazziotti G, Maffezzoni F, Giustina A. Vitamin D-binding protein: one more piece in the puzzle of acromegalic osteopathy? Endocrine. 2016;52:183–6.
101. Mazziotti G, Cimino V, De Menis E, Bonadonna S, Bugari G, De Marinis L, Veldhuis JD, Giustina A. Active acromegaly enhances spontaneous parathyroid hormone pulsatility. Metabolism. 2006;55:736–40.
102. Legovini P, De Menis E, Doroldi C, Carteri A, Billeci D, Roiter I, Breda F, Conte N. Parathormone levels during treatment of acromegaly with octreotide: one year follow-up. Curr Ther Res. 1993;53:360–6.
103. Kamenický P, Mazziotti G, Lombès M, Giustina A, Chanson P. Growth hormone, insulin-like growth factor-1, and the kidney: pathophysiological and clinical implications. Endocr Rev. 2014;35:234–81.
104. Shepherd JA, Schousboe JT, Broy SB, Engelke K, Leslie WD. Executive Summary of the 2015 ISCD position development conference on advanced measures from DXA and QCT: fracture prediction beyond BMD. J Clin Densitom. 2015;18:274–86.
105. Ueland T, Fougner SL, Godang K, Schreiner T, Bollerslev J. Serum GH and IGF-I are significant determinants of bone turnover but not bone mineral density in active acromegaly: a prospective study of more than 70 consecutive patients. Eur J Endocrinol. 2006;155: 709–15.
106. Ueland T, Ebbesen EN, Thomsen JS, Mosekilde L, Brixen K, Flyvbjerg A, Bollerslev J. Decreased trabecular bone biomechanical competence, apparent density, IGF-II and IGFBP-5 content in acromegaly. Eur J Clin Invest. 2002;32:122–8.
107. Diamond T, Nery L, Posen S. Spinal and peripheral bone mineral densities in acromegaly: the effects of excess growth hormone and hypogonadism. Ann Intern Med. 1989;111: 567–73.
108. Lesse GP, Fraser WD, Farquharson R, Hipkin L, Vora JP. Gonadal status is an important determinant of bone density in acromegaly. Clin Endocrinol (Oxf). 1998;48:59–65.
109. Griffith JF, Genant HK. New advances in imaging osteoporosis and its complications. Endocrine. 2012;42:39–51.
110. Frara S, Maffezzoni F, Mazziotti G, Giustina A. Current and emerging aspects of diabetes mellitus in acromegaly. Trends Endocrinol Metab. 2016;27:470–83.
111. Hong AR, Kim JH, Kim SW, Kim SY, Shin CS. Trabecular bone score as a skeletal fragility index in acromegalic patients. Osteoporos Int. 2016;27:1123–9.
112. Vestergaard P, Mosekilde L. Fracture risk is decreased in acromegaly – a potential beneficial effect of growth hormone. Osteoporos Int. 2004;15:155–9.
113. Mazziotti G, Bianchi A, Porcelli T, Mormando M, Maffezzoni F, Cristiano A, Giampietro A, De Marinis L, Giustina A. Vertebral fractures in patients with acromegaly: a 3-year prospective study. J Clin Endocrinol Metab. 2013;98:3402–10.
114. Genant HK, Jergas M, Palermo L, Nevitt M, Valentin RS, Black D, Cummings SR. Comparison of semiquantitative visual and quantitative morphometric assessment of prevalent and incident vertebral fractures in osteoporosis – The Study of Osteoporotic Fractures Research Group. J Bone Miner Res. 1996;11:984–96.
115. Bonadonna S, Mazziotti G, Nuzzo M, Bianchi A, Fusco A, De Marinis L, Giustina A. Increased prevalence of radiological spinal deformities in active acromegaly: a cross-sectional study in post-menopausal women. J Bone Miner Res. 2005;20:1837–44.
116. Mazziotti G, Bianchi A, Bonadonna S, Cimino V, Patelli I, Fusco A, Pontecorvi A, De Marinis L, Giustina A. Prevalence of vertebral fractures in men with acromegaly. J Clin Endocrinol Metab. 2008;93:4649–55.
117. Wassenaar MJ, Biermasz NR, Hamdy NA, Zillikens MC, van Meurs JB, Rivadeneira F, Hofman A, Uitterlinden AG, Stokkel MP, Roelfsema F, Kloppenburg M, Kroon HM, Romijn JA, Pereira AM. High prevalence of vertebral fractures despite normal bone mineral density in patients with long-term controlled acromegaly. Eur J Endocrinol. 2011;164: 475–83.

118. Battista C, Chiodini I, Muscarella S, Guglielmi G, Mascia ML, Carnevale V, Scillitani A. Spinal volumetric trabecular bone mass in acromegaly patients: a longitudinal study. Clin Endocrinol (Oxf). 2009;70:378–82.
119. Madeira M, Neto LV, Torres CH, de Mendonça LM, Gadelha MR, de Farias ML. Vertebral fracture assessment in acromegaly. J Clin Densitom. 2013;16:238–43.
120. Padova G, Borzì G, Incorvaia L, Siciliano G, Migliorino V, Vetri M, Tita P. Prevalence of osteoporosis and vertebral fractures in acromegalic patients. Clin Cases Miner Bone Metab. 2011;8:37–43.
121. Brzana J, Yedinak CG, Hameed N, Fleseriu M. FRAX score in acromegaly: does it tell the whole story? Clin Endocrinol (Oxf). 2014;80:614–6.
122. Claessen KM, Kroon HM, Pereira AM, Appelman-Dijkstra NM, Verstegen MJ, Kloppenburg M, Hamdy NA, Biermasz NR. Progression of vertebral fractures despite long-term biochemical control of acromegaly: a prospective follow-up study. J Clin Endocrinol Metab. 2013;98:4808–15.
123. Mazziotti G, Gola M, Bianchi A, Porcelli T, Giampietro A, Cimino V, Doga M, Gazzaruso C, De Marinis L, Giustina A. Influence of diabetes mellitus on vertebral fractures in men with acromegaly. Endocrine. 2011;40:102–8.
124. Johansson H, Odén A, McCloskey EV, Kanis JA. Mild morphometric vertebral fractures predict vertebral fractures bot not non-vertebral fractures. Osteoporos Int. 2014;25:235–41.
125. Mazziotti G, Porcelli T, Bianchi A, Cimino V, Patelli I, Mejia C, Fusco A, Giampietro A, De Marinis L, Giustina A. Glucocorticoid replacement therapy and vertebral fractures in hypopituitary adult males with GH deficiency. Eur J Endocrinol. 2010;163:15–20.
126. Mazziotti G, Mormando M, Cristiano A, Bianchi A, Porcelli T, Giampietro A, Maffezzoni F, Serra V, De Marinis L, Giustina A. Association between l-thyroxine treatment, GH deficiency, and radiological vertebral fractures in patients with adult-onset hypopituitarism. Eur J Endocrinol. 2014;170:893–9.
127. Orük G, Tarhan F, Argin M, Ozmen M. Is every joint symptom related to acromegaly? Endocrine. 2013;43:404–11.
128. Romijn JA. Acromegalic arthropathy: current perspectives. Endocrine. 2013;43:245–6.
129. Ben-Shlomo A, Sheppard MC, Stephens JM, Pulgar S, Melmed S. Clinical, quality of life, and economic value of acromegaly disease control. Pituitary. 2011;14:284–94.
130. Crespo I, Webb SM. Perception of health and cognitive dysfunction in acromegaly patients. Endocrine. 2014;46:365–7.
131. Melmed S. The pituitary. 3rd ed. London: Academic Press; 2011.
132. Rosén T, Edén S, Larsson G, Wilhelmsen L, Bengtsson BA. Cardiovascular risk factors in adult patients with growth hormone deficiency. Acta Endocrinol. 1993;129:195–200.
133. Doga M, Bonadonna S, Gola M, Mazziotti G, Nuzzo M, Giustina A. GH deficiency in the adult and bone. J Endocrinol Invest. 2005;28(8 Suppl):18–23.
134. Abdu TA, Neary R, Elhadd TA, Akber M, Clayton RN. Coronary risk in growth hormone deficient hypopituitary adults: increased predicted risk is due largely to lipid profile abnormalities. Clin Endocrinol (Oxf). 2001;55:209–16.
135. Møller N, Jørgensen JO. Effects of growth hormone on glucose, lipid, and protein metabolism in human subjects. Endocr Rev. 2009;30:152–77.
136. Jørgensen JO, Krag M, Jessen N, Nørrelund H, Vestergaard ET, Møller N, Christiansen JS. Growth hormone and glucose homeostasis. Horm Res. 2004;62(Suppl 3):51–5.
137. Gazzaruso C, Gola M, Karamouzis I, Giubbini R, Giustina A. Cardiovascular risk in adult patients with growth hormone (GH) deficiency and following substitution with GH – an update. J Clin Endocrinol Metab. 2014;99:18–29.
138. Chikani V, Cuneo RC, Hickman I, Ho KK. Impairment of anaerobic capacity in adults with growth hormone deficiency. J Clin Endocrinol Metab. 2015;100:1811–8.
139. Jørgensen AP, Fougner KJ, Ueland T, Gudmundsen O, Burman P, Schreiner T, Bollerslev J. Favorable long-term effects of growth hormone replacement therapy on quality of life, bone metabolism, body composition and lipid levels in patients with adult-onset growth hormone deficiency. Growth Horm IGF Res. 2011;21:69–75.

140. Corpas E, Harman SM, Blackman MR. Human growth hormone and aging. Endocr Rev. 1993;14:20–39.
141. Raisz LG. Local and systemic factors in the pathogenesis of osteoporosis. N Engl J Med. 1988;318:818–28.
142. Canalis E, Giustina A, Bilezikian JP. Medical progress: mechanisms of anabolic therapies for osteoporosis. N Engl J Med. 2007;357:905–16.
143. Lange M, Müller J, Svendsen OL, Kastrup KW, Juul A, Feldt-Rasmussen U. The impact of idiopathic childhood-onset growth hormone deficiency (GHD) on bone mass in subjects without adult GHD. Clin Endocrinol (Oxf). 2005;62:18–23.
144. de Boer H, Blok GJ, van Lingen A, Teule GJ, Lips P, van der Veen EA. Consequences of childhood-onset growth hormone deficiency for adult bone mass. J Bone Miner Res. 1994; 9:1319–26.
145. Toogood AA, Adams JE, O'Neill PA, Shalet SM. Elderly patients with adult onset growth hormone deficiency are not osteopenic. J Clin Endocrinol Metab. 1997;82:1462–6.
146. Murray RD, Columb B, Adams JE, Shalet SM. Low bone mass is an infrequent feature of the adult growth hormone deficiency syndrome in middle-age adults and the elderly. J Clin Endocrinol Metab. 2004;89:1124–30.
147. Ott SM. Attainment of peak bone mass. J Clin Endocrinol Metab. 1990;71:1082A–C.
148. Holmes SJ, Economou G, Whitehouse RW, Adams JE, Shalet SM. Reduced bone mineral density in patients with adult onset growth hormone deficiency. J Clin Endocrinol Metab. 1994;78:669–74.
149. Bravenboer N, Holzmann P, de Boer H, Blok GJ, Lips P. Histomorphometric analysis of bone mass and bone metabolism in growth hormone deficient adult men. Bone. 1996;18:551–7.
150. Lancer SR, Bowser EN, Hargis GK. The effect of growth hormone on parathyroid function in rats. Endocrinology. 1976;98:1289–93.
151. Hitz MF, Jensen JE, Eskildsen PC. Bone mineral density in patients with growth hormone deficiency: does a gender difference exist? Clin Endocrinol (Oxf). 2006;65:783–91.
152. Sartorio A, Conti A, Monzani M, Morabito F, Faglia G. Growth hormone treatment in adults with GH deficiency: effects on new biochemical markers of bone and collagen turnover. J Endocrinol Invest. 1993;16:893–8.
153. Delmas PD, Chatelain P, Malaval L, Bonne G. Serum bone GLA-protein in growth hormone deficient children. J Bone Miner Res. 1986;1:333–8.
154. Nielsen HK, Jørgensen JO, Brixen K, Christiansen JS. Serum osteocalcin and bone isoenzyme alkaline phosphatase in growth hormone-deficient patients: dose-response studies with biosynthetic human GH. Calcif Tissue Int. 1991;48:82–7.
155. Mazziotti G, Bianchi A, Cimino V, Bonadonna S, Martini P, Fusco A, De Marinis L, Giustina A. Effect of gonadal status on bone mineral density and radiological spinal deformities in adult patients with growth hormone deficiency. Pituitary. 2008;11:55–61.
156. Stall GM, Harris S, Sokoll LJ, Dawson-Hughes B. Accelerated bone loss in hypothyroid patients over-treated with L-thyroxine. Ann Intern Med. 1990;113:265–9.
157. Canalis E, Mazziotti G, Giustina A, Bilezikian JP. Glucocorticoid-induced osteoporosis: pathophysiology and therapy. Osteoporos Int. 2007;18:1319–28.
158. Wüster C, Slencza E, Ziegler R. Increased prevalence of osteoporosis and arteriosclerosis in conventionally substituted anterior pituitary insufficiency: need for additional growth hormone substitution? Klin Wochenschr. 1991;69:769–73.
159. Johansson AG, Burman P, Westermark K, Ljunghall S. The bone mineral density in acquired growth hormone deficiency correlates with circulating levels of insulin-like growth factor I. J Intern Med. 1992;232:447–52.
160. Beshyah SA, Freemantle C, Thomas E, Rutherford O, Page B, Murphy M. Abnormal body composition and reduced bone mass in growth hormone deficient hypopituitary adults. Clin Endocrinol (Oxf). 1995;42:179–89.
161. Degerblad M, Bengtsson BA, Bramnert M, Johnell O, Manhem P, Rosén T, Thorén M. Reduced bone mineral density in adults with growth hormone (GH) deficiency: increased bone turnover during 12-months of GH substitution therapy. Eur J Endocrinol. 1995;133:180–8.

162. Johansson AG, Eden Engstrom B, Ljunghall S, Karlsson FA, Burman P. Gender differences in the effects of long term growth hormone (GH) treatment on bone in adults with GH deficiency. J Clin Endocrinol Metab. 1999;84:2002–7.
163. Baum HB, Biller BM, Finkelstein JS, Cannistraro KB, Oppenheim DS, Schoenfeld DA, Michel TH, Wittink H, Klibanski A. Effects of physiologic growth hormone therapy on bone density and body composition in patients with adult-onset growth hormone deficiency. A randomized, placebo-controlled trial. Ann Intern Med. 1996;125:883–90.
164. Välimäki MJ, Salmela PI, Salmi J, Viikari J, Kataja M, Turunen H, Soppi E. Effects of GH treatment on bone mineral density and bone turn over in GH-deficient adults. Eur J Endocrinol. 1999;140:545–54.
165. Hansen TB, Brixen K, Vahl N, Jørgensen JO, Christiansen JS, Mosekilde L, Hagen C. Effects of 12 months of growth hormone (GH) treatment on calciotropic hormones, calcium homeostasis, and bone metabolism in adults with acquired GH deficiency: a double-blind, randomized, placebo-controlled study. J Clin Endocrinol Metab. 1996;81:3352–9.
166. Nilsson AG. Effects of growth hormone replacement therapy on bone markers and bone mineral density in growth hormone-deficient adults. Horm Res. 2000;54(Suppl 1):52–7.
167. Beshyah SA, Kyd P, Thomas E, Fairney A, Johnston DG. The effects of prolonged growth hormone replacement on bone metabolism and bone mineral density in hypopituitary adults. Clin Endocrinol (Oxf). 1995;42:249–54.
168. Beshyah SA, Thomas E, Kyd P, Sharp P, Fairney A, Johnston DG. The effect of growth hormone replacement therapy in hypopituitary adults on calcium and bone metabolism. Clin Endocrinol (Oxf). 1994;40:383–91.
169. Saggese G, Baroncelli GI, Bertelloni S, Cinquanta L, Di Nero G. Effects of long-term treatment with growth hormone on bone and mineral metabolism in children with growth hormone deficiency. J Pediatr. 1993;122:37–45.
170. Ueland T, Odgren PR, Yndestad A, Godang K, Schreiner T, Marks SC, Bollerslev J. Growth hormone substitution increases gene expression of members of the IGF family in cortical bone from women with adult onset growth hormone deficiency – relationship with bone turnover. Bone. 2003;33:638–45.
171. Johannsson G, Rosén T, Bosaeus I, Sjöström L, Bengtsson BA. Two years of growth hormone (GH) treatment increases bone mineral content and density in hypopituitary patients with adult onset GH deficiency. J Clin Endocrinol Metab. 1996;81:2865–73.
172. Götherström G, Svensson J, Koranyi J, Alpsten M, Bosaeus I, Bengtsson B, Johannsson G. A prospective study of 5 years of GH replacement therapy in GH-deficient adults: sustained effects on body composition, bone mass, and metabolic indices. J Clin Endocrinol Metab. 2001;86:4657–65.
173. Drake WM, Rodríguez-Arnao J, Weaver JU, James IT, Coyte D, Spector TD, Besser GM, Monson JP. The influence of gender on the short- and long-term effects of growth hormone replacement on bone metabolism and bone mineral density in hypopituitary adults: a 5-year study. Clin Endocrinol (Oxf). 2001;54:525–32.
174. Sneppen SB, Hoeck HC, Kollerup G, Sørensen OH, Laurberg P, Feldt-Rasmussen U. Bone mineral content and bone metabolism during physiological GH treatment in GH-deficient adults – an 18-month randomised, placebo-controlled, double-blinded trial. Eur J Endocrinol. 2002;146:187–95.
175. Janssen YJ, Hamdy NA, Frölich M, Roelfsema F. Skeletal effects of two years of treatment with low physiological doses of recombinant human growth hormone (GH) in patients with adult-onset GH deficiency. J Clin Endocrinol Metab. 1998;83:2143–8.
176. Abrahamsen B, Hangaard J, Horn HC, Hansen TB, Gregersen G, Hansen-Nord M, Vahl N, Junker P, Andersen M, Hagen C. Evaluation of the optimum dose of growth hormone (GH) for restoring bone mass in adult-onset GH deficiency: results from two 12-month randomized studies. Clin Endocrinol (Oxf). 2002;57:273–81.
177. Jensen LT, Jørgensen JOL, Risteli J, Christiansen JS, Lorenzen I. Type I and III procollagen propeptides in growth hormone-deficient patients: effects of increasing doses of GH. Acta Endocrinol (Copenh). 1991;124:278–82.

178. Thorén M, Soop M, Degerblad M, Sääf M. Preliminary study of the effects of growth hormone substitution therapy on bone mineral density and serum osteocalcin levels in adult growth hormone deficiency. Acta Endocrinol. 1993;128(Suppl 2):41–3.
179. Holmes SJ, Whitehouse RW, Swindell R, Economou G, Adams JE, Shalet SM. Effect of growth hormone replacement on bone mass in adults with adult onset growth hormone deficiency. Clin Endocrinol (Oxf). 1995;42:627–33.
180. Binnerts A, Swart GR, Wilson JHP, Hoogerbrugge N, Pols HA, Birkenhager JC, Lamberts SW. The effect of growth hormone administration in growth hormone-deficient adults on bone, protein, carbohydrate and lipid homeostasis, as well as body composition. Clin Endocrinol (Oxf). 1992;37:79–87.
181. Whitehead HM, Boreham C, McIlrath EM, Sheridan B, Kennedy L, Atkinson AB, Hadden DR. Growth hormone treatment of adults with growth hormone deficiency: results of a 13-month placebo-controlled cross-over study. Clin Endocrinol (Oxf). 1992;36:45–52.
182. Amato G, Carella C, Fazio S, La Montagna G, Cittadini A, Sabatini D, Marciano-Mone C, Sacca L, Bellastella A. Body composition, bone metabolism, and heart structure and function in growth hormone-deficient adults before and after GH replacement therapy at low doses. J Clin Endocrinol Metab. 1993;77:1671–6.
183. Vandeweghe M, Taelman P, Kaufman JM. Short and long-term effects of growth hormone treatment on bone turnover and bone mineral content in adult growth hormone-deficient males. Clin Endocrinol (Oxf). 1993;39:409–15.
184. Rodríguez-Arnao J, James I, Jabbar A, Trainer PJ, Perrett D, Besser GM, Ross RJ. Serum collagen crosslinks as markers of bone turn-over during GH replacement therapy in growth hormone-deficient adults. Clin Endocrinol (Oxf). 1998;48:455–62.
185. Bravenboer N, Holzmann P, de Boer H, Roos JC, van der Veen EA, Lips P. The effect of growth hormone (GH) on histomorphometric indices of bone structure and bone turnover in GH-deficient men. J Clin Endocrinol Metab. 1997;82:1818–22.
186. Finkenstedt G, Gasser RW, Höfle G, Watfah C, Fridrich L. Effects of growth hormone (GH) replacement on bone metabolism and mineral density in adult onset of GH deficiency: results of a double-blind placebo-controlled study with open follow-up. Eur J Endocrinol. 1997; 136:282–9.
187. Kotzmann H, Riedl M, Bernecker P, Clodi M, Kainberger F, Kaider A, Woloszczuk W, Luger A. Effect of long-term growth hormone substitution therapy on bone mineral density and parameters of bone metabolism in adult patients with growth hormone deficiency. Calcif Tissue Int. 1998;62:40–6.
188. Davidson P, Milne R, Chase D, Cooper C. Growth hormone replacement in adults and bone mineral density: a systematic review and meta-analysis. Clin Endocrinol (Oxf). 2004;60:92–8.
189. ter Maaten JC, de Boer H, Kamp O, Stuurman L, van der Veen EA. Long-term effects of growth hormone (GH) replacement in men with childhood-onset GH deficiency. J Clin Endocrinol Metab. 1999;84:2373–80.
190. Biermasz NR, Hamdy NA, Pereira AM, Romijn JA, Roelfsema F. Long-term skeletal effects of recombinant human growth hormone (rhGH) alone and rhGH combined with alendronate in GH-deficient adults: a seven-year follow-up study. Clin Endocrinol (Oxf). 2004;60:568–75.
191. Clanget C, Seck T, Hinke V, Wüster C, Ziegler R, Pfeilschifter J. Effects of 6 years of growth hormone (GH) treatment on bone mineral density in GH-deficient adults. Clin Endocrinol (Oxf). 2001;55:93–9.
192. Götherström G, Bengtsson BA, Bosaeus I, Johannsson G, Svensson J. Ten-year GH replacement increases bone mineral density in hypopituitary patients with adult onset GH deficiency. Eur J Endocrinol. 2007;156:55–64.
193. Bravenboer N, Holzmann PJ, ter Maaten JC, Stuurman LM, Roos JC, Lips P. Effect of long-term growth hormone treatment on bone mass and bone metabolism in growth hormone-deficient men. J Bone Miner Res. 2005;20:1778–84.
194. Arwert LI, Roos JC, Lips P, Twisk JW, Manoliu RA, Drent ML. Effects of 10 years of growth hormone (GH) replacement therapy in adult GH-deficient men. Clin Endocrinol (Oxf). 2005; 63:310–6.

195. Holmes SJ, Whitehouse RW, Economou G, O'Halloran DJ, Adams JE, Shalet SM. Further increase in forearm cortical bone mineral content after discontinuation of growth hormone replacement. Clin Endocrinol (Oxf). 1995;42:3–7.
196. Biller BM, Sesmilo G, Baum HB, Hayden D, Schoenfeld D, Klibanski A. Withdrawal of long-term physiological growth hormone (GH) administration: differential effects on bone density and body composition in men with adult-onset GH deficiency. J Clin Endocrinol Metab. 2000;85:970–6.
197. Wüster C, Abs R, Bengtsson BA, Bennmarker H, Feldt-Rasmussen U, Hernberg-Ståhl E, Monson JP, Westberg B, Wilton P, KIMS Study Group and the KIMS International Board. Pharmacia & Upjohn International Metabolic Database. The influence of growth hormone deficiency, growth hormone replacement therapy, and other aspects of hypopituitarism on fracture rate and bone mineral density. J Bone Miner Res. 2001;16:398–405.
198. Rosén T, Wilhelmsen L, Landin-Wilhelmsen K, Lappas G, Bengtsson BA. Increased fracture frequency in adult patients with hypopituitarism and GH deficiency. Eur J Endocrinol. 1997;137:240–5.
199. Bouillon R, Koledova E, Bezlepkina O, Nijs J, Shavrikhova E, Nagaeva E, Chikulaeva O, Peterkova V, Dedov I, Bakulin A, Oganov V, Attanasio AF. Bone status and fracture prevalence in Russian adults with childhood-onset growth hormone deficiency. J Clin Endocrinol Metab. 2004;89:4993–8.
200. Mazziotti G, Bianchi A, Bonadonna S, Nuzzo M, Cimino V, Fusco A, De Marinis L, Giustina A. Increased prevalence of radiological spinal deformities in adult patients with GH deficiency: influence of GH replacement therapy. J Bone Miner Res. 2006;21:520–8.
201. Giustina A, Mazziotti G. Growth hormone replacement therapy and fracture risk. Lancet Diabetes Endocrinol. 2015;3:307–8.
202. Van Staa P, Leufkens HG, Abenhaim L, Zhang B, Cooper C. Use of oral corticosteroids and risk of fracture. J Bone Miner Res. 2000;15:993–1000.
203. Mazziotti G, Delgado A, Maffezzoni F, Formenti AM, Giustina A. Skeletal fragility in endogenous hypercortisolism. Front Horm Res. 2016;46:66–73.
204. Mazziotti G, Formenti AM, Adler RA, Bilezikian JP, Grossman A, Sbardella E. Glucocorticoid-induced osteoporosis: pathophysiological role of GH/IGF-I and PTH/vitamin D axes, treatment options and guidelines. Endocrine. 2016;54:603–11. https://doi.org/10.1007/s12020-016-1146-8.
205. Lane NE, Yao W, Balooch M, Nalla RK, Balooch G, Habelitz S, Kinney JH, Bonewald LF. Glucocorticoid treated mice have localized changes in trabecular bone material properties and osteocyte lacunar size that are not observed in placebo-treated or estrogen-deficient mice. J Bone Miner Res. 2006;21:466–76.
206. Van Staa TP, Laan RF, Barton IP, Cohen S, Reid DM, Cooper C. Bone density threshold and other predictors of vertebral fracture in patients receiving oral glucocorticoid therapy. Arthritis Rheum. 2003;48:3224–9.
207. Devesa J, Barros MG, Gondar M, Tresquerres JA, Arce V. Regulation of hypothalamic somatostatin by glucocorticoids. J Steroid Biochem Mol Biol. 1995;53:277–82.
208. Tamura H, Kamegai J, Sugihara H, Kineman RD, Frohman LA, Wakabayashi I. Glucocorticoids regulate pituitary growth hormone secretagogue receptor gene expression. J Neuroendocrinol. 2000;12:481–5.
209. Miller TL, Mayo KE. Glucocorticoids regulate pituitary growth hormone-releasing hormone receptor messenger ribonucleic acid expression. Endocrinology. 1997;138:2458–65.
210. Fife SK, Brogan RS, Giustina A, Wehrenberg WB. Immunocytochemical and molecular analysis of the effects of glucocorticoid-treatment on the hypothalamic-somatotropic axis in the rat. Neuroendocrinology. 1996;64:131–8.
211. Malerba M, Bossoni S, Radaeli E, Mori S, Bonadonna S, Giustina A, Tantucci C. Growth hormone response to growth hormone-releasing hormone is reduced in adult asthmatic patients receiving long-term inhaled corticosteroid treatment. Chest. 2005;127:515–21.
212. Terzolo M, Bossoni S, Ali A, Doga M, Reimondo G, Milani G, Peretti P, Manelli F, Angeli A, Giustina A. Growth hormone (GH) response to GH-releasing hormone alone or combined with arginine in patients with adrenal incidentaloma: evidence for enhanced somatostatinergic tone. J Clin Endocrinol Metab. 2000;85:1310–5.

213. Wehrenberg WB, Bergman PJ, Stagg L, Ndon J, Giustina A. Glucocorticoid inhibition of growth in rats: partial reversal with somatostatin antibodies. Endocrinology. 1990;127: 2705–8.
214. Giustina A, Misitano V, Voltz D. Adrenergic and cholinergic involvement in basal and growth hormone-releasing hormone-stimulated growth hormone secretion in glucocorticoid-treated rats. Endocr Res. 1995;21:719–32.
215. Giustina A, Voltz DM, Teik J, Wehrenberg WB. Galanin counteracts the inhibitory effects of glucocorticoids on growth hormone secretion in the rat. Metabolism. 1995;44:224–7.
216. Benso A, Gramaglia E, Olivetti I, Tomelini M, Gigliardi VR, Frara S, Calvi E, Belcastro S, St Pierre DH, Ghigo E, Broglio F. The GH-releasing effect of acylated ghrelin in normal subjects is refractory to GH acute auto-feedback but is inhibited after short-term GH administration inducing IGF1 increase. Eur J Endocrinol. 2013;15:509–14.
217. Giustina A, Doga M, Bodini C, Girelli A, Legati F, Bossoni S, Romanelli G. Acute effects of cortisone acetate on growth hormone response to growth hormone-releasing hormone in normal adult subjects. Acta Endocrinol (Copenh). 1990;122:206–10.
218. Giustina A, Girelli A, Doga M, Bodini C, Bossoni S, Romanelli G, Wehrenberg WB. Pyridostigmine blocks the inhibitory effect of glucocorticoids on growth hormone releasing hormone stimulated growth hormone secretion in normal men. J Clin Endocrinol Metab. 1990;71:580–4.
219. Kaufmann S, Jones KL, Wehrenberg WB, Culler FL. Inhibition by prednisone of growth hormone (GH) response to GH-releasing hormone in normal men. J Clin Endocrinol Metab. 1988;67:1258–61.
220. Giustina A, Bussi AR, Doga M, Wehrenberg WB. Effect of hydrocortisone on the growth hormone (GH) response to GH-releasing hormone in acromegaly. Horm Res. 1994;41:33–7.
221. Magiakou MA, Mastorakos G, Gomez MT, Rose SR, Chrousos GP. Suppressed spontaneous and stimulated growth hormone secretion in patients with Cushing's disease before and after surgical cure. J Clin Endocrinol Metab. 1994;78:131–7.
222. Savage MO, Lienhardt A, Lebrethon MC, Johnston LB, Huebner A, Grossman AB, Afshar F, Plowman PN, Besser GM. Cushing's disease in childhood: presentation, investigation, treatment and long-term outcome. Horm Res. 2001;55(Suppl 1):24–30.
223. Lebrethon MC, Grossman AB, Afshar F, Plowman PN, Besser GM, Savage MO. Linear growth and final height after treatment for Cushing's disease in childhood. J Clin Endocrinol Metab. 2000;85:3262–5.
224. Lodish MB, Hsiao HP, Serbis A, Sinaii N, Rothenbuhler A, Keil MF, Boikos SA, Reynolds JC, Stratakis CA. Effects of Cushing disease on bone mineral density in a pediatric population. J Pediatr. 2010;156:1001–5.
225. Khanine V, Fournier JJ, Requeda E, Luton JP, Simon F, Crouzet J. Osteoporotic fractures at presentation of Cushing's disease: two case reports and a literature review. Joint Bone Spine. 2000;67:341–5.
226. Futo L, Toke J, Patocs A, Szappanos A, Varga I, Glaz E, Tulassay Z, Racz K, Toth M. Skeletal differences in bone mineral area and content before and after cure of endogenous Cushing's syndrome. Osteoporos Int. 2008;19:941–9.
227. Kawamata A, Iihara M, Okamoto T, Obara T. Bone mineral density before and after surgical cure of Cushing's syndrome due to adrenocortical adenoma: prospective study. World J Surg. 2008;32:890–6.
228. Di Somma C, Pivonello R, Loche S, Faggiano A, Marzullo P, Di Sarno A, Klain M, Salvatore M, Lombardi G, Colao A. Severe impairment of bone mass and turnover in Cushing's disease: comparison between childhood-onset and adulthood-onset disease. Clin Endocrinol (Oxf). 2002;56:153–8.
229. Scommegna S, Greening JP, Storr HL, Davies KM, Shaw NJ, Monson JP, Grossman AB, Savage MO. Bone mineral density at diagnosis and following successful treatment of pediatric Cushing's disease. J Endocrinol Invest. 2005;28:231–5.
230. Hochberg Z. Mechanisms of steroid impairment of growth. Horm Res. 2002;58:S33–8.
231. Filipsson H, Johannsson G. GH replacement in adults: interactions with other pituitary hormone deficiencies and replacement therapies. Eur J Endocrinol. 2009;161:S85–95.

232. Mazziotti G, Giustina A. Glucocorticoids and the regulation of growth hormone secretion. Nat Rev Endocrinol. 2013;9:265–76.
233. Giustina A, Bussi AR, Jacobello C, Wehrenberg WB. Effects of recombinant human growth hormone (GH) on bone and intermediary metabolism in patients receiving chronic glucocorticoid treatment with suppressed endogenous GH response to GH-releasing hormone. J Clin Endocrinol Metab. 1995;80:122–9.
234. Horber FF, Haymond MW. Human growth hormone prevents the protein catabolic side effects of prednisone in humans. J Clin Invest. 1990;86:265–72.
235. Mazziotti G, Frara S, Giustina A. Pituitary diseases and bone. Endocr Rev. 2018.; https://doi.org/10.1210/er.2018-00005

Adrenal Function and Skeletal Regulation

7

Iacopo Chiodini, Claudia Battista, Elisa Cairoli, Cristina Eller-Vainicher, Valentina Morelli, Serena Palmieri, Antonio Stefano Salcuni, and Alfredo Scillitani

7.1 Introduction

The hormones produced by the adrenal glands and in particular from its cortex (i.e., cortisol, aldosterone, and androgens) influence the skeletal tissue both in physiological and pathological conditions. Indeed, these adrenal hormones are important for the skeletal growth and development and for maintaining the skeletal health during the adult life, and their excess can lead to a reduction of bone mineral density and quality and to an increased fracture risk [1, 2].

Among the hormones secreted by the adrenal cortex, cortisol has the most significant effect on the bone, and the high sensitivity of the skeletal tissue to the cortisol excess explains why the occurrence of a fragility fracture can be the presenting manifestation of an otherwise asymptomatic hypercortisolism [3]. However, the different degree of cortisol secretion, though still in the normal range, is possibly

I. Chiodini (✉) · E. Cairoli
Unit for Bone Metabolism Diseases and Diabetes, IRCCS Istituto Auxologico Italiano, Milan, Italy

Department of Medical Sciences and Community Health, University of Milan, Milan, Italy
e-mail: iacopo.chiodini@unimi.it

C. Battista · A. Scillitani
Unit of Endocrinology, "Casa Sollievo della Sofferenza", Hospital, IRCCS, San Giovanni Rotondo, Foggia, Italy

C. Eller-Vainicher
Unit of Endocrinology, Fondazione Cà Granda IRCCS, Milan, Italy

V. Morelli · S. Palmieri
Department of Medical Sciences and Community Health, University of Milan, Milan, Italy

Unit of Endocrinology, Fondazione Cà Granda IRCCS, Milan, Italy

A. S. Salcuni
Endocrine Unit, Department of Medical Sciences, University of Cagliari, Cagliari, Italy

A. Lenzi, S. Migliaccio (eds.), *Multidisciplinary Approach to Osteoporosis*,
https://doi.org/10.1007/978-3-319-75110-8_7

associated with bone mineral density (BMD) in postmenopausal females [4], with the BMD changes in elderly subjects [5] and with fractures in diabetic postmenopausal women [6]. The sensitivity to glucocorticoids (GCs) varies among individuals due to the different polymorphisms of the glucocorticoid receptor (GR) gene and the different activity of the 11β-hydroxysteroid dehydrogenases (the enzyme responsible for the interconversion between the inactive cortisone and the active cortisol) [7]. The different GC sensitivities have been demonstrated to be possibly associated with bone health in patients with overt and subclinical cortisol excess and in osteoporotic patients without hypercortisolism [3, 7, 8].

The effect of the adrenal androgens on the bone is important particularly in women, in whom the adrenal is the main source of androgens, but evidences exist that the adrenal androgens influence the size and mineral content of the skeleton in both males and females [1]. Finally, the aldosterone excess has been suggested to be deleterious for the bone, probably with both direct effect on bone cells and indirect mechanisms.

This chapter will review the actions of the adrenal hormones on the bone in normal physiology and in the diseases characterized by their hypersecretion.

7.2 Adrenal Gland Hormones

The adult adrenal gland, situated immediately above the kidney, is composed of a cortex and a medulla. The adrenal cortex has a zona glomerulosa (15%), a zona fasciculata (75%), and a zona reticularis.

The main hormones produced by the adrenal cortex are cortisol, aldosterone, and adrenal androgens. Cholesterol, in particular the circulating low-density lipoprotein cholesterol, is the precursor for all adrenal steroidogenesis. Steroidogenesis requires the action of several enzymes expressed in a specific zonal manner. The adrenocorticotropic hormone (ACTH) controls the GC secretion from the zona fasciculata and adrenal androgens (DHEA, dehydroepiandrosterone sulfate [DHEAS], androstenedione) secretion from the zona reticularis; mineralocorticoids are secreted from the zona glomerulosa under the principal control of angiotensin II. DHEA and DHEAS represent an important amount (>50%) of circulating androgens in premenopausal females and exert their effects after conversion to testosterone.

GCs act on glucose, protein, and lipid metabolism; cause catabolic changes in the muscle, skin, and connective tissue; modulate bone and calcium metabolism; increase blood pressure; suppress immunologic responses; and inhibit TSH secretion, gonadotropin-releasing hormone pulsatility, and skeletal growth. Moreover GCs are involved in the pathogenesis of different gut and central nervous system diseases. In contrast to the diverse action of GCs, mineralocorticoids have a more restricted role, principally to stimulate epithelial sodium transport in the distal nephron, distal colon, and salivary glands.

Both free cortisol and aldosterone exert their effects binding the intracellular glucocorticoid and mineralocorticoid receptors (GR and MR, respectively).

The principal sites of cortisol and aldosterone metabolism are the liver and the kidney. The inactivation of cortisol to cortisone by 11β-hydroxysteroid dehydrogenase (11-HSD) is the main pathway. Furthermore, 11-HSD expressed in peripheral tissues plays a crucial role in regulating corticosteroid hormone action and in influencing individual variability. Two distinct 11-HSD isozymes have been reported: a type 1 (11-HSD1) that is expressed principally in the liver, which confers bioactivity to cortisone by converting it to cortisol, and a type 2 (11-HSD2), expressed in the kidney, colon, and salivary gland, that inactivates cortisol to cortisone. The main role of the 11-HSD2 is to protect the MR that shows the same affinity for cortisol and aldosterone, from the GCs excess.

The adrenal medulla, embryologically derived from neural crest tissue, mainly synthesizes and stores epinephrine. Catecholamines act widely in the body and affect many cardiovascular and metabolic processes [9].

7.3 Glucocorticoids and Bone Physiology

Although excessive GCs are a well-recognized cause of osteoporosis, little is known about the role of endogenous GCs in determining skeletal mass. The reason why the mechanisms of action of GCs on the bone are better known in pathological conditions than in physiological ones is linked to the fact that there are several difficulties with examining any relationships between endogenous GCs and bone physiology such as the natural diurnal and age-related variation of cortisol and the stress responses and problems in measuring free cortisol levels rather than total cortisol [1]. Moreover, besides the action of GCs through its receptor, specific enzymes modulate GC metabolism within the cell at the pre-receptor level [10, 11]. Two isoforms of 11β-hydroxysteroid dehydrogenase (11βHSD) modify intracellular GC concentrations independently of circulating levels: 11βHSD type 1 (11βHSD1) that increases intracellular GC concentrations by converting inactive cortisone to active cortisol and 11βHSD type 2 (11βHSD2) that catalyzes the conversion of active GCs to their inactive metabolites [10].

Endogenous GCs at physiological levels are essential for normal bone development and exert anabolic effects on the bone (Hartmann); in fact adrenalectomy in female rats causes significant loss of metaphyseal trabecular bone mass [12], and patients with Addison's disease are at a higher risk of hip fractures, independently of sex and age and association with other autoimmune diseases, indicating impaired bone quality [13].

Studies in mice models with cell-specific disruption of GC signaling or cell-specific deletion of the glucocorticoid receptor (GR) demonstrate that physiological levels of endogenous GCs are required to preserve full bone integrity under physiological conditions [14]. Targeted inactivation of GC signaling in transgenic mice overexpressing the 11βHSD2 (Col2.3–11βHSD2 transgenic mice) in osteoblasts (OBs) and osteocytes (OCs) resulted in reduced femoral cortical and vertebral trabecular bone mass and decreased mechanical bone strength [15–17]. In adult mice the disruption of the GR expression in OBs resulted in a lower bone mass and trabecular number (Rauch). Moreover, cultured OBs derived from GR-deficient mice show reduced proliferation and a diminished differentiation capacity with reduced expression of alkaline phosphatase (ALP), runt-related transcription factor 2 (Runx2), collagen type 1 (Col1a1), and osteocalcin (Bglap2) [18].

Wnt signaling by OBs is essential for mesenchymal progenitor cells to differentiate away from a default adipogenic into an osteoblastic lineage, and this process is GC-dependent. Dominant adipogenesis and reduced osteoblastogenesis were observed in calvarial cell cultures from Col2.3–11βHSD2 transgenic mice. This phenotypic shift was associated with a reduction in Wnt10b and Wnt7b mRNA and β-catenin protein levels and with an increase in the expression of secreted frizzled-related protein 1 (sFRP1), a Wnt inhibitor, compared with wild-type (WT) cultures [18]. Therefore, GCs stimulate differentiated OBs to produce Wnt, which activate the canonical Wnt-signaling cascade in mesenchymal progenitor cells [19]. However, these osteoblastogenesis-promoting actions of GCs appear to be independent of GR dimerization (Rauch). The effects of GCs are concentration-dependent; in fact Wnt signaling seems to be augmented by physiological but not by pharmacological GC concentrations [19, 20]. Indeed, dexamethasone inhibits OBs only at pharmacological levels (10–7, 10–6 M), whereas concentrations in the physiological range (10–8 M) are stimulatory [20]. In addition, GC-induced canonical Wnt signaling in OBs also affects the surrounding chondrocytes by augmenting the expression of matrix metalloproteinase 14, an enzyme implemented in the breakdown of the extracellular matrix during tissue development and remodeling [21].

Endogenous GC levels increase by 20–50% with age in humans [22–25] and in mice [26] because of blunting of the GC feedback inhibition of ACTH [27] as well as increased bone expression of 11β-HSD1 [22, 26]. Hence, in contrast to the anabolic effects of GCs seen in young and adult mice, endogenous GCs increase skeletal fragility in old mice [26]. This effect is abrogated in transgenic mice with impaired GC signaling in OBs [26]. Furthermore, cortisol concentration and the rate of bone loss are inversely related in a healthy aging population even after adjustments for possible interfering factors [25, 28].

Another potential element modifying the response of the bone to GCs is the sensitivity of GR to GCs. Some variants of GR have been described, and in particular, the N363S sequence variant and the BclI restriction site polymorphism of the GR gene have been associated with an increased sensitivity to GCs [29, 30].

Finally, GCs were shown to increase aromatase expression in human OBs in vitro, and current evidence suggests that extragonadal estrogens play an important role in bone metabolism [31, 32].

7.4 Androgens and Bone Physiology

Androgens play a role in bone physiology throughout life in both men and women, particularly at puberty and during adult life. The skeletal actions of androgens may be mediated directly via the androgen receptor or indirectly via the estrogen receptor after aromatization to estrogens [2].

First, androgen receptors are expressed in human epiphyseal chondrocytes and growth plate cartilage cells [33]. By their action on these cells, it is likely that androgens directly stimulate longitudinal bone growth during puberty and the subsequent epiphyseal growth plate closure; however androgens also influence pubertal bone growth indirectly by aromatization to estrogen [34] and by modulation of pituitary growth hormone secretion [35]. Second, androgen receptors are expressed in human osteoblasts [1]. Cortical human osteoblasts express higher androgen receptor mRNA levels and more androgen binding sites per cell than trabecular human osteoblasts of the same skeletal site [36], thus suggesting a prevalent effect of androgens on cortical compartment. Moreover, some studies showed that the expression of androgen receptors in osteoblasts is upregulated by androgens themselves [37]. Finally, androgen receptors have not been detected in human osteoclasts in vivo yet; therefore androgen effects on osteoclastogenesis and bone resorption are supposed to be carried out indirectly via osteoblasts and osteocytes, although several in vitro studies showed that androgens are able to directly induce osteoclast apoptosis [2].

The presence of androgen receptors on human osteoblasts [33] and the reduced bone mineral density (BMD) in individuals with complete androgen insensitivity syndrome [38] are demonstrative of direct effects of androgens on bone tissue. At the same time, however, men with inactivating mutations of estrogen receptor or enzyme aromatase genes have a severe skeletal involvement [39], thus implying that both androgens and estrogens, but mainly the second ones, are necessary for bone homeostasis.

The main androgens produced by the adrenal glands are dehydroepiandrosterone (DHEA) and androstenedione. Their production follows a specific pattern throughout life: it is low in childhood, then raises significantly during adrenarche, being still high in early adulthood, but finally declines deeply with age, with a decrease up to 40–70% at the age of 80 in comparison to the young adult. Androgen receptors bind testosterone and its more biologically active form, dihydrotestosterone, the latter with stronger affinity. Therefore, since at the moment there is no evidence that DHEA and androstenedione have specific receptors in the periphery, it is extremely likely that adrenal androgens act through their metabolites which bind the androgen or the estrogen receptor [1].

The contribution of adrenal glands to androgen effects on bone health can be considered variable according to sex and age. In male adults the role of adrenal androgens is likely very limited due to the gonadal origin of the majority of circulating androgens, whereas in female adults it is expected to be more important since that adrenal androgens are usually more abundant than the ovarian ones [1]. However, studies which explored the correlation between levels of adrenal androgens and BMD found no or only weak associations [40, 41], thus suggesting that in adults the role of these androgens in bone physiology is negligible.

A greater impact of adrenal androgens can be hypothesized during the physiological process of adrenarche before the beginning of the gonadal production of androgens. A prospective study of Remer and colleagues investigated the association between adrenal androgen metabolite excretion rates before the onset of puberty and several parameters of skeletal modeling in late puberty. They found that androstenediol, a direct metabolite of DHEA, was an early predictor of diaphyseal bone strength at the proximal radius measured by peripheral quantitative computed tomography in late puberty [42]. Although other factors, such as sex steroids in puberty and genetics, likely influence more than androstenediol skeletal geometry, a contribution of adrenal androgens to the bone accretion during growth may hence be asserted.

Finally, the decrease of adrenal androgens with aging has been supposed to be responsible of some age-related changes, included the reduced BMD. However, studies which investigated in the elderly the effect on bone health of restoring serum levels of DHEA back to those of young adults have given inconsistent results, suggesting that the skeletal impact of DHEA treatment is very limited [1].

7.5 Subclinical Hypercortisolism and the Bone

Subclinical hypercortisolism (SH) is a condition of cortisol excess in the absence of its classical signs and symptoms (i.e., striae rubrae, facial plethora, proximal myopathy, easy bruising) and may be of both exogenous (GCs, i.e., <5 mg/die prednisone equivalents) and endogenous origin [43]. The prevalence of SH, which in majority of cases is due to the presence of adrenal incidentaloma (AI; prevalence 4–7%) [44], is probably higher than previously suspected [43]. Less frequently, SH is due to a slight adrenocorticotropic hormone (ACTH) excess [45]. Nowadays SH prevalence is estimated between 0.2% and 2.0% [43]. SH has been suggested to be detrimental for the skeletal health, leading to an increased risk of vertebral fractures, only partially explained by bone mineral density (BMD) reduction and possibly associated with a decreased bone quality [46].

In SH an uncoupling between bone apposition and resorption is present, with the osteoblastic activity being predominantly affected, as happens in the overt form of hypercortisolism [1]. Most studies found a reduction of trabecular BMD; on the contrary, data regarding cortical bone are more discordant [43, 47, 48].

In SH, the prevalence of vertebral fractures varies between 46.3% and 82.4% [43, 47–51]. In addition, up to 48% of patients with AI and SH may experience a new asymptomatic vertebral fracture over time [49, 51], in spite of an almost stable BMD. On the other hand, patients surgically treated had a strong reduction of the probability of a new vertebral fracture [50].

The increased fracture risk in SH seems to be independent of gender and gonadal status [47]. Apparently surprising, the degree of fracture risk in SH is similar to that reported in overt cortisol excess [46]. However, SH is asymptomatic, and, therefore, at diagnosis, the duration of the hypercortisolism has been probably longer than that in patients with a clinically overt cortisol excess. In SH the degree of BMD reduction is scarcely predictive of the fracture risk. Indeed, up to 40% of vertebral fractures may be present in spite of a normal or only slightly reduced BMD [51], and the occurrence of a new vertebral fracture is independent of spinal BMD, age, and gender [49].

The reduced reliability of BMD in predicting the fracture risk in SH suggests, as in patients with overt cortisol excess [52], a reduction of bone quality (i.e., bone microarchitecture). Recently, a reduction of bone quality in SH has been indirectly evaluated using the trabecular bone score (TBS) and suggests a possible future role of TBS in predicting new vertebral fracture [48].

On the other hand, since SH is, by definition, asymptomatic, some authors investigated the prevalence of SH in patients with apparent primary osteoporosis.

Literature data suggest that the 1–10% of patients with apparently primary osteoporosis have in fact a SH, with the different inclusion criteria of the different studies accounting for the differences in the prevalence among studies [3, 53]. As for the different forms of secondary osteoporosis, SH should be suspected in subjects with BMD lower than expected for age and/or if BMD declines more rapidly than expected and/or if it fails to respond to appropriate therapy and/or in the presence of fragility fractures in eugonadal persons [54]. In these patients SH should be ruled out evaluating cortisol levels, between 8:00 and 9:00 a.m., after taking 1 mg dexamethasone at 11:00 p.m. of the previous day. The SH presence should be suspected in presence of cortisol level above 1.8–2.0 μg/dL (50–55 nmol/L) and should be confirmed by the commonly used additional second-line tests [3, 43]. The recovery from SH is necessary to favor the normalization of bone turnover with recovery of bone mass and reduction of fracture risk, but in some patients the fracture risk could not be normalized, and specific antiosteoporotic drugs should be given. Up to now, there are no specific guidelines for this disease, and data of literature do not allow performing an evidence-based approach, but a single-case evaluation is often needed. Vitamin D and calcium should be always given, while in this specific clinical context, other studies are needed to clarify role, effectiveness, and safety of antiresorptive and anabolic drugs [55].

7.6 Overt Hypercortisolism and the Bone

Cushing's syndrome (CS) is characterized by inappropriately high levels of cortisol produced by the adrenal glands due to a pituitary corticotroph tumor or ectopic ACTH production from tumor outside the pituitary or autonomous adrenal overproduction [56].

The prolonged exposure to this endogenous hypercortisolism exerts harmful effects to the bone, particularly inducing osteoporosis and increasing the incidence of low-energy fractures [57].

GC-induced osteoporosis (GIO) is the commonest cause of secondary osteoporosis. The prevalence of osteopenia and osteoporosis among patients with CS is usually estimated between 60 and 80% and 30 and 65%, respectively [58–60]. The increased incidence of fractures occurs within 2–3 years before diagnosis and treatment [61, 62] suggesting that prompt recognition and management of Cushing's syndrome are essential to reduce skeletal complications. Fractures occur most commonly at the thoracic and lumbar vertebrae, hip, ribs, and pelvis, not infrequently developing spontaneously or after low-energy trauma.

Male patients have a higher prevalence of osteoporosis (47% vs 32%) and vertebral fractures (52% vs 18%) [63] than female patients, suggesting that testosterone deficiency could negatively affect bone status in Cushing's syndrome. Most studies [64, 65], but not all [66], found that amenorrheic and eumenorrheic women with Cushing's syndrome have similar BMD values and fracture prevalence, suggesting that the harmful effects of GCs overcome estrogenic bone protection in Cushing's syndrome.

The pathogenesis of bone loss and fragility is multifactorial and depends on effects of GCs on both bone mineral density (BMD) and bone architecture, geometry, and rate of bone remodeling units (BRU). Moreover, the pathogenesis of GIO involves both skeletal and extraskeletal events.

Prolonged hypercortisolism induces an imbalance between bone formation and bone reabsorption, characterized by a rapid early phase of BMD reduction due to excessive bone resorption, which is followed later on by a slower phase of impaired bone formation [67].

Besides their direct effect on BRU, GCs reduce calcium absorption from the gastrointestinal tract and inhibit renal tubular calcium reabsorption [67]. GCs also influence the production and action of other hormones that regulate bone and calcium metabolism such as gonadotropins, adrenal androgens, estrogens, GH-IGF1 axis, and insulin [64, 68, 69].

In patients with CS, a significant reduction of lumbar spine BMD develops before involvement of the peripheral skeleton [66] because of a rapid loss of the trabecular bone [58]. The catabolic effects of GCs on the muscle also contribute to fracture risk due to an increased incidence of falls secondary to muscle weakness [67].

At tissue level, GCs inhibit osteoblast differentiation and function and promote osteoblast and osteocyte apoptosis, resulting in decreased bone formation and prolonged osteoclast lifespan.

The reduction of type I collagen synthesis by differentiated osteoblasts reduces the bone matrix available for mineralization [52].

Osteocytes are mechanosensors which function like a network transmitting information to the bone surface. Osteocyte apoptosis and the consequent disruption of the osteocyte canalicular network may result in a failure of signals that normally stimulate the replacement of the damaged bone [70] and in reducing bone surface turnover in response to mechanical forces [52]. Thus, a substantial effect of GCs on osteocytes might account for a disproportionate loss of bone strength in relation to reduction of bone mass.

At molecular level, glucocorticoid receptors and 11βHSD1 are present both in osteoblasts and in osteoclasts [71, 72]. Glucocorticoid-responsive elements are present in the promoter region of osteocalcin [73], a specific product of osteoblasts. GCs increase the expression of receptor activator of nuclear factor-κB ligand (RANKL), while the expression of osteoprotegerin (OPG) is decreased in osteoblasts [58], thus promoting increased osteoclastic activity [52, 74]. However, measurement of circulating RANKL and OPG concentrations does not reflect their bone tissue expression, with OPG levels increased in patients with chronic hypercortisolism [75] and persisting even after successful surgical treatment of CS [76]; the source of increased OPG level in patients with CS is probably the vascular endothelium [77].

Differential sensitivity of bone cells to glucocorticoid action has been described (see below) [52, 74].

In GIO fractures frequently occur in patients with normal or only slightly decreased BMD, due to a qualitative deterioration of bone tissue. Contrary to bone mineral content and density, bone quality remains poorly defined and relates to factors such as bone architecture and microarchitecture, bone turnover, degree of mineralization, and cellularity [78].

There are only few studies using DXA to evaluate the interference of hypogonadism on BMD of patients with CS, and the results are not concordant. Tauchmanovà et al. [5] found no differences in lumbar BMD and prevalence of vertebral fractures between amenorrheic and eumenorrheic women with overt endogenous CS, concluding that the deleterious effects of hypercortisolism on the spine cannot be counterbalanced by preserved menstrual cycles [64, 65]. In contrast, Karavitaki et al. [66] documented reduced forearm BMD in 16 postmenopausal but not in 13 premenopausal women with CS.

Sex steroids play a crucial role in maintaining the bone density and microstructure, particularly in trabecular bone. The deleterious effects of hypogonadism on the bone microstructure have been described in postmenopausal women, and they have been evaluated by high-resolution peripheral quantitative computed tomography (HR-pQCT) that allows the in vivo assessment of bone microarchitecture and volumetric BMD at the distal radius and tibia [79–81].

Two new noninvasive techniques have been recently introduced as surrogate marker of bone microarchitecture: (1) the spinal deformity index, an index measuring the number and the severity of vertebral fractures [82], and (2) the TBS, a texture parameter that evaluates pixel gray-level variations in two-dimensional images of the lumbar spine DEXA scan and correlates closely with the three-dimensional microarchitecture of the vertebrae [47].

Besides low bone mass and fractures, growth arrest is a specific feature of pediatric CS [83]. Bone age is delayed compared with the chronological age (mean delay 1.6 years) [84]. With ongoing remission, complete normalization of BMD occurred 3–4.5 years following successful surgical intervention [85, 86], although final height might be compromised by growth hormone deficiency if not actively treated [83, 84, 86].

The surgical treatment improved BMD in most studies [59, 87–92]. The studies highlight the potential reversibility of bone damage with cure of hypercortisolism, although the time to complete bone recovery is relatively long and variable. A greater increase in BMD after remission has been reported in male than in female patients [92]. Notably, the duration of glucocorticoid replacement was negatively correlated with lumbar spine BMD in women with Cushing's syndrome in long-term surgical remission [93], suggesting that several factors, including gender and glucocorticoid over-replacement, might affect the time to bone recovery. Few data regarding the effects of pharmacological treatment on bone disease are available [94–96].

Recommendations for the treatment of osteoporosis induced by exogenous hypercortisolism can be only partly translated to patients with endogenous Cushing's syndrome; therefore, specific guidelines for these patients are needed. Stratification of patients into two treatment subgroups—according to the cause of Cushing's syndrome, gonadal status, age, presence of fractures, and expected time for hypercortisolism resolution—has recently been suggested [55]. These subgroups are patients with less severe bone damage, needing only supplementation with calcium and vitamin D (e.g., those not presenting with prevalent fractures, premenopausal women, and men younger than 50 years), and patients with more severe bone damage requiring more aggressive treatment such as bone active therapy with teriparatide, denosumab, and bisphosphonates (e.g., those with severe hypercortisolism and prevalent hip or vertebral fractures and those older than 70 years) [55].

7.7 Glucocorticoid Sensitivity and the Bone

The effects of GCs in different subjects are variable in relation to their individual sensitivity.

The polymorphisms of the GR and gene and the 11βHSD shuttle are thought to play an important role in this variability. In particular some variants of the GR gene have been described, the N363S and BclI polymorphism associated with a relative increased sensitivity to GCs and the ER22/23EK GR polymorphism associated with a reduced sensitivity to GCs [97]. The role of this polymorphism in the development of glucocorticoid-related osteoporosis has become object of several studies. In the general population, BclI homozygous subjects showed lower trochanteric BMD, and heterozygous carriers of N363S polymorphism showed a decreased BMD at the lumbar spine [28, 29]. In postmenopausal diabetic patients, the N363S polymorphism was associated to the presence of vertebral fractures [98]. Another study carried on 800 Chinese patients found that both a single nucleotide polymorphism (SNP rs1866388) of GR and haplotype association (involving rs1866388 and rs2918419) are associated with extreme age-adjusted hip BMD *z*-score [99]. The possible role of these polymorphisms in influencing the bone consequences of hypercortisolism has been also evaluated. In patients with endogenous Cushing's syndrome, the results obtained have been conflicting. In a previous study, patients carrying the BclI polymorphism of the GR showed reduced femoral BMD as compared with patients carrying the wild-type GR [98], but in a subsequent study, this association was absent [100]. In both these studies, the N363S, ER22/23EK, and A3669G polymorphisms were not found to be related to BMD values. It is likely that in the presence of high cortisol levels, as in most patients with Cushing's syndrome, the role of the GR polymorphisms on glucocorticoid sensitivity may be limited. At variance in patients with a subtle cortisol excess as is the case of AI with SH, the impact of the GR polymorphism in modulating the skeletal sensitivity to the glucocorticoid excess could be greater. However, in AI patients, the few available data on this issue are not conclusive. In a previous study, the contemporary presence of homozygous BclI and heterozygous N363S GR polymorphism was associated with fragility vertebral fracture, but not with BMD levels [101]. However, in a further study, the association between the GR polymorphism and the BMD in AI patients was absent, but the small sample size and the lack of data about the presence of vertebral fractures could have influenced the results [102].

The 11βHSD1 activity, the other possible determinant of the individual bone sensitivity to GCs, seems to be important for the bone health in the conditions of both normal and increased cortisol levels [103]. Indeed, the 11βHSD1 enzyme, present in adult bone tissue and expressed primarily in osteoblast, regulates tissue levels of GCs independently of circulating cortisol levels [104]. The 11-HSD2 is not found in adult bone. The 11βHSD1 activity increase with age at the osteoblast level [27]. Therefore, the individual bone sensitivity to therapeutic GCs and age-related changes in bone are thought to be associated to the local enzyme activity [27, 105]. The expression of 11βHSD1 is mainly regulated by proinflammatory cytokines and GCs themselves [104]. In vitro studies have shown that the 11-HSD1 activity can be selectively inhibited enhancing osteoblastogenesis and inhibiting osteoclastogenesis [106] and that this inhibition seems to protect osteoblasts against glucocorticoid-induced damage [107]. In keeping with these data, some studies have evaluated the relation between the 11βHSD1 gene polymorphism and bone osteoporosis. A study conducted in Korean postmenopausal osteoporotic women without clinically apparent hypercortisolemia found that the presence of some 11-HSD1 polymorphism (+16374C > T and +27447G > C9) is associated with higher BMD levels and also with a reduced fracture risk [108]. Another polymorphic variant of the 11-HSD1 gene, the rs4844880 polymorphism responsible for a reduced expression of the enzyme, has been shown to be associated with higher BMD [109]. Moreover the SNP rs11811440 in intron 5 of the 11-HSD1 gene was positively associated with the spinal BMD and negatively associated with post-dexamethasone cortisol levels [8]. Few data are available about the role of the 11βHSD1 in patients with cortisol excess. Szappanos and coauthors showed that the 83,557insA variant of the 11-HSD1 gene was associated with serum osteocalcin levels in patients with endogenous Cushing's syndrome [110].

7.8 Congenital Adrenal Hyperplasia and the Bone

Congenital adrenal hyperplasia (CAH) is a disorder of the adrenal cortex characterized by impaired cortisol synthesis, with or without aldosterone deficiency, and adrenal androgen excess, due to an enzymatic defect in adrenal steroidogenesis. The most common form of CAH is caused by mutations in the gene encoding the adrenal steroid 21-hydroxylase enzyme. This enzymatic defect leads to the overproduction in the adrenal glands of precursors of cortisol and aldosterone which are diverted to androgen synthesis. Therefore, affected subjects are exposed to high levels of androgens of adrenal origin even from the intrauterine life. In females this high exposition results in variable degrees of virilization [111]. During postnatal life in both sexes, high levels of adrenal androgens imply accelerated longitudinal bone growth and premature epiphyseal growth plate closure, frequently resulting in a reduced final height. However the treatment of CAH is based on glucocorticoid (GC) replacement therapy, which is aimed to remedy cortisol deficiency and limit adrenal androgen synthesis by reducing pituitary ACTH secretion; therefore, a contribution of GC therapy on the reduced final stature must be taken into account [112].

Studies which explored bone health of patients affected with CAH have given conflicting results. Some studies found no differences in terms of BMD between patients with CAH and healthy subjects, especially in children and adolescents [11], whereas others showed a low BMD, especially when adult subjects were considered [113–116]. A conserved BMD despite chronic GC therapy could be explained by the anabolic effect of androgens which counteract the deleterious effect of GC on bone. However, it must be also considered that in children affected with CAH, the advancement of bone age induced by androgens could lead to an overestimation of BMD. In keeping with this, Garcia Alves Junior and colleagues found a reduced BMD in pediatric patients with CAH when bone age was taken into account rather than chronological age [117]. From an opposite point of view, the reduced stature commonly observed in CAH could bring to an underestimation of BMD, particularly at the spine, since that the areal BMD measured by DXA, which integrates cortical and trabecular bone mass divided by the two-dimensional projected skeletal area, is strictly influenced by bone size. After BMD correction for height, some authors found that only femoral neck BMD but not spine BMD resulted lower in adult patients affected with CAH [113].

In an attempt to understand the effect of the excess of adrenal androgens on the bone, an additional confounding factor comes from the GC replacement therapy which could vary in terms of type and dose of GCs used. Several studies found a negative correlation between BMD and cumulative doses of GCs [118], thus implying that the optimization of GC replacement therapy by using the lowest dose necessary is one of the goal of the treatment of CAH to preserve bone health. No correlations were generally found between androgen levels and BMD, probably because hormonal measurement from a single sample does not reflect the trend of the pathology across time.

Few studies explored the risk of fracture of patients affected with CAH. Falhammar and coworkers reported a significantly increased overall prevalence of fractures in adult women with CAH [114], whereas Raizada and colleagues did not find any differences in fracture frequency in a small sample of young adult females [115], but the younger age and the lower number of recruited patients could have contributed to this result. One study in adult males with CAH showed no differences in the prevalence of fractures between patients and healthy subjects [116]. Studies investigating prospectively the risk of fracture on large samples of patients with CAH are lacking and thus would be required in order to clarify the real skeletal effects of adrenal androgen excess and GC replacement therapy on these patients.

7.9 Aldosterone and the Bone

The renin-angiotensin system (RAS) is an endocrine system that governs body fluid and electrolyte balance and blood pressure, and it is also involved in bone metabolism.

In the classic endocrine RAS, renin produced by the juxtaglomerular apparatus of the kidney and secreted into the circulation cleaves angiotensinogen to the inactive decapeptide angiotensin I (Ang I), which is cleaved by angiotensin converting enzyme (ACE) to generate angiotensin II (Ang II).

Components of the RAS are expressed in the human bone cell [119] and can activate a local RAS response that leads to increased bone turnover and decreased BMD [120]. Several reports have been published on the effects of Ang II on bone cell function in vitro, including the inhibition of osteoblastic differentiation and mineralization [121], the stimulation of proliferation and collagen synthesis in osteoblasts [122], and the stimulation of osteoclastic bone resorption [119].

The majority of the studies on the effects of ACE inhibitors or Ang II type 1 receptor blockers on bone, including those in humans [123–126] and animal models [127–129], suggest that pharmacological inhibition of the RAS pathway can lead to decreased fracture risk and increased bone mass.

Some authors found that renin activity (PRA) was directly associated with bone mineral density (BMD) in highly selected samples of patients [130, 131]. Recently, Kuipers et al. [132] show that circulating RAS indexes, e.g., elevated PRA and low aldosterone to renin ratio (ARR), are associated with high BMD and low bone turnover independent of the confounding effect of hypertension. Association of PRA with BMD seems to be specific for the trabecular bone, and it has also been suggested in an animal model of osteoporosis [133, 134]. Both PRA and the relative levels of ARR could be important for skeletal health, although aldosterone levels alone seem not to be a significant factor [132]. In addition, there is evidence that there are shared genetic pathways underlying these associations [132].

Primary aldosteronism (PA), characterized by aldosterone excess, and renin and Ang II suppression, has probably another mechanism of action to impair bone health. In an animal model, as well as in humans, aldosterone excess was associated with an increased urinary and fecal loss of Ca++ and Mg++, in turn inducing hypocalcemia, hypomagnesemia, and secondary hyperparathyroidism [135–140], which was rescued by adrenalectomy or treatment with a mineralocorticoid receptor antagonist (MRA) [138, 139]. These alterations seem to lead to low bone mass and fragility fractures, whereas surgery or MRA therapy improved bone mass [138, 139]. Moreover, the possible relation between PA and bone was suggested by data coming from genome wide association between indexes of bone strength and some genes involved in aldosterone pathways [141]. In this regard it should be mentioned that the expression of mineralocorticoid receptor on bone cells [142, 143] could actually suggest a still unknown direct effect of mineralocorticoids on the skeletal tissue. Indeed, in an animal model, Fumoto et al. showed that pharmacological inhibition of mineralocorticoid function with eplerenone resulted in increased bone mass, with stimulation of bone formation and suppression of resorption [143]. The treatment with eplerenone as well as the specific deletion of mineralocorticoid receptor in osteocytes improved the cortical bone thinning caused by slow-release prednisolone pellets [143].

Finally, a recent study shows that mineralocorticoids may contribute to the regulation of FGF 23 transcription and release in vivo [144]. Many diseases, all complicated by low bone mass and high prevalence of fracture, such as chronic kidney disease, heart failure, diabetic nephropathy, and hepatic failure, are characterized by hyperaldosteronism [145–151], and the high FGF 23 plasma concentration that has been found in these diseases [152–157] could at least in part be secondary to the hyperaldosteronism. This association is intriguing, considering that PA is also associated with low phosphorus levels [156].

Conclusions

The hormones produced by the cortical adrenal gland contribute to the skeletal health during the growth and adult life. The effect of cortisol is modulated by polymorphic variants of GR gene that affect the sensitivity of bone tissue and by 11BHSD isoforms that regulates the final intracellular GCs concentration. In physiological concentrations, GCs stimulate osteoclastogenesis activating the canonical Wnt signaling, but in aged people, GCs increase till 50%, thus increasing skeletal fragility. Adrenal androgens affect the bone mainly at the beginning of puberty after their transformation in testosterone and estrogen.

Both subclinical and overt hypercortisolism are characterized by a high prevalence of vertebral fractures due mainly to worsening of bone quality, independent from the reduction of BMD. Moreover, the catabolic effect of GCs on skeletal muscles should be taken into account for estimating the risk of fractures in such patients. The prevalence of subclinical hypercortisolism is higher than previously hypothesized (i.e., up to 2% of general population), and consequently such a condition should be excluded in cases of unexpected diagnosis of osteoporosis and/or fractures.

Mineralocorticoid receptors have been identified in bone cells, and the excess of mineralocorticoids as in primary aldosteronism has been associated with osteoporosis and fractures.

Bone cells express receptors for catecholamines and are a target for the sympathetic nervous system, but a role of epinephrine delivered by the adrenal medulla on the bone has not been hypothesized nor the hypersecretion in pheochromocytoma or the lack of catecholamines after bilateral adrenalectomy seems to have an effect on the skeleton [1].

References

1. Hardy R, Cooper MS. Adrenal gland and bone. Arch Biochem Biophys. 2010;503:137–45.
2. Clarke BL, Khosla S. Androgens and bone. Steroids. 2009;74:296–305.
3. Chiodini I, Eller Vainicher C, Morelli V, Palmieri S, Cairoli E, Salcuni AS, Copetti M, Scillitani A. Mechanisms in endocrinology: endogenous subclinical hypercortisolism and bone: a clinical review. Eur J Endocrinol. 2016;175(6):R265–82.
4. Osella G, Ventura M, Ardito A, Allasino B, Termine A, Saba L, Vitetta R, Terzolo M, Angeli A. Cortisol secretion, bone health, and bone loss: a cross-sectional and prospective study in normal non-osteoporotic women in the early postmenopausal period. Eur J Endocrinol. 2012;166:855–60.
5. Cetin A, Gökçe-Kutsal Y, Celiker R. Predictors of bone mineral density in healthy males. Rheumatol Int. 2001;21:85–8.
6. Zhukouskaya VV, Eller-Vainicher C, Gaudio A, Cairoli E, Ulivieri FM, Palmieri S, Morelli V, Orsi E, Masserini B, Barbieri AM, Polledri E, Fustinoni S, Spada A, Fiore CE, Chiodini I.

In postmenopausal female subjects with type 2 diabetes mellitus, vertebral fractures are independently associated with cortisol secretion and sensitivity. J Clin Endocrinol Metab. 2015;100:1417–25.

7. Cain DW, Cidlowski JA. Specificity and sensitivity of glucocorticoid signaling in health and disease. Best Pract Res Clin Endocrinol Metab. 2015;29:545–56.
8. Siggelkow H, Etmanski M, Bozkurt S, Groβ P, Koepp R, Brockmöller J, Tzvetkov MV. Genetic polymorphisms in 11β-hydroxysteroid dehydrogenase type 1 correlate with the postdexamethasone cortisol levels and bone mineral density in patients evaluated for osteoporosis. J Clin Endocrinol Metab. 2014;99:293–302.
9. Larsen PR, et al. The adrenal cortex (chap. 14, adrenal cortex and endocrine hypertension by Paul M. Stewart). In: William textbook of endocrinology. 10th ed. New York: Elsevier; 2002. p. 492–506.
10. Draper N, Stewart PM. 11beta-hydroxysteroid dehydrogenase and the pre-receptor regulation of corticosteroid hormone action. J Endocrinol. 2005;186(2):251–71.
11. Durbridge TC, Morris HA, Parsons AM, Parkinson IH, Moore RJ, Porter S, Need AG, Nordin BE, Vernon-Roberts B. Progressive cancellous bone loss in rats after adrenalectomy and oophorectomy. Calcif Tissue Int. 1990;47(6):383–7.
12. Björnsdottir S, Sääf M, Bensing S, Kämpe O, Michaëlsson K, Ludvigsson JF. Risk of hip fracture in Addison's disease: a population-based cohort study. J Intern Med. 2011;270(2):187–95.
13. Hartmann K, Koenen M, Schauer S, Wittig-Blaich S, Ahmad M, Baschant U, Tuckermann JP. Molecular actions of glucocorticoids in cartilage and bone during health, disease, and steroid therapy. Physiol Rev. 2016;96(2):409–47.
14. Kalak R, Zhou H, Street J, Day RE, Modzelewski JR, Spies CM, Liu PY, Li G, Dunstan CR, Seibel MJ. Endogenous glucocorticoid signaling in osteoblasts is necessary to maintain normal bone structure in mice. Bone. 2009;45(1):61–7.
15. Sher LB, Woitge HW, Adams DJ, Gronowicz GA, Krozowski Z, Harrison JR, Kream BE. Transgenic expression of 11beta-hydroxysteroid dehydrogenase type 2 in osteoblasts reveals an anabolic role for endogenous glucocorticoids in bone. Endocrinology. 2004;145(2):922–9.
16. Sher LB, Harrison JR, Adams DJ, Kream BE. Impaired cortical bone acquisition and osteoblast differentiation in mice with osteoblast-targeted disruption of glucocorticoid signaling. Calcif Tissue Int. 2006;79(2):118–25.
17. Rauch A, Seitz S, Baschant U, Schilling AF, Illing A, Stride B, Kirilov M, Mandic V, Takacz A, Schmidt-Ullrich R, Ostermay S, Schinke T, Spanbroek R, Zaiss MM, Angel PE, Lerner UH, David JP, Reichardt HM, Amling M, Schütz G, Tuckermann JP. Glucocorticoids suppress bone formation by attenuating osteoblast differentiation via the monomeric glucocorticoid receptor. Cell Metab. 2010;11(6):517–31.
18. Zhou H, Mak W, Zheng Y, Dunstan CR, Seibel MJ. Osteoblasts directly control lineage commitment of mesenchymal progenitor cells through Wnt signaling. J Biol Chem. 2008;283(4):1936–45.
19. Leclerc N, Luppen CA, Ho VV, Nagpal S, Hacia JG, Smith E, Frenkel B. Gene expression profiling of glucocorticoid-inhibited osteoblasts. J Mol Endocrinol. 2004;33(1):175–93.
20. Zhou H, Mak W, Kalak R, Street J, Fong-Yee C, Zheng Y, Dunstan CR, Seibel MJ. Glucocorticoid-dependent Wnt signaling by mature osteoblasts is a key regulator of cranial skeletal development in mice. Development. 2009;136(3):427–36.
21. Van Cauter E, Leproult R, Kupfer DJ. Effects of gender and age on the levels and circadian rhythmicity of plasma cortisol. J Clin Endocrinol Metab. 1996;81:2468–73.
22. Dennison E, Hindmarsh P, Fall C, Kellingray S, Barker D, Phillips D, Cooper C. Profiles of endogenous circulating cortisol and bone mineral density in healthy elderly men. J Clin Endocrinol Metab. 1999;84:3058–63.
23. Purnell JQ, Brandon DD, Isabelle LM, Loriaux DL, Samuels MH. Association of 24-hour cortisol production rates, cortisol-binding globulin, and plasma-free cortisol levels with body composition, leptin levels, and aging in adult men and women. J Clin Endocrinol Metab. 2004;89:281–7.

24. Reynolds RM, Dennison EM, Walker BR, Syddall HE, Wood PJ, Andrew R, Phillips DI, Cooper C. Cortisol secretion and rate of bone loss in a population-based cohort of elderly men and women. Calcif Tissue Int. 2005;77:134–8.
25. Weinstein RS, Wan C, Liu Q, Wang Y, Almeida M, O'Brien CA, Thostenson J, Roberson PK, Boskey AL, Clemens TL, Manolagas SC. Endogenous glucocorticoids decrease skeletal angiogenesis, vascularity, hydration, and strength in aged mice. Aging Cell. 2010;9(2):147–61.
26. Wilkinson CW, Petrie EC, Murray SR, Colasurdo EA, Raskind MA, Peskind ER. Human glucocorticoid feedback inhibitions reduced in older individuals: evening study. J Clin Endocrinol Metab. 2001;86:545–50.
27. Cooper MS, Rabbitt EH, Goddard PE, Bartlett WA, Hewison M, Stewart PM. Osteoblastic 11beta-hydroxysteroid dehydrogenase type 1 activity increases with age and glucocorticoid exposure. J Bone Miner Res. 2002;17:979–86.
28. Huizenga NA, Koper JW, De Lange P, Pols HA, Stolk RP, Burger H, Grobbee DE, Brinkmann AO, De Jong FH, Lamberts SW. A polymorphism in the glucocorticoid receptor gene may be associated with and increased sensitivity to glucocorticoids in vivo. J Clin Endocrinol Metab. 1998;83(1):144–51.
29. van Schoor NM, Dennison E, Lips P, Uitterlinden AG, Cooper C. Serum fasting cortisol in relation to bone, and the role of genetic variations in the glucocorticoid receptor. Clin Endocrinol. 2007;67(6):871–8.
30. Enjuanes A, Garcia-Giralt N, Supervía A, Nogués X, Ruiz-Gaspà S, Bustamante M, Mellibovsky L, Grinberg D, Balcells S, Díez-Pérez A. Functional analysis of the I.3, I.6, pII and I.4 promoters of CYP19 (aromatase) gene in human osteoblasts and their role in vitamin D and dexamethasone stimulation. Eur J Endocrinol. 2005;153(6):981–8.
31. Watanabe M, Noda M, Nakajin S. Aromatase expression in a human osteoblastic cell line increases in response to prostaglandin E(2) in a dexamethasone-dependent fashion. Steroids. 2007;72(9–10):686–92.
32. Abu EO, Horner A, Kusec V, Triffitt JT, Compston JE. The localization of androgen receptors in human bone. J Clin Endocrinol Metab. 1997;82(10):3493–7.
33. Bord S, Horner A, Beavan S, Compston J. Estrogen receptors alpha and beta are differentially expressed in developing human bone. J Clin Endocrinol Metab. 2001;86(5):2309–14.
34. Kerrigan JR, Rogol AD. The impact of gonadal steroid hormone action on growth hormone secretion during childhood and adolescence. Endocr Rev. 1992;13(2):281–98.
35. Kasperk C, Helmboldt A, Börcsök I, Heuthe S, Cloos O, Niethard F, Ziegler R. Skeletal site-dependent expression of the androgen receptor in human osteoblastic cell populations. Calcif Tissue Int. 1997;61(6):464–73.
36. Wiren K, Keenan E, Zhang X, Ramsey B, Orwoll E. Homologous androgen receptor up-regulation in osteoblastic cells may be associated with enhanced functional androgen responsiveness. Endocrinology. 1999;140(7):3114–24.
37. Bertelloni S, Baroncelli GI, Federico G, Cappa M, Lala R, Saggese G. Altered bone mineral density in patients with complete androgen insensitivity syndrome. Horm Res. 1998; 50(6):309–14.
38. Jones ME, Boon WC, McInnes K, Maffei L, Carani C, Simpson ER. Recognizing rare disorders: aromatase deficiency. Nat Clin Pract Endocrinol Metab. 2007;3(5):414–21.
39. Barrett-Connor E, Kritz-Silverstein D, Edelstein SL. A prospective study of dehydroepiandrosterone sulfate (DHEAS) and bone mineral density in older men and women. Am J Epidemiol. 1993;137(2):201–6.
40. Greendale GA, Edelstein S, Barrett-Connor E. Endogenous sex steroids and bone mineral density in older women and men: the Rancho Bernardo Study. J Bone Miner Res. 1997;12(11): 1833–43.
41. Remer T, Manz F, Hartmann MF, Schoenau E, Wudy SA. Prepubertal healthy children's urinary androstenediol predicts diaphyseal bone strength in late puberty. J Clin Endocrinol Metab. 2009;94(2):575–8.

42. Chiodini I. Clinical review: diagnosis and treatment of subclinical hypercortisolism. J Clin Endocrinol Metab. 2011;96:1223–36.
43. Bovio S, Cataldi A, Reimondo G, Sperone P, Novello S, Berruti A, Borasio P, Fava C, Dogliotti L, Scagliotti GV, et al. Prevalence of adrenal incidentaloma in a contemporary computerized tomography series. J Endocrinol Investig. 2006;29:298–302.
44. Toini A, Dolci A, Ferrante E, Verrua E, Malchiodi E, Sala E, Lania AG, Chiodini I, Beck-Peccoz P, Arosio M, et al. Screening for ACTH-dependent hypercortisolism in patients affected with pituitary incidentaloma. Eur J Endocrinol. 2015;172:363–9.
45. Chiodini I, Torlontano M, Carnevale V, Trischitta V, Scillitani A. Skeletal involvement in adult patients with endogenous hypercortisolism. J Endocrinol Investig. 2008;31:267–76.
46. Chiodini I, Morelli V, Masserini B, Salcuni AS, Eller-Vainicher C, Viti R, Coletti F, Guglielmi G, Battista C, Carnevale V, et al. Bone mineral density, prevalence of vertebral fractures and bone quality in patients with adrenal incidentalomas with and without subclinical hypercortisolism: an Italian Multicenter Study. J Clin Endocrinol Metab. 2009;94:3207–14.
47. Eller-Vainicher C, Morelli V, Ulivieri FM, Palmieri S, Zhukouskaya VV, Cairoli E, Pino R, Naccarato A, Scillitani A, Beck-Peccoz P, et al. Bone quality, as measured by trabecular bone score in patients with adrenal incidentalomas with and without subclinical hypercortisolism. J Bone Miner Res. 2012;27:2223–30.
48. Morelli V, Eller-Vainicher C, Salcuni AS, Coletti F, Iorio L, Muscogiuri G, Della Casa S, Arosio M, Ambrosi B, Beck-Peccoz P, et al. Risk of new vertebral fractures in patients with adrenal incidentaloma with and without subclinical hypercortisolism: a multicenter longitudinal study. J Bone Miner Res. 2011;26:1816–21.
49. Salcuni AS, Morelli V, Eller-Vainicher C, Palmieri S, Cairoli E, Spada A, Scillitani A, Chiodini I. Adrenalectomy reduces the risk of vertebral fractures in patients with monolateral adrenal incidentalomas and subclinical hypercortisolism. Eur J Endocrinol. 2016;174:261–9.
50. Morelli V, Eller-Vainicher C, Palmieri S, Cairoli E, Salcuni AS, Scillitani A, Carnevale V, Corbetta S, Arosio M, Della Casa S, Muscogiuri G, Spada A, Chiodini I. Prediction of vertebral fractures in patients with monolateral adrenal incidentalomas. J Clin Endocrinol Metab. 2016;101(7):2768–75.
51. Chiodini I, Viti R, Coletti F, Guglielmi G, Battista C, Ermetici F, Morelli V, Salcuni A, Carnevale V, Urbano F, et al. Eugonadal male patients with adrenal incidentalomas and subclinical hypercortisolism have increased rate of vertebral fractures. Clin Endocrinol (Oxf). 2009;70:208–13.
52. Canalis E, Mazziotti G, Giustina A, Bilezikian JP. Glucocorticoid-induced osteoporosis: pathophysiology and therapy. Osteoporos Int. 2007;18:1319–28.
53. Chiodini I, Mascia ML, Muscarella S, Battista C, Minisola S, Arosio M, Santini SA, Guglielmi G, Carnevale V, Scillitani A. Subclinical hypercortisolism among outpatients referred for osteoporosis. Ann Intern Med. 2007;147:541–8.
54. Hofbauer LC, Hamann C, Ebeling PR. Approach to the patient with secondary osteoporosis. Eur J Endocrinol. 2010;162(6):1009–20.
55. Scillitani A, Mazziotti G, Di Somma C, Moretti S, Stigliano A, Pivonello R, Giustina A, Colao A, on behalf of ABC Group. Treatment of skeletal impairment in patients with endogenous hypercortisolism: when and how? Osteoporos Int. 2014;25:441–6.
56. Nieman LK, Biller BMK, Finding JW, Newell-Price J, Savage MO, Stewart PM, Montori VM. The diagnosis of Cushing's syndrome: an Endocrine Society clinical practice guideline. J Clin Endocrinol Metab. 2008;93:1526–40.
57. Chiodini I, Carnevale V, Torlontano M, Fusilli S, Guglielmi G, Pileri M, Modoni S, Di Giorgio A, Liuzzi A, Minisola S, Cammisa M, Trischitta V, Scillitani A. Alterations of bone turnover and bone mass at different skeletal sites due to pure glucocorticoid excess: study in eumenorrheic patients with Cushing's syndrome. J Clin Endocrinol Metab. 1998;83(6):1863–7.
58. Mancini T, Doga M, Mazziotti G, et al. Cushing's syndrome and bone. Pituitary. 2004;7:249–52.

59. Kawamata A, Iihara M, Okamoto T, et al. Bone mineral density before and after surgical cure of Cushing's syndrome due to adrenocortical adenoma: prospective study. World J Surg. 2008;32:890–6.
60. van der Eerden AW, den Heijer M, Oyen WJ, et al. Cushing's syndrome and bone mineral density: lowest Z scores in young patients. Neth J Med. 2007;65:137–41.
61. Dekkers OM, Horvath-Puho E, Jorgensen JO, et al. Multisystem morbidity and mortality in Cushing's syndrome: a cohort study. J Clin Endocrinol Metab. 2013;98:2277–84.
62. Vestergaard P, Lindholm J, Jorgensen JO, et al. Increased risk of osteoporotic fractures in patients with Cushing's syndrome. Eur J Endocrinol. 2002;146:51–6.
63. Valassi E, Santos A, Yaneva M, the ERCUSYN Study Group, et al. The European registry on Cushing's syndrome: 2-year experience. Baseline demographic and clinical characteristics. Eur J Endocrinol. 2011;165:383–92.
64. Tauchmanova L, Pivonello R, De Martino MC, et al. Effects of sex steroids on bone in women with subclinical or overt endogenous hypercortisolism. Eur J Endocrinol. 2007;157:359–66.
65. Tauchmanova L, Pivonello R, Di Somma C, et al. Bone demineralization and vertebral fractures in endogenous cortisol excess: role of disease etiology and gonadal status. J Clin Endocrinol Metab. 2006;91:1779–84.
66. Karavitaki N, Ioannidis G, Giannakopoulos F, Mavrokefalos P, Thalassinos N. Evaluation of bone mineral density of the peripheral skeleton in pre- and postmenopausal women with newly diagnosed endogenous Cushing's syndrome. Clin Endocrinol. 2004;60:264–70.
67. Mazziotti G, Angeli A, Bilezikian JP, Canalis E, Giustina A. Glucocorticoid-induced osteoporosis: an update. Trends Endocrinol Metab. 2006;17:144–9.
68. Pivonello R, De Leo M, Vitale P, et al. Pathophysiology of diabetes mellitus in Cushing's syndrome. Neuroendocrinology. 2010;92:77–81.
69. Thrailkill KM, Lumpkin CK Jr, Bunn RC, et al. Is insulin an anabolic agent in bone? Dissecting the diabetic bone for clues. Am J Phys Endocrinol Metab. 2005;289:E735–45.
70. Manolagas SC. Corticosteroids and fractures: a close encounter of the third cell kind. J Bone Miner Res. 2000;15:1001–5.
71. Abu EO, Horner A, Kusec V, et al. The localization of the functional glucocorticoid receptor alpha in human bone. J Clin Endocrinol Metab. 2000;85:883–9.
72. Cooper MS, Walker EA, Bland R, et al. Expression and functional consequences of 11beta-hydroxysteroid dehydrogenase activity in human bone. Bone. 2000;27:375–81.
73. Morrison NA, Shine J, Fragonas JC, et al. 1,25- dihydroxyvitamin D-responsive element and glucocorticoid repression in the osteocalcin gene. Science. 1989;246:1158–61.
74. Seibel MJ, Cooper MS, Zhou H. Glucocorticoid-induced osteoporosis: mechanisms, management, and future perspectives. Lancet Diabetes Endocrinol. 2013;1:59–70.
75. Yaneva M, Kalinov K, Zacharieva S. Mortality in Cushing's syndrome: data from 386 patients from a single tertiary referral center. Eur J Endocrinol. 2013;169:621–7.
76. Ntali G, Asimakopoulou A, Siamatras T, et al. Mortality in Cushing's syndrome: systematic analysis of a large series with prolonged follow-up. Eur J Endocrinol. 2013;169:715–23.
77. Hochberg Z, Pacak K, Chrousos GP. Endocrine withdrawal syndromes. Endocr Rev. 2003;24:523–38.
78. Brandi ML. Microarchitecture, the key to bone quality. Rheumatology (Oxford). 2009;48 (Suppl 4):iv3–8.
79. Nicks KM, Amin S, Atkinson EJ, et al. Relationship of age to bone microstructure independent of areal bone mineral density. J Bone Miner Res. 2012;27:637–44.
80. Nishiyama KK, Macdonald HM, Buie HR, et al. Postmenopausal women with osteopenia have higher cortical porosity and thinner cortices at the distal radius and tibia than women with normal aBMD: an in vivo HR-pQCT study. J Bone Miner Res. 2010;25:882–90.
81. Stein EM, Liu XS, Nickolas TL, et al. Abnormal microarchitecture and reduced stiffness at the radius and tibia in postmenopausal women with fractures. J Bone Miner Res. 2010; 25:2572–81.
82. Genant HK, Delmas PD, Chen P, et al. Severity of vertebral fracture reflects deterioration of bone microarchitecture. Osteoporos Int. 2007;18:69–76.

83. Scommegna S, Greening JP, Storr HL, et al. Bone mineral density at diagnosis and following successful treatment of pediatric Cushing's disease. J Endocrinol Investig. 2005;28:231–5.
84. Acharya SV, Gopal RA, Lila A, et al. Bone age and factors affecting skeletal maturation at diagnosis of paediatric Cushing's disease. Pituitary. 2010;13:355–60.
85. Lodish MB, Hsiao HP, Serbis A, et al. Effects of Cushing disease on bone mineral density in a pediatric population. J Pediatr. 2010;156:1001–5.
86. Leong GM, Abad V, Charmandari E, et al. Effects of child- and adolescent-onset endogenous Cushing syndrome on bone mass, body composition, and growth: a 7-year prospective study into young adulthood. J Bone Miner Res. 2007;22:110–8.
87. Bolland MJ, Holdaway IM, Berkeley JE, et al. Mortality and morbidity in Cushing's syndrome in New Zealand. Clin Endocrinol. 2011;75:436–42.
88. Di Somma C, Pivonello R, Loche S, et al. Effect of 2 years of cortisol normalization on the impaired bone mass and turnover in adolescent and adult patients with Cushing's disease: a prospective study. Clin Endocrinol. 2003;58:302–8.
89. Hermus AR, Smals AG, Swinkels LM, et al. Bone mineral density and bone turnover before and after surgical cure of Cushing's syndrome. J Clin Endocrinol Metab. 1995;80:2859–65.
90. Randazzo ME, Grossrubatscher E, Dalino Ciaramella P, Vanzulli A, Loli P. Spontaneous recovery of bone mass after cure of endogenous hypercortisolism. Pituitary. 2012;15:193–201.
91. Kristo C, Jemtland R, Ueland T, Godang K, Bollerslev J. Restoration of the coupling process and normalization of bone mass following successful treatment of endogenous Cushing's syndrome: a prospective, long-term study. Eur J Endocrinol. 2006;154:109–18.
92. Futo L, Toke J, Patocs A, et al. Skeletal differences in bone mineral area and content before and after cure of endogenous Cushing's syndrome. Osteoporos Int. 2008;19:941–9.
93. Barahona MJ, Sucunza N, Resmini E, et al. Deleterious effects of glucocorticoid replacement on bone in women after long-term remission of Cushing's syndrome. J Bone Miner Res. 2009;24:1841–6.
94. Castinetti F, Morange I, Jaquet P, Conte-Devolx B, Brue T. Ketoconazole revisited: a preoperative or postoperative treatment in Cushing's disease. Eur J Endocrinol. 2008;158:91–9.
95. Di Somma C, Colao A, Pivonello R, et al. Effectiveness of chronic treatment with alendronate in the osteoporosis of Cushing's disease. Clin Endocrinol. 1998;48:655–62.
96. Luisetto G, Zangari M, Camozzi V, Boscaro M, Sonino N, Fallo F. Recovery of bone mineral density after surgical cure, but not by ketoconazole treatment, in Cushing's syndrome. Osteoporos Int. 2001;12:956–60.
97. van Rossum EF, Voorhoeve PG, de Velde SJ, Koper JW, Delemarre-van de Waal HA, Kemper HC, Lamberts SW. The ER22/23EK polymorphism in the glucocorticoid receptor gene is associated with a beneficial body composition and muscle strength in young adults. J Clin Endocrinol Metab. 2004;89:4004–9.
98. Szappanos A, Patocs A, Toke J, Boyle B, Sereg M, Majnik J, Borgulya G, Varga I, Liko´ I, Racz K, et al. BclI polymorphism of the glucocorticoid receptor gene is associated with decreased bone mineral density in patients with endogenous hypercortisolism. Clin Endocrinol (Oxf). 2009;71:636–43.
99. Peng YM, Lei SF, Guo Y, Xiong DH, Yan H, Wang L, Guo YF, Deng HW. Sex-specific association of the glucocorticoid receptor gene with extreme BMD. J Bone Miner Res. 2008;23:247–52.
100. Trementino L, Appolloni G, Ceccoli L, Marcelli G, Concettoni C, Boscaro M, Arnaldi G. Bone complications in patients with Cushing's syndrome: looking for clinical, biochemical, and genetic determinants. Osteoporos Int. 2014;25:913–21.
101. Morelli V, Donadio F, Eller-Vainicher C, Cirello V, Olgiati L, Savoca C, Cairoli E, Salcuni AS, Beck-Peccoz P, Chiodini I. Role of glucocorticoid receptor polymorphism in adrenal incidentalomas. Eur J Clin Investig. 2010;40:803–11.
102. Tzanela M, Mantzou E, Saltiki K, Tampourlou M, Kalogeris N, Hadjidakis D, Tsagarakis S, Alevizaki M. Clinical and biochemical impact of BCL1 polymorphic genotype of the glucocorticoid receptor gene in patients with adrenal incidentalomas. J Endocrinol Investig. 2012;35:395–400.

103. Tomlinson JW, Walker EA, Bujalska IJ, Draper N, Lavery GG, Cooper MS, Hewison M, Stewart PM. 11β-Hydroxysteroid dehydrogenase type 1: a tissue specific regulator of glucocorticoid response. Endocr Rev. 2004;25:831–66.
104. Cooper MS. 11beta-Hydroxysteroid dehydrogenase: a regulator of glucocorticoid response in osteoporosis. J Endocrinol Investig. 2008;31:16–21.
105. Diederich S, Eigendorff E, Burkhardt P, et al. 11-Hydroxysteroid dehydrogenase types 1and 2:an important pharmacokinetic determinant for the activity of synthetic mineralo- and glucocorticoids. J Clin Endocrinol Metab. 2002;87:5695–701.
106. Park JS, Bae SJ, Choi SW, Son YH, Park SB, Rhee SD, Kim HY, Jung WH, Kang SK, Ahn JH, et al. A novel 11β-HSD1 inhibitor improves diabesity and osteoblast differentiation. J Mol Endocrinol. 2014;52:191–202.
107. Wu L, Qi H, Zhong Y, Lv S, Yu J, Liu J, Wang L, Bi J, Kong X, Di W, Zha J, et al. 11β-Hydroxysteroid dehydrogenase type 1 selective inhibitor BVT.2733 protects osteoblasts against endogenous glucocorticoid induced dysfunction. Endocr J. 2013;60:1047–58.
108. Hwang JY, Lee SH, Kim GS, Koh JM, Go MJ, Kim YJ, Kim HC, Kim TH, Hong JM, Park EK, et al. HSD11β1 polymorphisms predicted bone mineral density and fracture risk in postmenopausal women without clinically apparent hypercortisolemia. Bone. 2009;45: 1098–103.
109. Feldman K, Szappanos A, Butz H, Grolmusz V, Majnik J, Likó I, Kriszt B, Lakatos P, Tóth M, Rácz K, et al. The rs4844880 polymorphism in the promoter region of the HSD11B1 gene associates with bone mineral density in healthy and postmenopausal osteoporotic women. Steroids. 2012;77:1345–51.
110. Szappanos A, Patócs A, Gergics P, Bertalan R, Kerti A, Acs B, Feldmann K, Rácz K, Tóth M. The 83,557insA variant of the gene coding 11β-hydroxysteroid dehydrogenase type 1 enzyme associates with serum osteocalcin in patients with endogenous Cushing's syndrome. J Steroid Biochem Mol Biol. 2011;123:79–84.
111. Speiser PW, Azziz R, Baskin LS, Ghizzoni L, Hensle TW, Merke DP, Meyer-Bahlburg HF, Miller WL, Montori VM, Oberfield SE, Ritzen M, White PC, Endocrine Society. Congenital adrenal hyperplasia due to steroid 21-hydroxylase deficiency: an Endocrine Society clinical practice guideline. J Clin Endocrinol Metab. 2010;95(9):4133–60.
112. Mora S, Saggion F, Russo G, Weber G, Bellini A, Prinster C, Chiumello G. Bone density in young patients with congenital adrenal hyperplasia. Bone. 1996;18(4):337–40.
113. Ceccato F, Barbot M, Albiger N, Zilio M, De Toni P, Luisetto G, Zaninotto M, Greggio NA, Boscaro M, Scaroni C, Camozzi V. Long-term glucocorticoid effect on bone mineral density in patients with congenital adrenal hyperplasia due to 21-hydroxylase deficiency. Eur J Endocrinol. 2016;175(2):101–6.
114. Falhammar H, Filipsson H, Holmdahl G, Janson PO, Nordenskjöld A, Hagenfeldt K, Thorén M. Fractures and bone mineral density in adult women with 21-hydroxylase deficiency. J Clin Endocrinol Metab. 2007;92(12):4643–9.
115. Raizada N, Jyotsna VP, Upadhyay AD, Gupta N. Bone mineral density in young adult women with congenital adrenal hyperplasia. Indian J Endocrinol Metab. 2016;20(1):62–6.
116. Falhammar H, Filipsson Nyström H, Wedell A, Brismar K, Thorén M. Bone mineral density, bone markers, and fractures in adult males with congenital adrenal hyperplasia. Eur J Endocrinol. 2013;168(3):331–41.
117. Garcia Alves Junior PA, Schueftan DL, de Mendonça LM, Farias ML, Beserra IC. Bone mineral density in children and adolescents with congenital adrenal hyperplasia. Int J Endocrinol. 2014;2014:806895.
118. Zimmermann A, Sido PG, Schulze E, Al Khzouz C, Lazea C, Coldea C, Weber MM. Bone mineral density and bone turnover in Romanian children and young adults with classical 21-hydroxylase deficiency are influenced by glucocorticoid replacement therapy. Clin Endocrinol. 2009;71(4):477–84.
119. Hatton R, Stimpel M, Chambers TJ. Angiotensin II is generated from angiotensin I by bone cells and stimulates osteoclastic bone resorption in vitro. J Endocrinol. 1997;152: 5–10.

120. Asaba Y, Ito M, Fumoto T, Watanabe K, Fukuhara R, Takeshita S, Nimura Y, Ishida J, Fukamizu A, Ikeda K. Activation of renin-angiotensin system induces osteoporosis independently of hypertension. J Bone Miner Res. 2009;24:241–50.
121. Hagiwara H, Hiruma Y, Inoue A, Yamaguchi A, Hirose S. Deceleration by angiotensin II of the differentiation and bone formation of rat calvarial osteoblastic cells. J Endocrinol. 2006;156:543–50.
122. Lamparter S, Kling L, Schrader M, Ziegler R, Pfeilschifter J. Effects of angiotensin II on bone cells in vitro. J Cell Physiol. 1998;175:89–98.
123. Yamamoto S, Kido R, Onishi Y, Fukuma S, Akizawa T, Fukugawa M, Kazama JJ, Narita I, Fukuhara S. Use of renin-angiotensin system inhibitors is associated with reduction of fracture risk in hemodialysis patients. PLoS One. 2015;10:e01222691.
124. Aoki M, Kawahata H, Sotobayashi D, Yu H, Moriguchi A, Nakagami H, Ogihara T, Morishita R. Effect of angiotensin II receptor blocker, olmesartan, on turnover of bone metabolism in bedridden elderly hypertensive women with disuse syndrome. Geriatr Gerontol Int. 2015;15:1064–72.
125. Ghosh M, Majumda SR. Antihypertensive medications, bone mineral density, and fractures: a review of old cardiac drugs that provides new insights into osteoporosis. Endocrine. 2014;46:397–405.
126. Nakagami H, Osako MK, Morishita R. Potential effect of angiotensin II receptor blockade in adipose tissue and bone. Curr Pharm Des. 2013;19:3049–53.
127. Shimizu H, Nakagami H, Osako MK, Nakagami F, Kunugiza Y, Tomita T, Yoshikawa H, Rakugi H, Ogihara T, Morishita R. Prevention of osteoporosis by angiotensin-converting enzyme inhibitor in spontaneous hypertensive rats. Hypertens Res. 2009;32:786–90.
128. Donmez BO, Ozdemir S, Sarikanat M, Yaras N, Koc P, Demir N, Karayalcin B, Oguz N. Effect of angiotensin II type 1 receptor blocker on osteoporotic rat femurs. Pharmacol Rep. 2012;64:878–88.
129. Garcia P, Schwenzer S, Slotta JE, Scheuer C, Tami AE, Holstein JH, Histing T, Burkhardt M, Pohlemann T, Menge MD. Inhibition of angiotensin-converting enzyme stimulates fracture healing and periosteal callus formation – role of a local renin-angiotensin system. Br J Pharmacol. 2010;159:1672–80.
130. Tylavsky FA, Johnson KC, Wan JY, Harshfield G. Plasma renin activity is associated with bone mineral density in premenopausal women. Osteoporos Int. 1998;8:136–40.
131. Altun B, Kiykim AA, Seyrantepe V, Usalana C, Arici M, Çağlar M, Erdem Y, Yasavul U, Turgan C, Çağlar S. Association between activated renin angiotensin system and bone formation in hemodialysis patients: is the bone mass genetically determined by ACE gene polymorphism? Ren Fail. 2004;26:425–31.
132. Kuipers AL, Kammerer CM, Pratt JH, Bunker CH, Wheeler VW, Patrick AL, Zmuda JM. Association of circulating renin and aldosterone with osteocalcin and bone mineral density in African ancestry families. Hypertension. 2016;67:977–82.
133. Gu SS, Zhang Y, Li HL, Wu SY, Diao TY, Hai R, Deng HW. Involvement of the skeletal renin-angiotensin system in age-related osteoporosis of ageing mice. Biosci Biotechnol Biochem. 2012;76:1367–71.
134. Yongtao Z, Kunzheng W, Jingjing Z, Hu S, Jianqiang K, Ruiyu L, Chunsheng W. Glucocorticoids activate the local renin–angiotensin system in bone: possible mechanism for glucocorticoid-induced osteoporosis. Endocrine. 2014;47:598–608.
135. Chhokar VS, Sun Y, Bhattacharya SK, Ahokas RA, Myers LK, Xing Z, Smith RA, Gerling IC, Weber KT. Loss of bone minerals and strength in rats with aldosteronism. Am J Physiol Heart Circ Physiol. 2004;287:H2023–6.
136. Pilz S, Kienreich K, Drechsler C, Ritz E, Fahrleitner-Pammer A, Gaksch M, Meinitzer A, März W, Pieber TR, Tomaschitz A. Hyperparathyroidism in patients with primary aldosteronism: cross-sectional and interventional data from the GECOH study. J Clin Endocrinol Metab. 2012;97:E75–9.
137. Law PH, Sun Y, Bhattacharya SK, Chhokar VS, Weber KT. Diuretics and bone loss in rats with aldosteronism. J Am Coll Cardiol. 2005;46:142–6.

138. Salcuni AS, Palmieri S, Carnevale V, Morelli V, Battista C, Guarnieri V, Guglielmi G, Desina G, Eller-Vainicher C, Beck-Peccoz P, Scillitani A, Chiodini I. Bone involvement in aldosteronism. J Bone Miner Res. 2012;27:2217–22.
139. Ceccoli L, Ronconi V, Giovannini L, Marcheggiani M, Turchi F, Boscaro M, Giacchetti G. Bone health and aldosterone excess. Osteoporos Int. 2013;24:2801–7.
140. Petramala L, Zinnamosca L, Settevendemmie A, Marinelli C, Nardi M, Concistrè A, Corpaci F, Tonnarini G, De Toma G, Letizia C. Bone and mineral metabolism in patients with primary aldosteronism. Int J Endocrinol. 2014;2014:836529.
141. Gupta M, Cheung CL, Hsu YH, Demissie S, Cupples LA, Kiel DP, Karasi D. Identification of homogeneous genetic architecture of multiple genetically correlated traits by block clustering of genome-wide associations. J Bone Miner Res. 2011;26:1261–71.
142. Beavan S, Horner A, Bord S, Ireland D, Compston J. Colocalization of glucocorticoid and mineralocorticoid receptors in human bone. J Bone Miner Res. 2001;16:1496–504.
143. Fumoto T, Ishii KA, Ito M, Berger S, Schütz G, Ikeda K. Mineralocorticoid receptor function in bone metabolism and its role in glucocorticoid-induced osteopenia. Biochem Biophys Res Commun. 2014;447:407–12.
144. Zhang B, Umbach AT, Chen H, Yana J, Fakhri H, Fajol A, Salker MS, Spichtig D, Daryadel A, Wagner CA, Föller M, Lang F. Up-regulation of FGF23 release by aldosterone. Biochem Biophys Res Commun. 2016;470:384–90.
145. Lang F, Ritz E, Voelkl J, Alesutan I. Vascular calcification—is aldosterone a culprit? Nephrol Dial Transplant. 2013;28:1080–4.
146. Ma TK, Szeto CC. Mineralocorticoid receptor antagonist for renal protection. Ren Fail. 2012;34:810–7.
147. Ritz E, Koleganova N, Piecha G. Is there an obesity-metabolic syndrome related glomerulopathy? Curr Opin Nephrol Hypertens. 2011;20:44–9.
148. Mihailidou AS. Aldosterone in heart disease. Curr Hypertens Rep. 2012;14:125–9.
149. Sarraf M, Masoumi A, Schrier RW. Cardiorenal syndrome in acute decompensated heart failure. Clin J Am Soc Nephrol. 2009;4:2013–26.
150. Schrier RW. Water and sodium retention in edematous disorders: role of vasopressin and aldosterone. Am J Med. 2006;119:S47–53.
151. Schrier RW, Masoumi A, Elhassan E. Aldosterone: role in edematous disorders, hypertension, chronic renal failure, and metabolic syndrome. Clin J Am Soc Nephrol. 2010;5:1132–40.
152. Imazu M, Takahama H, Asanuma H, Funada A, Sugano Y, Ohara T, Hasegawa T, Asakura M, Kanzaki H, Anzai T, Kitakaze M. Pathophysiological impact of serum fibroblast growth factor 23 in patients with non-ischemic cardiac disease and early chronic kidney disease. Am J Physiol Heart Circ Physiol. 2014;307:H1504–11.
153. Hu MC, Shiizaki K, Kuro-o M, Moe OW. Fibroblast growth factor 23 and Klotho: physiology and pathophysiology of an endocrine network of mineral metabolism. Annu Rev Physiol. 2013;75:503–33.
154. Evenepoel P, Meijers B, Viaene L, Bammens B, Claes K, Kuypers D, Vanderschueren D, Vanrenterghem Y. Fibroblast growth factor-23 in early chronic kidney disease: additional support in favor of a phosphate-centric paradigm for the pathogenesis of secondary hyperparathyroidism. Clin J Am Soc Nephrol. 2010;5:1268–76.
155. Faul C, Amaral AP, Oskouei B, Hu MC, Sloan A, Isakova T, Gutierrez OM, Aguillon-Prada R, Lincoln J, Hare JM, Mundel P, Morales A, Scialla J, Fischer M, Soliman EZ, Chen J, Go AS, Rosas SE, Nessel L, Townsend RR, Feldman HI, St John Sutton M, Ojo A, Gadegbeku C, Di Marco GS, Reuter S, Kentrup D, Tiemann K, Brand M, Hill JA, Moe OW, Kuro OM, Kusek JW, Keane MG, Wolf M. FGF23 induces left ventricular hypertrophy. J Clin Invest. 2011;121:4393–408.
156. Zanchi C, Locatelli M, Benigni A, Corna D, Tomasoni S, Rottoli D, Gaspari F, Remuzzi G, Zoja C. Renal expression of FGF23 in progressive renal disease of diabetes and the effect of ace inhibitor. PLoS One. 2013;8:e70775.
157. Prie D, Forand A, Francoz C, Elie C, Cohen I, Courbebaisse M, Eladari D, Lebrec D, Durand F, Friedlander G. Plasma fibroblast growth factor 23 concentration is increased and predicts mortality in patients on the liver-transplant waiting list. PLoS One. 2013;8:e66182.

Skeletal Tissue and Ovarian Function: Puberty and Menopause

8

Annamaria Colao, Carolina Di Somma,
and Volha V. Zhukouskaya

8.1 Introduction

During their life-span, women live through three critical phases—the reproductive, menopausal transition, and postmenopausal phases—all of which are characterized by the complex interactions between hypothalamic, pituitary, and ovarian function. Throughout these phases, ovarian function, in particular estrogens (E), plays a central role not only in female reproduction but also in the skeletal homeostasis, in the regulation of bone mass from puberty till menopause. Why are the sex steroids rather than the primary calcitrophic hormones the major regulators of bone mass? It can be explained from a biological point of view. When the new function is needed, the evolutionary process adapts an existing mechanism rather than developing a completely new one. It is speculated that the major role of E in regulating bone mass evolved from their primary role in supporting reproduction. For example, in birds, bone mineral content is mobilized to supply calcium for eggshell mineralization. With evolution, in mammals this earlier system was co-opted to provide calcium for mineralizing the fetal skeleton and for subsequent lactation. Even the role of the sex steroids in inducing and supporting the pubertal growth spurt can be understood in evolutionary terms. The tight coupling between the onset of puberty and the skeletal growth spurt ensures that reproduction cannot occur until there is sufficient skeletal mass to support pregnancy. Therefore, since reproductive success is the keystone of natural selection, the surprising complexity of sex steroid regulation of bone mass in mammals can be explained by its evolutionary linkage to ancient reproductive mechanisms [1].

A. Colao (✉) · V. V. Zhukouskaya
Department of Clinical Medicine and Surgery, Division of Endocrinology,
University of Naples Federico II, Naples, Italy
e-mail: colao@unina.it

C. Di Somma
IRCCS SDN, Naples, Italy

A. Lenzi, S. Migliaccio (eds.), *Multidisciplinary Approach to Osteoporosis*,
https://doi.org/10.1007/978-3-319-75110-8_8

8.2 Ovarian Sex Steroids

Ovaries secrete both steroid hormones and different peptides. Steroid hormones produced by the ovary include C18- (estradiol, estron), C19- (dehydroepiandrosterone, androstenedione, testosterone), and C21-carbon (pregnenolone, progesterone, 17α-hydroxyprogesterone) steroids, among which estradiol and progesterone are the major steroid products synthesized by granulosa and theca ovary cells, respectively. Different peptides secreted by the ovary represent growth factors (e.g., insulin-like growth factors), cytokines (e.g., interleukin-1), activin, inhibin, and follistatin [2].

E derive not only from ovarian but also from extraovarian secretion. In premenopausal women more than 95% of E are derived from the ovary, and peripheral conversion of steroids represents only the minor part as a source for E. After menopause, the latter becomes the main source for E in postmenopausal women [1]. The peripheral conversion of steroids takes place in subcutaneous fat, skin, and other physiological (e.g., the brain, breast) and pathological estrogen-dependent tissues (e.g., breast cancer cells, endometrial cancer cells), and it is possible due to aromatization of androstenedione that arises from the ovary and the adrenal gland in premenopausal women and primarily forms the adrenal gland in postmenopausal women. The main product of this reaction is estron, weaker E, which is further converted to the biologically active estradiol in target tissues. Although only small part of E is produced by individual adipocyte or skin fibroblast, these cell types contribute to circulating estradiol level in the relevant manner because of their relative abundance, and this effect is more pronounced in obese women due to increased mass of the adipose tissue and skin [2] (see Fig. 8.1).

Sex steroid hormones act on their target cells by binding to member of the nuclear hormone receptor superfamily: E bind to estrogen receptor (ER) α or β, and progesterone binds to its progesterone receptor. Members of this superfamily of receptors are located in the nucleus and represent zinc-finger-containing transcription factors characterized by an N-terminal domain, a central DNA-binding domain, and a C-terminal, ligand-binding domain. Binding of E or progesterone to their receptors in the nucleus stimulates transcription of target genes resulting from direct interaction of the receptor proteins with DNA or from interactions with other transcription factors. Additionally, besides nuclear-initiated signaling, nongenomic mode of action of sex steroids also exists. In particular, through binding to sex steroid receptors in the plasma membrane, E can initiate signal transduction by triggering the production of cyclic nucleotides and calcium flux and activation of cytoplasmic kinases. Activation of these kinases, in turn, leads to the phosphorylation of substrate proteins and transcription factors (such as AP-1 and Elk1), which mediate some of the gene-regulatory effects of E. Interestingly, a lot of genes are regulated by ERα through this indirect mode of action than are regulated via the direct association of E with DNA [3] (see Fig. 8.1).

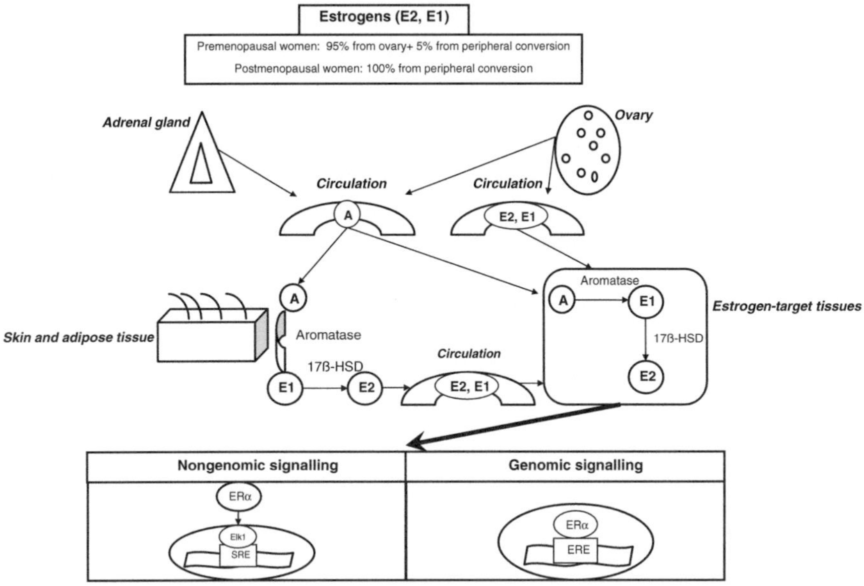

Fig. 8.1 Schematic illustration of sources of estrogens in women and its principal of action: E derives from ovarian and extraovarian secretion (peripheral conversion of steroids). In premenopausal women more than 95% of E is derived from the ovary, and peripheral conversion of steroids represents only the minor part as a source for E, whereas in postmenopausal women peripheral conversion is the principal source of E. The peripheral conversion of steroids takes place in subcutaneous fat, skin, and other physiological/pathological estrogen-dependent tissues, and it is possible due to aromatization of androstenedione that arises from the ovary and the adrenal gland in premenopausal women and primarily forms the adrenal gland in postmenopausal women. The main product of this reaction is estron, which is further converted to the biologically active estradiol with the help of 17β-HSD enzyme in target tissues. Sex steroid hormones act on their target cells by binding to estrogen receptor α or β. There are two principal mode of E action: genomic (direct) and nongenomic (indirect) one. Binding of E to its receptors in the nucleus stimulates transcription of target genes resulting from direct interaction of the receptor proteins with DNA or from interactions with other transcription factors. Through binding to sex steroid receptors in the plasma membrane, E can initiate signal transduction by triggering transcription factors (e.g., Elk1), which mediate some of the gene-regulatory effects of E. *A* androstenedione, *E* estrogens, *E1* estrone, *E2* estradiol, *ERα* estrogen receptor, *ERE* estrogen response element, *Elk1* ETS domain-containing protein Elk1, *SRE* serum response element, *17β-HSD* 17β-hydroxysteroid dehydrogenase

8.3 Physiological Effects of Sex Steroids, Its Receptors, and Other Ovarian Peptides on the Bone

8.3.1 Estrogens and Bone

Having multiple functions, E and ERα influence not solely the cells directly regulating bone remodeling (osteoblasts (OB), osteoclasts (OC), and osteocytes) but also the cells connected to skeletal tissue such as chondrocytes and immune system cells, T- and B-lymphocytes, which, in turn, participate in bone growth and remodeling too. All these effects were explored on mice models with deletion of the ERα which provided the functional role of E and their receptor in specific cell types (see Table 8.1).

Osteoclasts There is strong evidence that E restrain osteoclastogenesis and OC survival through direct inhibitory action on OC and their progenitors because deletion of ERα in the entire macrophage-monocyte lineage and in mature OC led to the notable increase in OC numbers and its survival. Interestingly, this effect is demonstrated only in trabecular bone in female mice, but not in cortical bone and not in male mice [3, 4].

Table 8.1 Physiological effects of sex steroids, its receptors, and other ovarian peptides on different cell types in women

Estrogens/estrogen receptor α		
	Trabecular bone	Cortical bone
Osteoblasts	–	• ↑ Osteoblastogenesis → ↓ bone resorption on endocortical surface
		• ↓ Osteoblastogenesis → ↓ periosteal bone formation
		• Estrogen receptor α, independent of estrogens, potentiates the responsiveness of osteoblast progenitors/osteocytes to mechanical forces at the beginning of puberty → ↑ bone accrual and periosteal bone formation
Osteoclasts	• ↓ Osteoclastogenesis	–
	• ↓ Osteoclast apoptosis	
	• ↓ Bone resorption	
Osteocyte	• ↓ Osteocyte apoptosis	
Chondrocytes	• Closure of epiphyseal growth plates	
T-/B--lymphocytes	• ↓ T-/B-lymphocytes → ↓ proosteoclastogenic cytokines (tumor necrosis factor-α, IL-1, IL-6, IL-7, IL-17, receptor activator of NF-κB ligand (RANKL)) → ↓ bone resorption	
Progesterone/progesterone receptor		
Osteoblasts	• Potential stimulatory effect on osteoblastogenesis	
Osteoclasts	–	
Osteocytes	–	
Inhibin A/B		
Osteoblasts	• Biphasic effect on osteoblastogenesis: cyclic/short-term action → ↓ osteoblastogenesis, continuous action → ↑ osteoblastogenesis	
Osteoclasts	• ↓ Osteoclastogenesis	
Osteocytes	–	
Activins		
Osteoblasts	• Potential stimulatory effect on osteoblastogenesis	
Osteoclasts	• Potential stimulatory effect on osteoclastogenesis	
Osteocytes	–	

Osteoblasts The effect of E on OB is more complex in comparison to its effect on OC. On the one hand, E have direct stimulatory action on the OB progenitors attenuating osteoclastic resorption in the endocortical surface. On the other hand, E decrease osteoblastogenesis in periosteum leading to the attenuation of periosteal apposition [3]. This effect of E is typical for cortical bone in female.

Osteocytes The direct action of E on osteocytes is still unclear. A lot of studies have demonstrated that E deficiency leads to an increase of OB and osteocyte apoptosis in both trabecular and cortical compartment. In the other studies, the deletion of ERα brought to OB and osteocyte apoptosis but bone mass was not altered in these mice models, suggesting that effect of E on osteocytes is only additive, and OB/osteocyte apoptosis alone due to E deficiency is not enough for bone loss [3].

It has been recently hypothesized that osteocytes may have a role for sensing and responding to mechanical forces during growth and adult life [1, 3]. At the same time, the presence of ERα stimulates periosteal bone formation in response to the mechanical forces. These data suggest that osteocytes and ERα work in coordinated way responding to mechanical stimuli. Probably, ERα can potentiate responsiveness of bone cells, in particular osteocytes, to mechanical strain, stimulating, in this way, periosteal bone formation [3].

Chondrocytes Not tightly belonging to the skeletal tissue, chondrocytes are also under control of E. Endochondral ossification, when the cartilage is formed and then replaced by the bone, is essential for longitudinal bone growth, and E play crucial role in the closure of the growth plate at the late stage of puberty. As the demonstration of that, lack of ERα on the chondrocytes leads to continued longitudinal growth [3].

T-/B-Lymphocytes OC are differentiated cells which are derived from hematopoietic cells of monocyte-macrophage lineage, and their function is strongly connected to the other cells of immune system. T- and B-lymphocytes during their activity produce a lot of cytokines, among which are proinflammatory and, at the same time, proosteoclastogenic factors (IL-1, IL-6, IL-7, IL-17), tumor necrosis factor (TNF)-α, and receptor activator of NF-κB ligand (RANKL) [5]. E are the key regulator of immune function as demonstrated both in animals and humans [3, 5]. E loss promotes T-cell activation with subsequent increase of osteoclastogenic cytokines, which in turn activate OC formation and survival. Also B-cells are directly implicated in the regulation of bone resorption because they produce both RANKL and osteoprotegerin (OPG, binding to RANKL, prevents the connection of RANKL to its receptor RANK causing inhibition of osteoclastogenesis). However, activated B-lymphocytes due to E loss and activation of T-cells overexpress RANKL, rather than OPG, and promote in this way osteoclastogenesis [5].

8.3.2 Progesterone and Bone

Although the major focus has been directed to E, progesterone is a critical sex steroid which is required for ovulation, and its responses are modulated by E. OB expresses receptors of progesterone, and the level of progesterone receptor can be stimulated by E. Low doses of progesterone increase expression of growth factor and proteins which can locally promote osteoblastogenesis [6]. However, this effect is not absolutely necessary for normal bone growth, considering that mice models lacking progesterone receptor did not show largely compromised bone phenotype [6, 7].

8.3.3 Activins/Inhibins and Bone

Inhibins and activins, peptides secreted by the ovary, can potentially take part in the regulation of bone homeostasis too.

Inhibin is produced by many tissues; however, the main source of inhibin is granulosa cells in the ovary. It has two isoforms, inhibin A and inhibin B, and its main function is to suppress follicle-stimulating hormone (FSH). Activin is produced by granulosa cells too, and it has opposed function to inhibin, stimulation of FSH [2]. It has been demonstrated that both hormones could be implicated in the bone homeostasis, stimulatory effect in case of activin and inhibitory effect in case of inhibin. In fact, activin is produced and stored also in the bone, exerting the effect on OB and OC development [6, 8]. As regards inhibin, it has biphasic effect on the bone, depending upon exposure: in cyclic/short-term administration, inhibin has negative, inhibitory influence on the bone; vice versa, in continuous administration it has positive, anabolic effect on bone metabolism [6, 9]. In vitro studies showed that normal cyclic levels of inhibin (as in normal physiological conditions) suppress both osteobasto- and osteoclastogenesis, leading to decreased bone turnover [6, 9]. As the demonstration of inhibitory effect of inhibin on bone differentiation, there is evidence of increased bone turnover and bone loss much before the menopause when the levels of E are still maintaining at the normal level, and it happens, probably, due to initial loss of ovarian inhibin secretion [6, 9].

8.4 Role of Sex Steroids in Skeletal Maturation During Puberty

The bone mass acquisition follows complex pattern which starts straight after the birth when children experience the greatest postnatal growth during the infancy. Thereafter, the growth and the gaining of bone mass decrease to the nadir known as the minimal prespurt velocity, the slowest period of growth in childhood, immediately before the pubertal growth spurt. The beginning of puberty is the time of the most rapid growth and bone acquisition followed by decreasing of velocity and cessation of growth at epiphyseal fusion at the end of puberty [10]. Skeletal maturation during puberty is a crucial moment because properly this period, when children achieve the peak of bone mass, represents the possibility to reach that much bone quantity and bone strength which will be able to meet and to resist to all the load-bearing demands throughout of the individual's lifetime. Additionally, the accrual of bone mass and size during growth is a critical determinant of the risk for development of osteoporosis later in life.

The peak bone mineral accretion rate occurs at about 12.5 years at stage 2–3 of sexual maturity in girls and at about 14.1 years at stage 3–4 of sexual maturity in boys. During the 4 years surrounding the peak in bone accretion, 39% of total body mineral content is acquired; by 4 years following the peak, 95% of adult bone mass has been achieved [11].

Skeletal growth occurs mainly by modeling, coordinated action of bone deposition and resorption, which allows increasing the size and shape of bones. Linear bone growth occurs by ossification of the endochondral growth plate. Radial bone growth occurs by periosteal apposition, and the marrow cavity size increases by endosteal resorption. The excess of periosteal bone apposition over endosteal bone resorption that occurs during the pubertal growth spurt increases both the size and the volumetric bone mineral density of extremities [1]. Distinct increase in the trabecular bone of the spine and long bones occurs between sexual maturity at stages 3–4. Cortical bone growth, instead, is lower in adolescent period that may bring to increased intracortical porosity since the rapid pubertal phase of growth exceeds the cortical bone acquisition [11]. At the time of epiphyseal plate closure, bones have reached about 90–95% of peak mass after which the process named as "consolidation" or "plateau" begins. Period of "consolidation" is characterized by stabilization and achievement of maximal values of skeletal mass and decline of the intracortical porosity due to continued periosteal apposition and, probably, continued trabecular thickening [1, 11]. How long does "consolidation" last? It still remains disputed, and, probably, it depends on the skeletal site. Some found that for women it can last till the third decade for trabecular bone and till the second decade for cortical bone [11, 12].

Sex steroids (E in girls and both E and testosterone in boys) are a clue component in skeletal maturation. E act through different mechanisms during puberty. Firstly, direct action of E on bone modeling, stimulating formation and inhibiting resorption, increases bone mass during skeletal maturation [3]. Secondly, E act indirectly through growth hormone (GH)/insulin-like growth factor-1 (IGF-1) axis. Puberty is triggered by increase in pulsatile secretion of gonadotropin-releasing hormone (GnRH) by the hypothalamus which promotes the increase of gonadotropins and sex steroids, consequently. Rising levels of E potentiate secretion of GH and IGF-1 which, in turn, stimulate periosteal bone apposition. Levels of GH and IGF-1 remain elevated during the 3–4 years of rapid growth; thereafter, they gradually return to the prepubertal levels [1, 3]. Finally, ERα, independent of E levels, potentiates responsiveness of osteoblast progenitors and osteocytes on mechanical forces, enhancing in this way bone accrual and periosteal bone formation [3]. At the end of puberty when E reach their peak level, they induce epiphyseal plate closure leading to growth cessation [1, 3]. Thus, it appears that E both initiate the pubertal growth spurt and then it ends it.

Girls experience different pattern of growth in comparison with boys which explains the differences in the final height and peak bone mass between two sexes. Since boys enter puberty 2 years later than girls and their pubertal growth spurt lasts for 4 years rather than 3 years like in girls, it accounts for 10% higher final height and for 25% greater peak bone mass in males. Moreover, there are the differences also in bone dimension between two sexes. Boys have larger bones with thicker cortex which are opposite to girls having smaller bones with thinner cortex [1, 11]. In the latter phenomenon, sex steroids are responsible for gender dimorphism of skeleton. In males, E together with testosterone cause stimulatory effect on both trabecular and cortical bone, promoting in this way periosteal apposition and thicker cortex [1, 3]. In females, E might have both stimulatory and inhibitory effect on the bone, according to their blood levels. At the beginning of puberty, low E levels upregulate the expression of ERα which is the predominant clue when E levels remain low. ERα, in turn, amplifies the responsiveness of bone cells to mechanical strain and increased periosteal bone apposition, making cortex thicker. The dramatic rise of E levels at later stages of puberty restrains periosteal bone formation which leads to smaller diameter and thinner cortex preventing bones from becoming excessively large and heavy [3]. This restraining effect of high levels of E on periosteum remains predominant till the menopause.

The schematic illustration of women's bone mass changes during life is presented on Fig. 8.2.

8.5 Role of Sex Steroids in Bone Loss After Menopause

As it was mentioned before, after completion of growth and after reaching of 90–95% of peak bone mass, the phase of "consolidation" or "plateau" starts, and it continues approximately till the third decade of life. As it has been demonstrated by large epidemiological studies [13], immediately after this period and long before any change in sex steroid production, in both women and men, bone loss begins. In women after menopause, bone loss accelerates, and it follows two major phases: an early accelerated, but transient, phase that begins at menopause and lasts about 4–8 years and a slow, continuous phase [1]. During the early accelerated phase, there is a loss predominantly of trabecular bone, whereas cortical bone declines substantially during the slow continuous phase [1, 3, 13]. There are several mechanisms which explain the present pattern of bone dynamic after peak bone mass, and E deficiency plays a role during all the phases of bone decline, especially in the early accelerated phase.

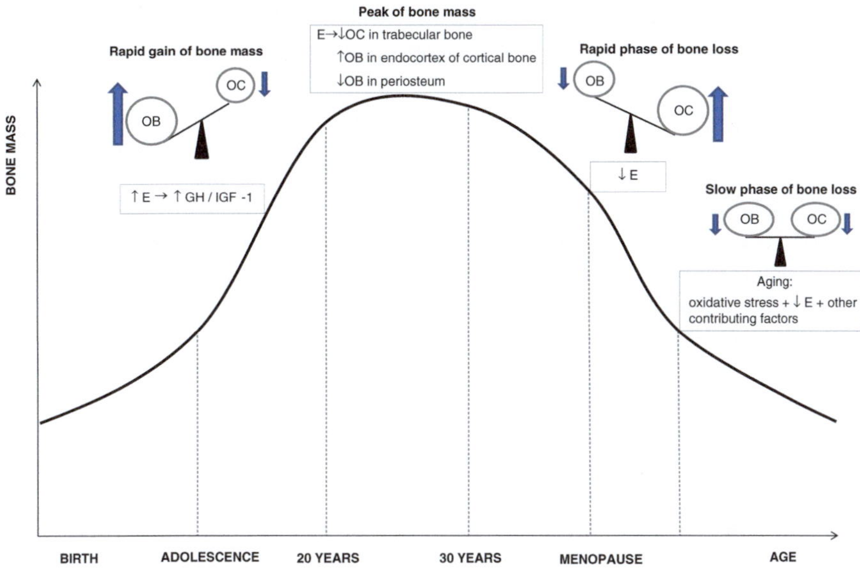

Fig. 8.2 Schematic illustration of changes of bone mass in women during life: in adolescence, during the phase of rapid bone gain, rising levels of E act directly and indirectly through GH/IGF-1 axis on bone formation, leading to accumulation of bone mineral content and rapid bone accrual. At the end of puberty in girls, after reaching of peak bone mass, high levels of E restrain periosteal bone formation and promote closure of epiphyseal plate, leading to growth cessation and balance between bone formation and resorption. During the peak of bone mass in adult life, E maintains the balance in bone turnover, suppress osteoclastogenesis in trabecular bone, increase osteoblastogenesis on endocortical surface and reduce osteoblastogenesis on periosteum of cortical bone, reduce apoptosis of osteocytes, and decrease T- and B-cell activation with consequent inhibition of osteoclastogenesis. After menopause, acute E decline causes rapid bone loss, especially in trabecular bone, due to imbalance between bone formation and resorption toward the latter one. The rapid bone loss is followed by the slow bone loss which happens especially in cortical bone. The slow bone loss is caused by predominant process of aging (oxidative stress, lipid, FoxO and PPARγ activation) and other age-related changes (increased GC production/sensitivity, calcium negative balance, reduced levels of IGF-1, muscle mass, bone hydration, and vascularity) which all together suppress bone formation. E deficiency worsens age-related changes, lowering antioxidant defenses of bone cells and contributing to calcium negative balance. *E* estrogens, *GC* glucocorticosteroids, *GH* growth hormone, *FoxO* forkhead box protein, *IGF-1* insulin-like growth factor-1, *OB* osteoblasts, *OC* osteoclasts, *PPARγ* peroxisome proliferator-activated receptor-γ

8.5.1 The Early Accelerated Phase of Bone Loss

The early accelerated phase of bone loss starts after menopause with cessation of ovarian E production. The rapid decline of E levels leads to the loss of inhibitory effect of E on osteoclastogenesis, promoting OC life-span. Additionally, E deficiency activates T- and B-lymphocytes with subsequent releasing of proosteoclastogenic cytokines, such as TNF-α, IL-1, IL-6, IL-7, IL-17, and RANKL, which, in turn, maintain OC formation. Altogether these factors dramatically increase bone resorption that occurs especially in trabecular bone. As regards the cells of bone formation, E deficiency causes OB/osteocyte apoptosis and decreased osteoblastogenesis. The latter process of decreased osteoblastogenesis happens on endocortical surface of cortical bone which leads to the increased bone resorption in this area. At the same time, E deficiency brings to the cessation of restraining effect of E on osteoblastogenesis on periosteum of cortical bone, increasing periosteal bone formation. However, it appears insufficient to maintain balance of bone remodeling, and bone resorption exceeds bone formation causing the rapid decline of bone mass. Thus, during the early phase of bone loss, trabecular bone undergoes fast changes such as trabecular perforation and loss of connectivity, whereas cortical bone becomes thinner as a result of an increase in the medullary diameter due to increases of bone resorption on endocortical surface [1, 3, 13].

8.5.2 The Slow Continuous Phase of Bone Loss

The slow continuous phase of bone loss, following the early rapid phase, involves primarily the cortical bone and is distinguished from the rapid phase by lower and continuous rates of bone loss and by decreased rates of both bone formation and resorption [1, 3]. How can the high rates of bone loss with high turnover during the early rapid phase be converted to the condition of low bone turnover during the slow phase? There are multiple factors contributing to bone loss during the latter phase, and the majority of them are associated with aging.

Aging, Oxidative Stress, and Estrogen Deficiency Oxidative stress and the formation of reactive oxygen species (ROS) are inescapable consequences of life in an oxygen-rich environment. Evolutionary, our organism developed different defense mechanisms to detoxify ROS. The most important ones are antioxidant enzymes (superoxide dismutases), thiol-containing oligopeptides (glutathione, thioredoxin), and FoxO transcription factors. FoxOs belong to a large family of forkhead proteins, and their activation due to increased oxidative stress leads to enhanced transcription of antioxidant enzymes and other genes involved in cell cycle, DNA repair, and life-span [13]. At the skeletal level, in particular in OB, in order to decrease ROS concentration, FoxOs activated by oxidative stress bind to β-catenin (the important transcription factor of bone differentiation), promoting FoxO-mediated transcription at the expense of β-catenin-mediated transcription and decreasing in this way osteoblastogenesis [13].

With aging, there is a decline of antioxidant mechanisms which inevitably increases oxidative stress, formation of ROS, and FoxO activation and decreases bone formation. Scientific evidence demonstrated that E deficiency directly takes part in the lowering of antioxidant defenses. In fact, ovariectomy in rats decreases antioxidant substances and increases ROS and lipid peroxidation which normalized after

E replacement. Additionally, administration of antioxidants such as N-acetylcysteine prevented ovariectomy-induced bone loss as effectively as the replacement with E did [13–15]. At the molecular level in OB, E reduces phosphorylation of $p66^{shc}$ (the important mediator of oxidative stress-induced apoptosis), causing antiapoptotic effect on OB/osteocytes [13, 16]. In OC, E stimulates the synthesis of glutathione and thioredoxin reductases which increase the pool of antioxidant substances able to capture and decrease ROS production, normally essential for osteoclastogenesis through activation of RANKL and TNF-α expression. In this way, E causes proapoptotic effect on OC [13, 14, 16].

Taking together all the data, increased oxidative stress and decreased antioxidant defenses with aging per se suppress bone metabolism. It worsens by E deficiency which further decreases antioxidant capacities of bone cells, enhancing cellular oxidative stress and leading, in this way, to apoptosis of OB/osteocytes and survival of OC.

Aging, Lipid Oxidation, and PPARγ Another process activated and increased with age is lipid oxidation. Due to the lack of defense mechanism with aging, during lipid oxidations there is a notable generation of ROS and other forms of fatty acid derivatives which bind and activate peroxisome proliferator-activated receptor-γ (PPAR-γ). Activation of PPAR-γ increases adipogenesis at the expense of osteoblastogenesis in the bone marrow. Additionally, ROS generated during lipid oxidation activates FoxO-mediated gene transcription at the expense of β-catenin-mediated transcription, thus ultimately, decreasing in this way osteoblastogenesis [13].

Aging and Glucocorticoids Cortisol is rather essential for normal bone metabolism, but it is well known how glucocorticoid (GC) excess has deleterious influence on the bone causing reduced osteoblastogenesis, strong and rapid OB/osteocyte apoptosis, and transient increased OC survival followed by suppressed osteoclastogenesis. All these changes lead to low bone state (reduction of both bone formation and resorption) which is something similar to what happens during the process of aging [17]. There is evidence that aging is associated with GC endogenous availability and production. In fact, aging in humans blunts GC feedback inhibition of ACTH, stimulates conversion of inactive cortisone to active cortisol, and increases endogenous GC production [18]. Therefore, aging-associated state of hypercortisolism inevitably contributes to suppression of bone remodeling.

Aging, Calcium Metabolism, and Estrogen Deficiency There are a lot of changes in calcium metabolism associated with aging. Aging impairs intestinal calcium absorption and renal calcium conservation leading to external calcium wasting. Unless dietary calcium is substantially increased to offset this lost, PTH level increases to maintain normal levels of serum ionic calcium by resorption of the bone that contain 99% of body calcium stores. Progressive increase of PTH levels can lead to secondary hyperparathyroidism which ultimately damages bone metabolism [1, 19].

Moreover, E acting through its ER increases intestinal calcium absorption and renal conservation, trying to maintain normal blood calcium levels [1, 19]. Thus, when the menopause comes, E deficiency worsens all these processes which normally happen with aging (reduced intestinal calcium absorption and renal conservation with consequent secondary hyperparathyroidism).

Other Age-Related Contributing Factors Among the other factors which contribute to age-associated bone loss, there is reduction of growth factors such as IGF-1, of muscle mass and mechanical strain due to decreased physical activity, and of bone vascularity and hydration. The normal levels of these factors are required for adequate function of bone metabolism, and its reduction is additional contributing factor to major age-related factors of bone damage [3, 13].

The schematic illustration of women's bone mass changes during life is presented on Fig. 8.2.

8.6 Summary

In summary, E play one of the most important roles in bone metabolism, and it is evidenced during the entire women's life-span, from the phase of bone gain in puberty, during the phase of bone maintenance in adult life, and during the phase of bone loss in either menopause or, thereafter, aging.

E have multiple functions. Normally, they suppress osteoclastogenesis in trabecular bone, increase osteoblastogenesis on endocortical surface and reduce osteoblastogenesis on periosteum of cortical bone, reduce apoptosis of osteocytes, and decrease T- and B-cell activation with consequent inhibition of osteoclastogenesis. Additionally, they possess antioxidant properties, protecting bone cells from oxidative stress, and participate in intestinal calcium absorption and renal conservation. In adolescence, during the phase of rapid bone gain, rising levels of E act directly and indirectly through GH/IGF-1 axis on bone formation, leading to accumulation of bone mineral content and rapid bone accrual. At the end of puberty in girls, after reaching of peak bone mass, high levels of E restrain periosteal bone formation and promote closure of epiphyseal plate, leading to growth cessation and balance between bone formation and resorption. After menopause, acute E decline causes rapid bone loss, especially in trabecular bone, due to imbalance between bone formation and resorption toward the latter one. The rapid bone loss is followed by the slow bone loss which happens especially in cortical bone. The slow bone loss is caused by predominant process of aging. Age-related increased oxidative stress, lipid oxidation, and ROS concentration initiate cascade of processes as FoxO and PPARγ activation. FoxO activation sequesters β-catenin to promote the gene transcription of antioxidant defenses. PPARγ activation stimulates formation of adipocytes instead of OB. Together these processes suppress normal osteoblastogenesis diverting it to formation of other substances (antioxidants) and cells (adipocytes). Age-related increased GC production/sensitivity and other age-related changes (calcium negative balance, reduced levels of IGF-1, muscle mass, bone hydration and vascularity) ultimately contribute to suppressed bone formation and bone loss. In this slow phase, E deficiency worsens age-related changes. It lowers antioxidant defenses of bone cells and contributes in calcium negative balance.

References

1. Riggs BL, Khosla S, Melton LJ III. Sex steroids and the construction and conservation of the adult skeleton. Endocr Rev. 2002;23:279–302.
2. Melmed S, Polonsky KS, Larsen PR, Kronenberg HM. Williams textbook of endocrinology. In: Bulun SE, editor. Physiology and pathology of female reproductive axis. 12th ed. Philadelphia: Elsevier; 2011. p. 581–644.
3. Manolagas SC, O'Brien CA, Almeida M. The role of estrogen and androgen receptors in bone health and disease. Nat Rev Endocrinol. 2013;9:699–712.
4. Martin-Millan M, Almeida M, Ambrogini E, Han L, Zhao H, Weinstein RS, Jilka RL, O'Brien CA, Manolagas SC. The estrogen receptor α in osteoclasts mediates the protective effects of estrogens on cancellous but not cortical bone. Mol Endocrinol. 2010;24:323–34.
5. Mori G, D'Amelio P, Faccio R, Brunetti G. Bone-immune cell crosstalk: bone diseases. J Immunol Res. 2015;2015:108451. https://doi.org/10.1155/2015108451.
6. Nicks KM, Fowler TW, Gaddy D. Reproductive hormones and bone. Curr Osteoporos Rep. 2010;8:60–7.
7. Chappell PE, Lydon JP, Conneely OM, O'Malley BW, Levine JE. Endocrine defects in mice carrying a null mutation for the progesterone receptor gene. Endocrinology. 1997;138:4147–52.
8. Nicks KM, Perrien DS, Akel NS, Suva LJ, Gaddy D. Regulation of osteoblastogenesis and osteoclastogenesis by the other reproductive hormones, activinand inhibin. Mol Cell Endocrino. 2009;310:11–20.
9. Perrien DS, Akel NS, Edwards PK, Carver AA, Bendre MS, Swain FL, Skinner RA, Hogue WR, Nicks KM, Pierson TM, Suva LJ, Gaddy D. Inhibin A is an endocrine stimulator of bone mass and strength. Endocrinology. 2007;148:1654–65.
10. Melmed S, Polonsky KS, Larsen PR, Kronenberg HM. Williams textbook of endocrinology. In: Styne DM, Grumbach MM, editors. Puberty: ontogeny, neuroendocrinology, physiology, and disorders. 12th ed. Philadelphia: Elsevier; 2011. p. 1055–108.
11. Weaver CM, Gordon CM, Janz KF, et al. The National Osteoporosis Foundation's position statement on peak bone mass development and lifestyle factors: a systematic review and implementation recommendations. Osteoporos Int. 2016;27:1281–386.
12. Berger C, Goltzman D, Langsetmo L, Joseph L, Jackson S, Kreiger N, Tenenhouse A, Davison KS, Josse RG, Prior JC, Hanley DA. Peakbonemassfromlongitudinal data: implications for the prevalence, pathophysiology, and diagnosis of osteoporosis. J Bone Miner Res. 2010;25:1948–57.
13. Manolagas SC. Fromestrogen-centric to aging and oxidative stress: a revised perspective of the pathogenesis of osteoporosis. Endocr Rev. 2010;31(3):266–300.
14. Lean JM, Davies JT, Fuller K, Jagger CJ, Kirstein B, Partington GA, Urry ZL, Chambers TJ. A crucial role forthiolantioxidantsinestrogen-deficiencyboneloss. J Clin Invest. 2003;112:915–23.
15. Muthusami S, Ramachandran I, Muthusamy B, Vasudevan G, Prabhu V, Subramaniam V, Jagadeesan A, Narasimhan S. Ovariectomyinducesoxidativestressandimpairsbone antioxidantsysteminadultrats. Clin Chim Acta. 2005;360:81–6.
16. Almeida M, Han L, Martin-Millan M, Plotkin LI, Stewart SA, Roberson PK, Kousteni S, O'Brien CA, Bellido T, Parfitt AM, Weinstein RS, Jilka RL, Manolagas SC. Skeletal involution by age-associated oxidative stress and its acceleration by loss of sex steroids. J Biol Chem. 2007;282:27285–97.

17. Rizzoli R, Adachi JD, Cooper C, et al. Management of glucocorticoid-induced osteoporosis. Calcif Tissue Int. 2012;91:225–43.
18. Gathercole LL, Lavery GG, Morgan SA, et al. 11β-hydroxysteroid dehydrogenase 1: translational and therapeutic aspects. Endocr Rev. 2013;34(4):525–55.
19. Diaz de Barboza G, Guizzardi S, Tolosa de Talamoni N. Molecular aspects of intestinal calcium absorption. World J Gastroenterol. 2015;21(23):7142–54.

9 Obesity and Osteoporosis: Is the Paradigm Changing?

Emanuela A. Greco, Rachele Fornari, Andrea Lenzi, and Silvia Migliaccio

9.1 Introduction

During the last decades, obesity and osteoporosis have become important global health problems with an increasing prevalence worldwide [1–4], and the belief that obesity is protective against osteoporosis has recently come into question. In fact, the latest epidemiologic and clinical studies have shown that a high level of fat mass might be a risk factor for osteoporosis and fragility fractures [5–8].

Several potential mechanisms have been proposed to explain the complex relationship between the adipose tissue and bone.

For instance, fat has long been viewed as a passive energy reservoir, but since the discovery of leptin and the identification of other adipose tissue-derived hormones and serum mediators [9–11], it has come to be considered as an active endocrine organ involved in the modulation of the energy homeostasis. Adipose tissue, in fact, secretes various inflammatory cytokines, including interleukin (IL)-6, tumor necrosis factor-alpha (TNF-α) resistin, leptin, and adiponectin, which affect human energy and metabolic homeostasis and are involved in bone metabolism [12–15]. Moreover, fat tissue is one of the major sources of aromatase, an enzyme also expressed in the gonads, which synthesizes estrogens from androgen precursors. As known estrogens are steroid hormones which play a pivotal role in the maintenance of skeletal homeostasis, protecting against osteoporosis by reducing bone resorption and stimulating bone formation, and in obese postmenopausal women, increased

E. A. Greco (✉) · R. Fornari · A. Lenzi
Department of Experimental Medicine, Section of Medical Pathophysiology, Endocrinology and Nutrition, Sapienza University of Rome, Rome, Italy
e-mail: emanuela.greco@uniroma1.it

S. Migliaccio
Department of Movement, Human and Health Science, Unit of Endocrinology, University of Foro Italico, Rome, Italy

A. Lenzi, S. Migliaccio (eds.), *Multidisciplinary Approach to Osteoporosis*, https://doi.org/10.1007/978-3-319-75110-8_9

estrogen synthesis by adipose tissue has been suggested as one of the potential mechanisms for the protective effect of fat mass on the bone. Thus, the pathophysiological role of adipose tissue in skeletal homeostasis lies in the production of several adipokines and hormones which modulate bone remodeling via their effects on either bone formation or resorption.

On the other hand, since the demonstration that bone cells express several specific hormone receptors, the skeleton is considered an endocrine target organ [13–16], and since recent observations have shown that bone-derived factors, such as osteocalcin and osteopontin, affect body weight control and glucose homeostasis [17–19], the bone has come to be considered an endocrine organ itself [20]. These considerations suggest a possible role of the bone as a player of a potential feedback mechanism between the skeleton and the other endocrine organs [20]. Thus, the cross talk between fat and bone likely constitutes a homeostatic feedback system in which adipokines and bone-derived molecules represent the link of an active bone-adipose axis.

Finally, adipocytes and osteoblasts originate from a common progenitor, a pluripotential mesenchymal stem cell (MSC) [21], which has an equal propensity for differentiation into adipocytes or osteoblasts (or other lines) under the influence of several cell-derived transcription factors. This process is complex, suggesting significant plasticity and multifaceted mechanism(s) of regulation within different cell lineages, among which are adipocytes and osteoblasts [22, 23].

9.2 Obesity and Osteoporosis: Fat and Bone Metabolism Interplay

Obesity is recognized as a risk factor for metabolic and cardiovascular diseases [2]. However, it has been considered a protective factor for bone loss and osteoporosis, which is defined as a bone metabolic disease, characterized by a decrease in bone strength leading to an increased risk of developing spontaneous and traumatic fractures. Even though body fat and lean mass are linked with bone mineral density (BMD), with obesity apparently exerting protection against bone loss, especially after menopause, during the last decades numerous evidences have described an opposite event, suggesting an inverse relationship between obesity and osteoporosis. In fact recent studies have shown that an increased abdominal fat tissue might be considered a risk factor for osteoporosis [5, 7, 8].

The mechanisms whereby increased central adiposity leads to metabolic alterations, cardiovascular morbidity, and bone loss have been largely based on the demonstration that adipose tissue secretes a number of cytokines and bioactive compounds, named adipokines.

The adipokines, which include a variety of pro-inflammatory peptides, are involved in many physiological or pathological processes, and their disregulation is a strong determinant of the low-grade inflammatory state of obesity, which promotes a cascade of metabolic alterations leading to cardiovascular complications, insulin resistance or diabetes mellitus, and bone loss [9, 11].

Leptin, the first identified adipose tissue-derived factor, is an anorexigenic hormone secreted by adipocytes in proportion to body fat content. Leptin levels are typically elevated in obesity, which is considered a leptin-resistant state [24]. In obese subjects hyperleptinemia has been widely recognized as an independent cardiovascular risk factor associated with hyperinsulinemia and insulin resistance [25] while its effect on the bone is complex, and both negative and positive actions have been reported on BMD [26, 27]. Leptin-deficient ob/ob mice and leptin receptor-deficient db/db mice are extremely obese, with increased vertebral trabecular bone volume due to increased bone formation [28]. Interestingly, intracerebroventricular infusion of leptin in both ob/ob and wild-type mice was shown to decrease vertebral trabecular bone mass [28]. In vivo studies indicate that the effect of leptin might depend on its site and mode of action [29], and it has been proposed that peripheral administration of leptin could increase bone mass by inhibiting bone resorption and increasing bone formation, while inhibiting bone formation through a central nervous system effect [26]. In vitro studies also found that leptin can act directly on bone marrow-derived mesenchymal stem cells (BMSCs) to enhance their differentiation into osteoblasts and to inhibit their differentiation into adipocytes [30]. Finally, leptin inhibits the expression of neuropeptide Y (NPY), a hypothalamus-derived peptide, essential for the regulation of food consumption, energy homeostasis, and bone remodeling [31]. Specific NPY-knockout mice show a significant decrease in body weight, a significant increase in food intake, and twofold increase in trabecular bone volume compared with wild-type animals [32].

Adiponectin exerts a protective role on cardiovascular system and glucose metabolism, and in contrast with leptin, serum adiponectin levels are reduced in obese and diabetic subjects and increase after weight loss [33]. Low levels of adiponectin are a common feature of obesity and correlate with insulin resistance [34]. Adiponectin levels are inversely related to the circulating levels of C-reactive protein (CRP), TNF-α, and IL-6, which are powerful inhibitors of adiponectin expression and secretion in cultured human adipose cells [35]. Human osteoblasts express adiponectin and its receptors, and in vivo and in vitro studies show that adiponectin increases bone mass by suppressing osteoclastogenesis and activating osteoblastogenesis [36], likely indicating that a rise in adiponectin levels, caused by fat reduction, could have a beneficial effect on BMD.

Resistin is produced by macrophages and visceral adipocytes. It is elevated in obesity and regulates insulin sensitivity in the skeletal muscle and liver, and it is positively associated with insulin resistance and glucose tolerance in both human and animal models [37]. Resistin might also play a role in bone remodeling, increasing osteoblast proliferation, cytokine release, and osteoclast differentiation [38].

TNF-α is a pro-inflammatory cytokine which plays important regulatory effects on lipid metabolism, adipocyte function, insulin signaling, and bone remodeling [39]. Its expression has been shown to correlate with percent body fat and insulin resistance in humans [40], and it was further recognized that inflammatory processes predispose to bone loss, giving rise to speculation that inflammatory cytokines, such as IL-6 and TNF-α, may play critical roles in osteoclast activity [41]. Osteoclasts are the unique cells of the body tasked with resorbing the bone, and in the late 1990s, the identification of three different molecules built the bases of the modern bone biology: an osteoclastogenic cytokine, the receptor activator of NF-kB ligand (RANKL), its receptor (RANK), and its inhibitor osteoprotegerin (OPG) [42]. It is now clear that RANKL is the key osteoclastogenic cytokine effector, inducing osteoclast formation and promoting osteoclast resorptive activity, while OPG functions as a decoy receptor, preventing association of RANKL with RANK receptor, thus moderating osteoclastogenesis and bone resorption [43]. It has also become clear that TNF-α promotes RANKL production by BMSCs and mature osteoblasts, reduces OPG production, and upregulates the receptor RANK on osteoclast precursors, increasing their sensitivity to prevailing RANKL concentrations [44]. Additionally, TNF-α turns out to have another property that is relatively unique among the inflammatory cytokines; it has potent effects on osteoclastogenesis as it not only promotes RANKL production but synergizes with RANKL to amplify osteoclastogenesis and to intensify osteoclastic resorption by directly modulating RANKL-induced signal transduction pathways [45]. These effects are likely a consequence of the fact that RANKL is a TNF-superfamily member and functions through many of the same pathways induced by TNF-α itself.

IL-6 is a cytokine, which has a wide range of actions; it is secreted by several cell types, including fibroblast, endothelial cells, and adipocytes; and its plasma levels are significantly upregulated in human obesity and insulin resistance [46]. As TNF-α also IL-6 is a well-recognized stimulator of osteoclastogenesis and bone resorption. Several data show that IL-6 mRNA is expressed in preosteoblasts and osteoblasts [47] and that it stimulates osteoblast proliferation and differentiation by controlling the production of local factor [48]. In addition, IL-6 may play a role in bone formation in conditions of high bone turnover [49].

Emerging evidence points to a critical role for the skeleton in several homeostatic processes including energy balance and adipose metabolism, and the connection between fuel utilization and skeletal remodeling seems to begin in the bone marrow with lineage allocation of MSCs into adipocytes or osteoblasts.

Mature bone cells secrete factors that modulate insulin sensitivity and glucose metabolism, such as osteocalcin (OCN), by which the skeleton could function as an endocrine organ itself [50]. OCN is an osteoblast-specific protein and a major noncollagenous protein in the extracellular matrix. Karsenty and colleagues recently demonstrated that uncarboxylated OCN, acting as a prohormone, can increase β-cell proliferation, insulin secretion, insulin sensitivity, and adiponectin expression [51]. Thus, osteoblasts may be able to regulate glucose metabolism by modulating the bioactivity of OCN. In addition, more recent studies showed that OCN bioactivity is modulated by enhanced sympathetic tone driven by leptin, which has been shown to suppress insulin secretion by β-cells [52], and three recent studies have demonstrated an inverse correlation between serum OCN and plasma glucose levels, supporting a role for this pathway in humans [53]. Thus, a novel picture has emerged linking glucose metabolism, adipose stores, and skeletal activity.

Since its first description more than 20 years ago, osteopontin (OPN) has emerged as an active player in many physiological and pathological processes, including biomineralization, tissue remodeling, and inflammation. Modulation of immune cell response by OPN has been associated with various inflammatory diseases and may play a pivotal role in the development of adipose tissue inflammation, insulin resistance, and diabetes [54]. OPN expression is significantly upregulated by 40- and 80-fold in adipose tissue from diet-induced and genetically obese mice, respectively [55]. Moreover, it has been demonstrated that OPN expression in adipose tissue and circulating OPN levels were substantially elevated in obese, diabetic, and insulin-resistant patients compared with lean subjects and conversely that dietary weight loss significantly decreased OPN concentrations [56, 57].

9.3 Fat Bone Marrow and Osteoporosis: Cause or Consequence?

Adipocytes and osteoblasts originate from a common progenitor, a pluripotential MSC [58], which has an equal propensity for differentiation into adipocytes or osteoblasts or other lines, such as chondrocytes, fibroblast, and endothelial cells, under the influence of several cell-derived transcription factors. This process is complex, suggesting significant plasticity and multifaceted mechanism(s) of regulation within different cell lineages, among which are adipocytes and osteoblasts [24, 59].

Transdifferentiation is the irreversible switching of differentiated cells that sometimes occurs during disease [60], and it interests partially differentiated cells (e.g., preosteoblasts) that switches to another lineage (e.g., adipocytes) [61].

Fat bone marrow is indicative of aging and it is frequently observed in the presence of osteoporosis, especially in postmenopausal women [62]. One possible cause of bone marrow fat deposition is the aberrant commitment of BMMSCs into adipocytes due to their inability to differentiate into other cell lineages, such as osteoblasts. There exists an inverse relationship between bone marrow fat production and bone formation during osteoporosis; in fact an inhibited adipogenesis in patients with a high bone mass has been observed [63].

Recently, a correlation between the osteo-adipogenic transdifferentiation of bone marrow cells and numerous bone metabolism diseases has been established. Human BMMSC-derived osteoblasts, adipocytes, and chondrocytes had the potential to transdifferentiate to each lineage, and these findings provided new insights on the pathogenesis of skeletal diseases such as osteoporosis [64].

Estrogens can regulate several molecular signals within bone metabolism and play an important role in the development of bone marrow fat [65–68]. After menopause an increase in adipogenic switches in bone marrow and a decrease in bone mass have been observed [69, 70]. Several human and animal studies have examined the function of adipocytes in bone marrow. Mesenchymal stem cells isolated from bone marrow in postmenopausal osteoporotic patients express more adipose differentiation markers than those from subjects with normal bone mass [25], and pronounced fatty infiltration in the bone marrow of rats following oophorectomy has been observed, suggesting a pivotal role of estrogen in regulating adipocyte and osteoblast recruitment [26]. More recent studies have shown that estrogens are negative regulators of adipogenesis, and they are essential for osteogenic commitment; in particular, it seems that estrogens simultaneously induce osteogenesis and inhibits adipogenesis both in vivo and in vitro [71–73], and it has been demonstrated that estrogens suppress osteo-adipogenic transdifferentiation via canonical Wnt signaling, an important system which regulates bone development, adipogenic differentiation, and gene expression in whole process of bone metabolism [63, 74]. Specifically, canonical Wnt/β-catenin signaling is highly expressed in mesenchymal precursor cells and pluripotent cells, especially toward the osteoblast lineage, while it inhibits adipogenic differentiation [75]. Canonical Wnt signaling stabilizes and promotes cellular and nuclear β-catenin levels, which inhibits adipogenesis [75], and the suppression of Wnt signaling is essential for PPARγ induction and preadipocyte differentiation [76].

PPARγ plays a central role in initiating adipogenesis, and mutations of the PPARγ gene are associated with an altered balance between bone and fat formation in the bone marrow [59]. PPARγ insufficiency led to increased osteoblastogenesis in vitro and higher trabecular bone volume in vivo, confirming the key role of mesenchymal stem cell lineage allocation in the skeleton [58]. Interestingly, aged mice exhibit fat infiltration into bone marrow and enhanced expression of PPARγ, along with reduced mRNA expression of bone differentiation factors [77], and mice with premature aging (the SAM-P/6 model) show nearly identical patterns of adipocyte infiltration, with impaired osteoblastogenesis [78], indicating that aging or events that accelerate aging result in significant bone marrow adiposity and a defect in osteoblastogenesis in mice [79].

Conclusions

Body fat and bone interplay through several adipokines and bone-derived molecules, which modulate bone remodeling, adipogenesis, body weight control, and glucose homeostasis.

Thus, the existence of a cross talk between fat and the skeleton suggests a homeostatic feedback system in which adipokines and bone-derived molecules form part of an active bone-adipose axis, which due also its peculiarity to the common origin of osteoblasts and adipocytes from a pluripotent mesenchymal stem cell.

When specific conditions occur, such as aging, menopause, or diseases as osteoporosis, obesity, or metabolic alterations, it has been observed an osteo-adipogenic transdifferentiation and an aberrant commitment of BMMSCs into adipocytes because of their inability to differentiate into other cell lineages, such as osteoblasts.

However, the mechanism(s) by which all these events occur remains unclear, and this molecular control could be crucial to understand the pathogenesis of both obesity and osteoporosis.

References

1. Kado DM, Huang MH, Karlamangla AS, Barrett-Connor E, Greendale GA. Hyperkyphotic posture predicts mortality in older community-dwelling men and women: a prospective study. J Am Geriatr Soc. 2004;52:1662–7.
2. Rossner S. Obesity: the disease of the twenty-first century. Int J Obes Relat Metab Disord. 2002;26(Suppl 4):S2–4.

3. Hu FB. Overweight and obesity in women: health risks and consequences. J Women Health (Larchmt). 2003;12(2):163–72.
4. Obesity: preventing and managing the global epidemic. Report of a WHO consultation. World Health Organ Tech Rep Ser. 2000;894:1–253.
5. Greco EA, Fornari R, Rossi F, Santiemma V, Prossomariti G, Annoscia C, Aversa A, Brama M, Marini M, Donini LM, Spera G, Lenzi A, Lubrano C, Migliaccio S. Is obesity protective for osteoporosis? Evaluation of bone mineral density in individuals with high body mass index. Int J Clin Pract. 2010;64(6):817–20.
6. Kim KC, Shin DH, Lee SY, Im JA, Lee DC. Relation between obesity and bone mineral density and vertebral fractures in Korean postmenopausal women. Yonsei Med J. 2010;51(6):857–63.
7. Greco EA, Francomano D, Fornari R, Marocco C, Lubrano C, Papa V, Wannenes F, Di Luigi L, Donini LM, Lenzi A, Aversa A, Migliaccio S. Negative association between trunk fat, insulin resistance and skeleton in obese women. World J Diabetes. 2013;4(2):31–9.
8. Compston JE, Flahive J, Hosmer DV, Watts NB, Siris ES, Silverman S, Saag KG, Roux C, Rossini M, Pfeilschiffer J, Nieves JW, Netelenbos JC, March L, LaCroix AZ, Hooven FH, Greenspan SL, Gehlbach SH, Diez-Perez A, Cooper C, Chapurlat RD, Boonen S, Anderson FA Jr, Adami S, Adachi JD, GLOW Investigators. Relationship of weight, height, and body mass index with fracture risk at different sites in postmenopausal women: the Global Longitudinal study of Osteoporosis in Women (GLOW). J Bone Miner Res. 2014;29(2):487–93.
9. Kadowaki T, Yamauchi T. Adiponectin and adiponectin receptors. Endocr Rev. 2005;26:439–51.
10. Steppan CM, Crawford DT, Chidsey-Frink KL, Ke H, Swick AG. Leptin is a potent stimulator of bone growth in ob/ob mice. Regul Pept. 2000;92:73–8.
11. Vendrell J, Broch M, Vilarrasa N, Molina A, Gomez JM, Gutierrez C, Simon I, Soler J, Richart C. Resistin, adiponectin, ghrelin, leptin, and proinflammatory cytokines: relationships in obesity. Obes Res. 2004;12:962–71.
12. Magni P, Dozio E, Galliera E, Ruscica M, Corsi MM. Molecular aspects of adipokine-bone interactions. Curr Mol Med. 2010;10(6):522–32.
13. Eriksen EF, Colvard DS, Berg NJ, Graham ML, Mann KG, Spelsberg TC, Riggs BL. Evidence of estrogen receptors in normal human osteoblast-like cells. Science. 1988;241(4861):84–6.
14. Kim HJ. New understanding of glucocorticoid action in bone cells. BMB Rep. 2010;43(8):524–9.
15. Komm BS, Terpening CM, Benz DJ, Graeme KA, Gallegos A, Korc M, Greene GL, O'Malley BW, Haussler MR. Estrogen binding, receptor mRNA, and biologic response in osteoblast-like osteosarcoma cells. Science. 1988;241(4861):81–4.
16. Migliaccio S, Davis VL, Gibson MK, Gray TK, Korach KS. Estrogens modulate the responsiveness of osteoblast-like cells (ROS 17/2.8) stably transfected with estrogen receptor. Endocrinology. 1992;130(5):2617–24.
17. Gomez-Ambrosi J, Rodrıguez A, Catalan V, Fruhbeck G. The bone-adipose axis in obesity and weight loss. Obes Surg. 2008;18:1134–43.
18. Takeda S. Effect of obesity on bone metabolism. Clin Calcium. 2008;18:632–7.
19. Gimble JM, Zvonic S, Floyd ZE, Kassem M, Nuttall ME. Playing with bone and fat. J Cell Biochem. 2006;98:251–66.
20. Fukumoto S, Martrin TJ. Bone as an endocrine organ. Trends Endocrinol Metab. 2009; 20(5):230–6.
21. Akune T, Ohba S, Kamekura S, Yamaguchi M, Chung UI, Kubota N, Terauchi Y, Harada Y, Azuma Y, Nakamura K, Kadowaki T, Kawaguchi H. PPARγ insufficiency enhances osteogenesis through osteoblast formation from bone marrow progenitors. J Clin Invest. 2004; 113:846–55.
22. Gimble JM, Robinson CE, Wu X, Kelly KA, Rodriguez BR, Kliewer SA, Lehmann JM, Morris DC. Peroxisome proliferator activated receptor-gamma activation by thiazolidinediones induces adipogenesis in bone marrow stromal cells. Mol Pharmacol. 1996;50:1087–94.
23. Rodriguez JP, Montecinos L, Rios S, Reyes P, Martinez J. Mesenchymal stem cells from osteoporotic patients produce a type I collagen-deficient extracellular matrix favoring adipogenic differentiation. J Cell Biochem. 2000;79:557–65.
24. Considine RV, Sinha MK, Heiman ML, Kriauciunas A, Stephens TW, Nyce MR, Ohannesian JP, Marco CC, McKee LJ, Bauer TL, Caro JF. Serum immunoreactive leptin concentrations in normal-weight and obese humans. N Engl J Med. 1996;34:292–5.

25. Martin SS, Qasim A, Reilly MP. Leptin resistance: a possible interface of inflammation and metabolism in obesity-related cardiovascular disease. J Am Coll Cardiol. 2008;52:1201–10.
26. Kontogianni MD, Dafni UG, Routsias JG, Skopouli FN. Blood leptin and adiponectin as possible mediators of the relation between fat mass and BMD in perimenopausal women. J Bone Miner Res. 2004;19:546–55.
27. Goulding A, Taylor RW. Plasma leptin values in relation to bone mass and density and to dynamic biochemical markers of bone resorption and formation in postmenopausal women. Calcif Tissue Int. 1998;63:456–8.
28. Ducy P, Amling M, Takeda S, Priemel M, Schilling AF, Beil FT, Shen J, Vinson C, Rueger JM, Karsenty G. Leptin inhibits bone formation through a hypothalamic relay: a central control of bone mass. Cell. 2000;100:197–207.
29. Thomas T. The complex effects of leptin on bone metabolism through multiple pathways. Curr Opin Pharmacol. 2004;4:295–300.
30. Thomas T, Gori F, Khosla S, Jensen MD, Burguera B, Riggs BL. Leptin acts on human marrow stromal cells to enhance differentiation to osteoblasts and to inhibit differentiation to adipocytes. Endocrinology. 1999;140:1630–8.
31. Baldock PA, Sainsbury A, Couzens M, Enriquez RF, Thomas GP, Gardiner EM, Herzog H. Hypothalamic Y2 receptors regulate bone formation. J Clin Invest. 2002;109:915–21.
32. Sainsbury A, Schwarzer C, Couzens M, Fetissov S, Furtinger S, Jenkins A, cox HM, Sperk G, Hokfelt T, Herzog H. Important role of hypothalamic Y2 receptors in body weight regulation revealed in conditional knockout mice. Proc Natl Acad Sci U S A. 2002;99:8938–43.
33. Pajvani UB, Du X, Combs TP, Berg AH, Rajala MW, Schulthess T, Engel J, Brownlee M, Scherer PE. Structure-function studies of the adipocytes-secreted hormone Acrp30/adiponectin. Implications for metabolic regulation and bioactivity. J Biol Chem. 2003;278:9073–85.
34. Yamauchi T, Kamon J, Waki H, Terauchi Y, Kubota N, Hara K, Mori Y, Ide T, Murakami K, Tsuboyama-Kasaoka N, Ezaki O, Akanuma Y, Gavrilova O, Vinson C, Reitman ML, Kagechika H, Shudio K, Yoda M, Nakano Y, Tobe K, Nagai R, Kimura S, Tomita M, Froguel P, Kadowaki T. The fat-derived hormone adiponectin reverses insulin resistance associated with body lipoatrophy and obesity. Nat Med. 2001;7:941–6.
35. Fasshauer M, Klein J, Neumann S, Eszlinger M, Paschke R. Hormonal regulation of adiponectin gene expression in 3T3-L1 adipocytes. Biochem Biophys Res Commun. 2002;290: 1084–9.
36. Jurimae J, Rembel K, Jurimae T, Rehand M. Adiponectin is associated with bone mineral density in perimenopausal women. Horm Metab Res. 2005;37:297–302.
37. Ukkola O. Resistin–a mediator of obesity-associated insulin resistance or an innocent bystander? Eur J Endocrinol. 2002;147:571–4.
38. Thommesen L, Stunes AK, Monjo M, Grosvik K, Tamburstuen MV, Kjobli E, Lyngstadaas SP, Reseland JE, Syversen U. Expression and regulation of resistin in osteoblasts and osteoclasts indicate a role in bone metabolism. J Cell Biochem. 2006;99(3):824–34.
39. Fasshauer M, Klein J, Krahlisch S, Lossner U, Klier M, Bluher M, Paschke R. GH is a positive regulator of tumor necrosis factor-alpha-induced adipose related protein in 3T3-L1 adipocytes. J Endocrinol. 2003;178:523–31.
40. Hotamisligil G, Arner P, Caro J, Atkinson R, Spiegelman B. Increased adipose tissue expression of tumor necrosis factor-alpha in human obesity and insulin resistance. J Clin Invest. 1995;95:2409–15.
41. Pacifici R, Brown C, Puscheck E, Friedrich E, Slatopolsky E, Maggio D, McCracken R, Avioli LV. Effect of surgical menopause and estrogen replacement on cytokine release from human blood mononuclear cells. Proc Natl Acad Sci U S A. 1991;88(12):5134–8.
42. Simonet WS, Lacey DL, Dunstan CR, Kelley M, Chang MS, Luthy R, Nguyen HQ, Wooden S, Bennet L, Boone T, Shimamoto G, DeRose M, Elliot R, Colombero A, Tan HL, Trail G, Sullivan J, Davy E, Bucay N, Renshaw-Gegg L, Hughes TM, Hill D, Pattison W, Campbell P, Sander S, Van G, Tarpley J, Derby P, Lee R, Boyle WJ. Osteoprotegerin: a novel secreted protein involved in the regulation of bone density. Cell. 1997;89(2):309–19.

43. Anderson DM, Maraskovsky E, Billingsley WL, Dougall WC, Tometsko ME, Roux ER, Teepe MC, DuBose RF, Cosman D, Galibert L. A homologue of the TNF receptor and its ligand enhance T-cell growth and dendritic-cell function. Nature. 1997;390(6656):175–9.
44. Wei S, Kitaura H, Zhou P, Ross P, Teitelbaum SL. IL-1 mediates TNFα-induce osteoclastogenesis. J Clin Invest. 2005;115(2):282–90.
45. Cenci S, Weitzmann MN, Roggia C, Namba N, Novack D, Woodring J, Pacifici R. Estrogen deficiency induces bone loss by enhancing T-cell production of TNF-α. J Clin Invest. 2000;106(10):1229–37.
46. Vozarova B, Weyer C, Hanson K, Tataranni PA, Bogardus C, Pratley RE. Circulating IL-6 in relation to adiposity, insulin action and insulin secretion. Obes Res. 2001;9:414–7.
47. Dodds A, Merry K, Littlewood A, Gowen M. Expression of mRNA for IL1 beta, IL6 and TGF beta 1 in developing human bone and cartilage. J Histochem Cytochem. 1994;42:733–44.
48. Taguchi Y, Yamamoto M, Yamate T, Lin SC, Mocharla H, DeTogni P, Nakayama N, Boyce BF, Abe E, Manolagas SC. Interleukin-6-type cytokines stimulate mesenchymal progenitor differentiation toward the osteoblastic lineage. Proc Assoc Am Physicians. 1998;110:559–74.
49. Sims NA, Jenkins BJ, Quinn JM, Nakamura A, Glatt M, Gillespie MT, Ernst M, Martin TJ. Glycoprotein 130 regulates bone turnover and bone size by distinct downstream signaling pathways. J Clin Invest. 2004;113:379–89.
50. Lee NK, Sowa H, Hinoi E, Ferron M, Ahn JD, Confavreux C, Dacquin R, Mee PJ, McKee MD, Jung DY, Zhang Z, Kim JK, Mauvais-Jarvis F, Ducy P, Karsenty G. Endocrine regulation of energy metabolism by the skeleton. Cell. 2007;130:456–69.
51. Ferron M, Hinoi E, Karsenty G, Ducy P. Osteocalcin differentially regulates beta cell and dipocyte gene expression and affects the development of metabolic diseases in wild-type mice. Proc Natl Acad Sci U S A. 2008;105:5266–70.
52. Hinoi E, Gao N, Jung DY, Yadav V, Yoshizawa T, Myers MG Jr, Chua SC Jr, Kim JK, Kaestner KH, Karsenty G. The sympathetic tone mediates leptin's inhibition of insulin secretion by modulating osteocalcin bioactivity. J Cell Biol. 2008;183:1235–42.
53. Covey SD, Wideman RD, McDonald C, Unniappan S, Huynh F, Asadi A, Speck M, Webber T, Chua SC, Kieffer TJ. The pancreatic beta cell is a key site for mediating the effects of leptin on glucose homeostasis. Cell Metab. 2006;4:291–302.
54. Scatena M, Liaw L, Giachelli CM. Osteopontin: a multifunctional molecule regulating chronic inflammation and vascular disease. Arterioscler Thromb Vasc Biol. 2007;27:2302–9.
55. Kiefer FW, Zeyda M, Todoric J, Huber J, Geyeregger R, Weichhart T, Aszmann O, Ludvik B, Silberhumer GR, Prager G, Stulnig TM. Osteopontin expression in human and murine obesity: extensive local up-regulation in adipose tissue but minimal systemic alterations. Endocrinology. 2008;149:1350–7.
56. Sarac F, Basoglu OK, Gunduz C, Bayrak H, Biray Avci C, Akcicek F. Association of osteopontin and tumor necrosis factor-alpha levels with insulin resistance in obese patients with obstructive sleep apnea syndrome. J Endocrinol Invest. 2011;34:528–33.
57. You JS, Ji HI, Chang KJ, Yoo MC, Yang HI, Jeong IK, Kim KS. Serum osteopontin concentration is decreased by exercise-induced fat loss but is not correlated with body fat percentage in obese humans. Mol Med Rep. 2013;8:579–84.
58. Sekiya I, Larson BL, Vuoristo JT, Cui JG, Prockop DJ. Adipogenic differentiation of human adult stem cells from bone marrow stroma (MSCs). J Bone Miner Res. 2004;19:256–64.
59. Martin RB, Zissimos SL. Relationships between marrow fat and bone turnover in ovariectomized and intact rats. Bone. 1991;12:123–31.
60. Burke ZD, Tosh D. Therapeutic potential of transdifferentiated cells. Clin Sci (Lond). 2005; 108:309–21.
61. Schilling T, Kuffner R, Klein-Hitpass L, Zimmer R, Jakob F, Schutze N. Microarray analyses of transdifferentiated mesenchymal stem cells. J Cell Biochem. 2008;103:413–33.
62. Menagh PJ, Turner RT, Jump DB, Wong CP, Lowry MB, Yakar S, Rosen CJ, Iwaniec UT. Growth hormone regulates the balance between bone formation and bone marrow adiposity. J Bone Miner Res. 2010;25:757–68.

63. Gao B, Huang Q, Lin Y-S, Wei B-Y, Guo Y-S, Sun Z, Wang L, Fan J, Zhang H-Y, Han Y-H, Li X-J, Shi J, Liu J, Yang L, Luo Z-J. Dose-dependent effect of estrogen suppresses the osteo-adipogenic transdifferentiation of osteoblasts via canonical wnt signaling pathway. PLoS One. 2014;9(6):e-99137.
64. Song L, Tuan RS. Transdifferentiation potential of human mesenchymal stem cells derived from bone marrow. FASEB J. 2004;18:980–2.
65. Abdallah BM, Ditzel N, Mahmood A, Isa A, Traustadottir GA, Schilling AF, ruiz-hidalgo MJ, Laborda J, Amling M, Kassem M. DLK1 is a novel regulator of bone mass that mediates estrogen deficiency induced bone loss in mice. J Bone Miner Res. 2011;26:1457–71.
66. Kamiya Y, Chen J, Xu M, Utreja A, Choi T, Drissi H, Wadhwa S. Increased mandibular condylar growth in mice with estrogen receptor beta deficiency. J Bone Miner Res. 2013;28:1127–34.
67. Song L, Zhao J, Zhang X, Li H, Zhou Y. Icariin induces osteoblast proliferation, differentiation and mineralization through estrogen receptor mediated ERK and JNK signal activation. Eur J Pharmacol. 2013;714:15–22.
68. Pierroz DD, Rufo A, Bianchi EN, Glatt V, Capulli M, Rucci N, Cavat F, Rizzoli R, Teti A, Bouxsein ML, Ferrari SL. Beta Arrestin2 regulates RANKL and ephrins gene expression in response to bone remodeling in mice. J Bone Miner Res. 2009;24:775–84.
69. Justesen J, Stenderup K, Ebbesen EN, Mosekilde L, Steiniche T, Kassem M. Adipocyte tissue volume in bone marrow is increased with aging and in patients with osteoporosis. Biogerontology. 2001;2:165–71.
70. Gambacciani M, Ciaponi M, Cappagli B, Piaggesi L, De Simone L, Orlandi R, genazzani AR. Body weight, body fat distribution, and hormonal replacement therapy in early postmenopausal women. J Clin Endocrinol Metab. 1997;82:414–7.
71. Guo YF, Xiong DH, Shen H, Zhao LJ, Xiao P, guo Y, Wang W, Yang TL, Recker RR, Deng HW. Polymorphisms of the low-density lipoprotein receptor-related protein 5 (LRP5) gene are associated with obesity phenotypes in a large family-based association study. J Med Genet. 2006;43:798–803.
72. Mani A, Radhakrishnan J, Wang H, Mani A, Mani MA, Nelson-William C, Carew KS, Mane S, Najmabadi H, Wu D, Lifton RP. LRP6 mutation in a family with early coronary disease and metabolic risk factors. Science. 2007;315:1278–82.
73. Grant SF, Thorleifsson G, Reynisdottir I, Benediktsson R, Manolescu A, Sainz J, Helgason A, Stefansson H, Emilsson V, Helgadottir A, Styrkarsdottir U, Magnusson KP, walters GB, Palsdottir E, Jonsdottir T, Gudmundsdottir T, Gylfason A, Saemundsdottir J, Wilensky RL, Reilly MP, Rader DJ, Bagger Y, Christiansen C, Gudnason V, Sigurdsson G, Thorsteinsdottir U, Gulcher JR, Kong A, Stefansson K. Variant of transcription factor 7-like 2 (TCF7L2) gene confers risk of type 2 diabetes. Nat Genet. 2006;38:320–3.
74. Colaianni G, Brunetti G, Faienza MF, Colucci S, Grano M. Osteoporosis and obesity: role of Wnt pathway in human and murine models. World J Orthop. 2014;5(3):242–6.
75. Krishnan V, Bryant HU, Macdougald OA. Regulation of bone mass by Wnt signaling. J Clin Invest. 2006;116:1202–9.
76. Qiu W, Chen L, Kassem M. Activation of non-canonical Wnt/JNK pathway by Wnt3a is associated with differentiation fate determination of human bone marrow stromal (mesenchymal) stem cells. Biochem Biophys Res Commun. 2011;413:98–104.
77. Moerman EJ, Teng K, Lipschitz DA, Lecka-Czernik B. Aging activates adipogenic and suppresses osteogenic programs in mesenchymal marrow stroma/stem cells: the role of PPAR-γ^2-transcription factor and TGF-β/BMP signaling pathways. Aging Cell. 2004;3:379–89.
78. Kajkenova O, Lecka-Czernik B, Gubrij I, Hauser SP, Takahashi K, Parfitt AM, Jilka RL, Manolagas SC, Lipschitz DA. Increased adipogenesis and myelopoiesis in the bone marrow of SAMP6: a murine model of defective osteoblastogenesis and low turnover osteopenia. J Bone Miner Res. 1997;12:1772–9.
79. Duque G, Macoritto M, Kremer R. Vitamin D treatment of senescence accelerated mice (SAM-P/6) induces several regulators of stromal cell plasticity. Biogerontology. 2004;5:421–9.

Bone and Diabetes

10

Andrea Palermo, Anda Mihaela Naciu, Gaia Tabacco, Luca D'Onofrio, and Nicola Napoli

10.1 Introduction

Diabetes is a metabolic disease characterized by high blood glucose levels resulting from impaired insulin production or insulin resistance or both. It has been well established that bone fragility is a new complication of diabetes, particularly of type 1 diabetes (T1D) [1]. Diabetes may negatively affect bone health by unbalancing several processes and systems: bone formation, bone resorption, collagen formation and collagen cross-linking, secretion of inflammatory cytokines, skeletal muscle, incretin system, bone marrow adiposity, calcium metabolism, etc.

Lower bone mass in T1D and compromised skeletal quality despite preserved bone density in type 2 (T2D) diabetes identified two different bone phenotypes that may reflect the peculiar pathophysiological background of the two types of diabetes. Indeed, although T1D and T2D share hyperglycaemia as their main hallmark, they are heterogeneous diseases whose aetiology and clinical presentation differ considerably. T1D is an autoimmune disease characterized by beta-cell destruction (usually leading to absolute insulin deficiency), and inflammation related to the autoimmune activation. T2D is due to a progressive loss of insulin secretion on the background of insulin resistance. In T2D, there is a "chronic low grade inflammation" that is directly related to "visceral obesity" and insulin resistance. Moreover, several anti-diabetic drugs can affect the bone strength.

A. Palermo · A. M. Naciu · G. Tabacco · N. Napoli (✉)
Unit of Endocrinology and Diabetes, Campus Bio-Medico University, Rome, Italy

L. D'Onofrio
Department of Experimental Medicine, "Sapienza" University of Rome, Rome, Italy

A. Lenzi, S. Migliaccio (eds.), *Multidisciplinary Approach to Osteoporosis*,
https://doi.org/10.1007/978-3-319-75110-8_10

10.2 Fracture Risk in Diabetes Mellitus

10.2.1 Type 1 Diabetes

Between 1927 and 1964, it has been published some papers that suggested an increased prevalence of fragility fractures in T1D [1]. One of the first important proofs of the diabetes induced bone fragility is represented by the results of the Iowa Women's Health Study, an 11-year follow-up of 32,089 postmenopausal women [2]. Hip fractures were found to be 12-times more common in women with T1DM compared to matched controls. Instead, men with T1D were found to have a 17.8 fold increased risk of hip fractures in a 6-year follow-up of a large cohort of Norwegian subjects [3]. These findings were confirmed by Miao et al. with 8–12 fold increase in hip fracture risk in a Swedish cohort of more than 99 24,000 patients with T1D [4]. In 2007, Vestergaard [5] and Janghorbani [6] published two large meta-analyses that reported, respectively, 6.9 and 6.3 fold increase in hip fracture risk in patients with T1D compared to subjects without diabetes. Although no large studies have evaluated the risk of vertebral fracture in T1D, there is data suggesting higher prevalence of clinical (OR = 2.5 95% CI: 1.3–4.6) [7] and morphometric vertebral fractures [8]. A more recent meta-analysis showed that T1D was associated with a three-fold higher risk of any fracture [9]. Moreover, a retrospective cohort study from the THIN database in the UK established the association between T1D and increased risk of fracture of lower extremities [10].

10.2.2 Type 2 Diabetes

Although T2D is less strong characterized by fragility fractures compared to T1D [11], evidence accumulated during the past two decades suggests that there is a three times increased risk of hip and other non-vertebral fractures [5, 6]. In particular, large studies such as the Health, Ageing, And Body Composition Study [12] and Women's Health Initiative Observational Study [13] reported that type 2 diabetes was associated, respectively, with 64% and 20% increase in fractures at all sites compared with non-diabetic subjects, despite a higher baseline BMD. Furthermore, in a systematic review of 16 independent observational studies, T2D was associated with two to three times greater risk of hip fracture in both men and women than individuals without diabetes [6]. Chinese [14] and Mexican-American and non-Hispanic black individuals [15] have also shown an increased risk of hip fracture in those with type 2 diabetes compared with non-diabetics. Contrasting evidence has been provided regarding the association between vertebral fracture and T2D, although a significant or a trend towards an increased vertebral fracture risk has been recorded [12, 13, 16].

Moreover, it is still not fully elucidated the impact of T2D on non-axial bones. Indeed, many studies have shown an increased risk of ankle, humerus and foot fractures [17, 18] instead, a meta-analysis published in 2007 [6] has documented no change in fracture risk.

10.3 Pathophysiology of Bone Fragility in Patients with Diabetes

10.3.1 Type 1 and Type 2 Diabetes: Insulin Deficiency, Hyperinsulinaemia and Insulin Resistance

10.3.1.1 Insulin Deficiency

Insulin has a key role in bone metabolism. Insulin receptor (IR) is expressed on osteoblasts and osteoclasts surface. Particularly, in vitro [19] and in vivo [20] studies showed that insulin increased osteoblast proliferation and upgrade osteoblast differentiation, with a better bone formation rate. Insulin stimulation works by activating the substrate of the insulin receptor (IRS), which activates the intracellular MAPK and PI3-K/Akt pathways that are necessary for osteoblasts growth, osteoblast differentiation and survival of osteoblasts. Therefore, dysfunction of osteoblasts may result from impaired insulin signaling. Indirectly, insulin may also affect osteoclast function, across the insulin signaling pathway inside the osteoblast.

Particularly, IRS-1, which is located only on the osteoblast surface, is required to develop osteoclast differentiation factors such as the receptor activator of nuclear factor kappa-B ligand (RANKL)/osteoclast differentiation factor (ODF) [21].

Some in vivo studies evidence that insulin could restore the damage of osteoclast and osteoblast function in association with diabetes. In fact, up-regulation of osteoclastogenesis and down-regulation of osteoblastogenesis were inverted by insulin therapy, in STZ induced diabetic rats [22]. This observation was also confirmed in human, in a study that included 62 patients with new onset T1D, in whom stabilization of bone mineral density (BMD) at all sites was associated with insulin therapy for 7 years [23]. Moreover, studies in humans indicate a prospective interplay between insulin and the osteoclastic pathway. Another study demonstrated that in newly diagnosed T1D patients insulin therapy significantly decreases OPG levels [24]. An upgrade in endothelium-dependent arterial dilation was associated with changes in OPG levels. Unluckily, this outcome does not provide an idea in what way insulin affects bone resorption in vivo.

C-peptide is another factor that can also affect bone strength. It has been previously proved that C-peptide can exert extra-pancreatic effects on various metabolic pathways connected to cancer development and to the cardiovascular system [25]. There were conducted a couple of population-based cross-sectional studies to explore the association between BMD and c-peptide, with contradictory results. Particularly, Hsu et al. showed that C-peptide serum levels were notably negatively associated with most regional BMD in more than 6000 subjects without diabetes. The majority of these associations remained significant following stratification based on insulin levels in the serum [25]. In another study, Montalcini et al. showed that lumbar BMD was positively associated with C-peptide levels, unrelated with insulin levels [26]. In the only one cross-sectional study conducted in men and postmenopausal women with TD2, urinary C-peptide (a marker of insulin secretion) was positively correlated with femoral BMD in both genders; in women, it was negatively related with vertebral fractures presence [27].

10.3.1.2 IGF-1

Insulin-like growth factor 1 (IGF-1), also called somatomedin C and IR pathways are necessary for bone health [28]. In fact, the IGF receptor is expressed on osteoblasts surface [29], and IRS-1 and IRS-2 are important mediators in the IGF signaling cascade [30].

Teen T1D patients have low levels of IGF-1 confronted with healthy control subjects [28]. Other factors such as earlier age at diagnosis and poor metabolic control were predictive of lower IGF-1 in these patients [28]. It has also been proved that the reduction of IGF-1 is associated with low femoral and lumbar spine BMD.

Despite the fact that low levels of IGF-1 seems to be a hallmark of T1D, some studies have reported a relationship between decreased serum IGF-1 and vertebral fractures in post-menopausal women with T2D [31].

10.3.1.3 Hyperinsulinaemia and Insulin Resistance

Hyperinsulinaemia and insulin resistance are the features of T2D. Relative increase in BMD observed in T2D patients compared to subjects without diabetes might be explained by high levels of insulin. In some cross-sectional studies has been demonstrated the positive correlation between insulin and BMD [32, 33]. In fact, conditions such as metabolic syndrome, polycystic ovary syndrome or lipodystrophy, that are associated with hyperinsulinaemia, are characterized by high BMD levels.

On the other hand, some investigators have demonstrated that insulin may be negatively correlated with bone mass, despite the fact that this was probably due to insulin resistance rather than to a "harmful" effect of insulin itself [34]. This report is supported by the evidence that insulin appears to be positively correlated with bone mass, but this correlation is inverted after adjusting for body weight [34].

However, insulin resistance may have a significant role in the bone impairment observed in T2D. In several studies has been already shown that a damage in insulin signaling in osteoblasts can negatively affect bone mass and bone quality (cortical porosity) [21, 35], and insulin resistance may change insulin signaling in osteoblasts. Particularly, insulin resistance was correlated with higher BMD with no dependence and after adjustment for BMI [36].

This outcome was confirmed by Shin and colleagues, who have demonstrated that insulin resistance (evaluated by HOMA-IR) and fasting plasma insulin levels were negatively correlated with BMD in a large cohort of more than 3000 Korean men aged ≥20 years [37]. Furthermore, insulin resistance caused by elevated levels of free saturated fatty acids is correlated with decreased circulating levels of osteocalcin (OC), which in turn brings to a declined insulin sensitivity in skeletal muscle.

10.3.2 Type 1 and Type 2 Diabetes and Bone Health: Common Pathways for the Bone Fragility

10.3.2.1 Glucose Toxicity on Bone Formation

Osteoblast

Hyperglycaemia exercises destructive effects on *osteoblastogenesis* from the first differentiation step. Osteoblasts derive from mesenchymal stem cells (MSC), and

MSC viability and clonogenicity may be reduced by high glucose concentrations. Hyperglycaemia exerts an unfavourable effect on *Wnt/β-catenin signalling*. Some studies made on STZ diabetic rats have demonstrated a reduction of β-catenin and an increased expression of the Wnt signalling inhibitors SOST and Dickkopf-related protein 1 (Dkk1) [38]. Bone marrow stromal cells (BMSC) faced to high glucose show increased adipogenic pathway. Consequently, diabetes correlated to hyperglycaemia may increase proliferator-activated receptor γ (PPARγ 2) expression and decrease runt-related transcription factor 2 (RUNX2), ALP and OC expression in osteoblasts. Adipogenesis appears to be precipitated by chronic rather than acute hyperglycaemia.

One of the mechanisms that can describe the stimulation of adipogenesis over osteoblastogenesis involves the PI3K/Akt pathway, which is stimulated by reactive oxygen species (ROS) correlated with hyperglycaemia. Additionally, advanced glycation end-products (AGEs) owing to prolonged hyperglycaemia could decrease RUNX2, OC and osterix expression [39].

The impairment in osteoblast function may also be explained by the unbalanced protein synthesis process. Some investigators have demonstrated that high glucose levels minimized tyrosyl-tRNA synthetase expression and production in osteoblast-like UMR-106 cells, emerging in reduced protein synthesis [40]. Endoplasmic reticulum function is essential to osteoblast differentiation and activity, and it may be suppressed by AGEs. The osteoblast death rate may be increased by high glucose levels. In fact, AGEs can decrease osteoblast growth and increase apoptotic death [39]. In several in vitro studies it has been showed the impairment of bone formation in human osteoblasts.

Osteocyte

A significant contribution of osteocytes on bone fragility in DM was highlighted in several studies. Sclerostin is one of the most important proteins counteracting bone formation. It operates as an antagonist of the WNT/β catenin canonical signalling pathway. Increased osteocyte apoptosis can lead to decreased osteocyte density [41] and numbers as showed in several studies on STZ diabetic mice. An important role of sclerostin in diabetic bone metabolism is also sustained by the observation that treatment with sclerostin antibodies ameliorates bone mass and strength in rats with T2D and STZ diabetic mice. Homogeneous evidences were indicated in cross-sectional studies in humans. In patients with diabetes have been observed increased serum levels of sclerostin. Particularly, Gennari et al. reported higher sclerostin levels in T2D patients compared to controls and T1D patients [42]. Additionally, sclerostin levels were higher in T1D patients confronted with healthy controls [43]. Diabetes may have negative effect on the Wnt pathway, leading to impaired osteocyte function with decreased bone formation as suggested by these evidences reported.

10.3.2.2 Glucose Toxicity on Bone Resorption

Osteoclast

Hyperglycaemia may negatively affect osteoclastogenesis, resulting in an impairment of bone resorption. Physiological glucose levels promote differentiation of embryonic stem cells (ESCs) into osteoclasts, and hyperglycaemia may impair this process. Anyway, the effects of hyperglycaemia on osteoclasts are controversial as reported in several studies. The majority of in vitro studies have showed a decrease in osteoclast function. High glucose levels seems to reduce nuclear factor κB (NF-κB) activity, resulting in reduced osteoclast formation [44]. Several studies have demonstrated that elevated TRAP activity [45], cathepsin K activity [45] and RANKL levels in diabetic mice may support an increased osteoclast activity. In different T2D mouse models have been reported contrasting data on osteoclast activity. Hyperglycaemia can affect both osteoclastogenesis and osteoclast function with contrasting evidence as reported by both in vitro and in vivo studies. On the one hand, hyperglycaemia can raise bone resorption, as confirmed by RANKL elevation, but on the other hand may reduce bone turnover, that might be the essential driver of bone fragility.

10.3.3 AGEs and "Diabetic Collagenopathy"

A damage of tissue material properties may have a significant role in the development of bone fragility, as diabetes may be characterized by an important impairment in bone strength that is not fully described by BMD.

It is renowned that bone ductility, hardness and strength are based on the type of cross-links between adjacent collagen molecules, while the mineral constituent of the bone matrix provides stiffness.

To stabilize the newly formed collagen fibres it has been described that are required two types of covalent cross-links: *enzymatic* cross-links (lysyl oxidase (LOX)-mediated cross-linking) [46] and *non-enzymatic* cross-links (glycation or oxidation-induced AGEs cross-linking) [47]. The quantity of *enzymatic cross-links* in bone is strictly controlled by the expression of LOX, which plays the role to prevent imprudent accumulation of enzymatic cross-links in the physiological process of mineralization [46]. It has been showed that to ensure osteoblastic differentiation, proper enzymatic cross-link formation is also required [48]. Across the homocysteine pathway, diabetes is one of the conditions that may indirectly interest LOX activity. In fact, diabetes is correlated with elevated plasma levels of homocysteine, which successively can down-regulate gene expression and enzymatic activity of LOX [49].

Chronic hyperglycaemia is correlated with the production of AGEs. AGEs form spontaneously across non-enzymatic glycation or oxidation, and a substantial body of evidence indicates that production of AGEs within collagen fibres has a negative effect on bone strength. In fact, whereas enzymatic cross-links are crucial to preserve bone strength, *non-enzymatic AGEs cross-links* looks to injure bone quality [47]. Furthermore, AGEs form irrevocable cross-links among the fibres in the triple helix, and competitively forbid enzymatic cross-link formation because AGEs cross-links are made between Lys residues, which are key sites of enzymatic cross-linking in collagen molecules. The decelerate turnover of collagen leads to storage of a big quantity of altered type 1 collagen, which can cause biomechanical changes either in cortical and trabecular bone [50].

Furthermore, in vitro and in vivo animal and human studies showed that cancellous bone is vulnerable to the storage of non-enzymatic glycation, which raises its propensity to fracture and reduced post-yield strain and energy.

Anyway, AGEs may also have a negative effect on bone health by causing cellular disorders. In fact, important and quite clear studies have been issued that the interplay of AGEs with their receptor RAGE (also expressed on osteoblasts and immune cells) decreases *osteoblast activity* [51].

In spite of the fact that the osteoblast system is negatively influenced by AGEs, their impact on osteoclast pathway is debatable. In fact, while some investigators have found that AGEs can raise osteoclast activity [52]. The inhibition of bone resorption was established by a significant decrease in the release of type I collagen fragments produced by the collagenolytic enzymes secreted by osteoclasts in the culture medium of AGE-modified mineralized matrices.

A few in vivo clinical trials have proved to confirm the significance of AGEs on the damage of bone health in diabetes, concentrating on pentosidine. In fact, *pentosidine* is one of the most usual non-enzymatic cross-links in bone, and it has been suggested as a specific marker of AGEs in bone. Some studies on animal models with diabetes [53, 54] and, importantly, in TD2 patients [55], pentosidine levels are elevated. An important increase in pentosidine bone level, probably responsible for low material properties, has been demonstrated in STZ diabetic rats [54]. Taking into consideration these observations, plasma and/or urinary pentosidine has been studied as a potential new marker of bone impairment in diabetes. Particularly, Yamamoto et al. have observed the relation among serum pentosidine levels and vertebral fractures in Japanese T2D patients; Pentosidine levels were notably increased in post-menopausal women with vertebral fractures confronted to the control group [56]. In spite of the fact that glycaemic control and renal function may influence plasma pentosidine levels, in this cross-sectional study pentosidine was correlated with fractures independent of BMD, diabetic status, risk factors for osteoporosis, and renal function [56].

In spite of the fact that these observations indicate that the injury in collagen cross-links and AGE formation could explain the link among bone fragility and diabetes, sizable studies are needed to confirm this theory. Furthermore, the immunoassay necessary to identify and measure pentosidine has a reduced grade of sensitivity and specificity owing to various factors in blood and urine that interfere with immunoassay standardization [57], consequently it needs to be ameliorated.

10.3.4 Incretin System

The incretin system includes a high number of peptides but more than 90% of its physiological effects are realized by glucose-dependent insulinotropic peptide (GIP) and glucagon-like peptide-1 (GLP-1). Many studies demonstrated that the vastness of nutrient-stimulated insulin secretion is decreased in patients with T2D, which prompted investigations to find out whether endogenous secretion and/or incretin action is decreased in diabetic individuals. GIP plasma levels seem to be normal or even increased in T2D subjects, while meal-stimulated GLP-1 plasma levels are mildly but significantly decreased in patients with reduced glucose tolerance or T2D. Instead, T1D subjects can have normal incretin responses to meals [58].

Generally, GIP and GLP-1 have short half-lives and are rapidly degraded by dipeptidyl peptidase-4 (DPP-4). This system is altered in T2D subjects, and drugs currently used to ameliorate glucose control, such as GLP-1 receptor analogs (resistant to DPP-4 degradation) and DPP-4 inhibitors (which decelerate the enzymatic cleavage of GLP-1), amplify the half-life of these native hormones.

GIP bring to bear its functions by activating a particular G protein-coupled receptor (*GIPR*) expressed by different cells, including pancreatic beta-cells and adipocytes, and seemingly also by osteoclasts [59], osteoblasts [60], osteocytes and chondrocytes [61].

GLP-1 exercises its effects across interplay with the GLP-1 receptor found in pancreatic islets, lung, hypothalamus, stomach, heart and kidney. GLP-1 may also have a functional link with osteoblastic cells, probably across a GPI/IPG-coupled receptor (GLP-1R), as well showed for the first time by Nuche-Berenguer et al. [62].

By increasing the expression of collagen type I and the activity of alkaline phosphatase [58], *GIP* stimulates osteoblast proliferation. Moreover, GIP seems to inhibit osteoclast activity among cyclic adenosine monophosphate (cAMP).

Although GLP-1 on osteoblasts has not been completely explained, there are some evidence showing that it can induce osteogenic differentiation in bone [63]. In fact, some authors described the expression of GLP-1R pending osteogenic differentiation of adipose-derived stem cells [63]. GLP-1 appears to be able to repress osteoclasts across a calcitonin-dependent pathway [62].

Some in vivo researches, using diverse animal models, have demonstrated a significant role for incretin hormones in bone metabolism, but there are only limited data relating to the impact of DPP-4 inhibitors and GLP-1 agonists on bone health in humans [64].

Administration of GLP-1 (or its analog enzyme-resistant variant, like exendin-4) to normal and diabetics rats seems to rise trabecular bone mass and the expression of osteoblast markers. These results validate the probable anabolic effect of GLP-1 on trabecular bone [65].

Furthermore, the administration of GLP-1 to T2D and insulin resistance mice had a favorable effect on bone mass, while administration to WT mice had no consequence on bone structure [65].

Recent studies also show a favorable effect of GIP and GLP-1 analogs on bone quality in T1D. In STZ diabetic mice, GIP and GLP-1 were capable to conserve cortical microarchitecture and to avoid the whole bone strength loss [66].

10.3.5 Acute and Chronic Diabetic Complications

Some large studies have indicated that hypoglycaemia is strictly correlated with risk of falls in T2D patients [67].

There is robust evidence sustaining a link among chronic diabetes complications and risk of fracture in either T1D or T2D. A few studies found no relation between HbA1c and BMD. Patients with complications of diabetes were distinguished by increased fracture risk and decreased BMD values [5]. In fact, chronic diabetes complications can influence the risk fracture by various mechanisms [68].

Especially, retinopathy, macrovascular disease and neuropathy can raise the risk of fracture by growing the probability of falls [68, 69]. In addition, in T1D diabetic kidney disease there is a significant growth in the risk of fractures, maybe due to altered vitamin D and parathyroid hormone (PTH) levels [68].

In a recent cross-sectional study, was demonstrated only a subgroup of T2D subjects with microvascular complications had deficiencies of cortical bone confronted with T2D subjects without microvascular complications or control subjects, but the investigators were not able to clear this feature [70]. Alternatively, no notable distinction in trabecular bone parameters and trabecular microarchitecture was recorded in patients with microvascular complications [70].

10.3.6 Inflammation

Differently, either TD1 or TD2 can be contemplated as inflammatory diseases. Susceptibility to T1D demands an intricate interaction among genetic and environmental factors, but there is now higher testimony for a role of natural inflammation. Especially, IL-1, a pro-inflammatory cytokine central to innate immunity, and tumor necrosis factor-α (TNF-α) have been involved in T1D onset and beta cell damage having a negative effect on insulin bio-synthesis. Either cytokines may encourage the osteoclastogenic process and increase osteoclast activity by causing the expression of RANKL and by exercising an anti-apoptotic effect [71].

In addition it has been suggested that TNF-α may down-regulate RUNX2 and osterix, consequently growing the expression of sclerostin and Dkk1 [72]. Systematically, reduced levels of TNF-α or suppression of TNF-α by TNF soluble binding protein or an anti-TNF-α [73] decrease the RANKL-induced osteoclast formation, repressing bone resorption.

It has been shown that a low-grade chronic inflammation is associated with the pathogenic processes determining TD2 [74]. IL-6 is one of the cytokines most strictly related to obesity and T2D, as it is released from the adipose tissue [74]. In fact, either insulin resistance or hyperglycaemia is correlated with increased levels of IL-6. Recent studies have confirmed the relationship among IL-6 and bone metabolism. IL-6 is able to increase osteoclastogenesis, and some investigators have suggested that serum IL-6 [75] and gene polymorphism in IL-6 seems to have a role in decreasing BMD and affecting muscle strength [75]. Anyway, contrasting results were obtained about the role of this cytokin on bone metabolism. Some authors showed that IL-6 stimulates mesenchymal progenitor differentiation on the way to the osteoblastic lineage, and has a positive effect on bone formation in conditions of higher bone turnover [76].

10.3.7 Marrow Adiposity

Fat cells occupy the bone marrow along with osteoblasts and their usual mesenchymal precursors. In the bone marrow, constitutional transformations happen continuously with ageing and various environmental and health conditions [77]. Transformation of marrow adiposity is a physiological age-related phenomenon that includes the transformation of an active marrow (hematopoietic/red marrow, status at birth) into a less active one (fat/yellow). This phenomenon finishes around the age of 25–30 years [77].

Many studies have demonstrated several pathophysiological correlations among adipose tissue and bone that are sustained by the common mesenchymal origin of osteoblasts and adipocytes [78].

Subcutaneous adipose tissue, visceral fat and bone marrow fat have typical tissue properties and consequently distinct metabolic activity. Fat bone marrow appears to be an insulin-sensitive tissue, closely in relation to systemic energy metabolism, because of brown adipose tissue (expression of genetic and metabolic features) [78].

Many studies have suggested that composition of bone marrow fat could be not normal in subjects with osteoporosis and/or T2D [78]. A few studies in humans have discovered an opposite association among bone marrow adiposity and BMD [78]. These observations propose that bone marrow microenvironment disruption may elevate adipogenesis at the expense of osteoclastogenesis [79].

10.3.8 Muscle

10.3.8.1 Sarcopenia

Diabetes exerts effect on all musculoskeletal system elements, including muscle, bone and connective tissue. Some musculoskeletal affections like diabetic myonecrosis, diabetic amyotrophy and osteoporosis are contemplated as diabetic chronic complications, confirming diabetes capability to affect the musculoskeletal system. In addition, diabetes is one of the states that may determine sarcopenia. In T1D subjects, "diabetic myopathy" is featured by decreased muscle growth and strength [80] and damaged stem cell differentiation regarding the myogenic lineage [81]. Some studies in humans have demonstrated a decrease in muscle mass and fibre size. Some investigators have calculated that the risk of developing sarcopenia is three-fold higher in T2D patients compared to non-diabetic individuals after adjusting for many risk factors [82]. It has been confirmed that sarcopenia expands the risk of falls and fractures. In spite of the fact that the mechanism supporting the association among sarcopenia and diabetes has not been fully described, a decrease in muscle protein synthesis and a growth in protein destruction owed to insulin resistance appear to have a significant role [83]. In postmenopausal women with T2D, pentosidine is negatively correlated with relative skeletal muscle mass index and could be an independent risk factor for reduced muscle mass. In summary, diabetes can induce muscle impairment and reduced muscle strength that may increase the risk of falls [84].

10.3.8.2 Irisin

Irisin might be a further link within diabetes, increased risk of fracture and skeletal muscle. Irisin is an exercise-induced myokine that can trigger "browning" of white adipose tissue. In vitro and in vivo studies evidenced that irisin may have a positive effect on bone health. Some cross-sectional studies have demonstrated that low levels of irisin are correlated with vertebral fractures in post-menopausal women [85]. Diabetic patients have lower irisin serum levels as compared to control healthy individuals [86]. Animal models lacking irisin might aid to understand the processes underlying the damage of cortical bone that is generally seen in diabetes.

10.4 Oral Anti-Diabetic Drugs and Fracture Risk

10.4.1 Metformin

The biguanide, metformin, is globally accepted as first line therapy in the treatment of T2DM. The available preclinical and clinical data seemed to indicate that metformin had a good safety profile regarding the bone. Indeed, in preclinical studies both bone mass and bone quality are improved by the use of metformin but there were not clearly data in clinical studies: some trials supported a beneficial effect of metformin on fracture risk, other reported a neutral effect. Prospective RCTs are needed to demonstrate its potential protective role.

10.4.1.1 Preclinical Data

Many studies evaluated the potential anabolic role of metformin on bone [87–89] and they have found that metformin increases cellular proliferation, ALP activity, calcium deposition and the number of nodules formed in rat primary osteoblasts, effects that may counteract the detrimental effects of hyperglycaemia on osteoblast function [89]. Another bone anabolic pathway increased by metformin is differentiation towards the osteoblast line of bone marrow mesenchymal cell progenitors (BMPCs) [89, 90]. Both bone mass and bone quality are improved by the use of metformin [91, 92]. In particular, a recent study conducted in vitro, in vivo and ex vivo has shown that metformin may prevent the decrease in trabecular area, the reduction in osteocyte density, and the reduction in TRAP activity induced by high glucose levels [93]. Anyway, a number of preclinical studies have failed to confirm the anabolic role of metformin on bone [94, 95].

Some studies have demonstrated that metformin modulates the receptor activator of nuclear factor κB (RANK)/receptor activator of nuclear factor κB ligand (RANKL)/osteoprotegerin (OPG) pathway resulting in reduction of bone resorption [96, 97]. In contrast, a number of studies conducted in vitro and one conducted in vivo have found no effect of metformin on bone metabolism [98–100].

10.4.1.2 Clinical Data

Observational studies have found a reduction in fracture risk in patients treated with metformin. Vestergaard et al. in one of the larger case control studies (mean age

43 ± 27 years old (y.o.); 41.8% women) have shown that treatment with biguanide was associated with a decreased risk of any fractures (HR 0.81; 95% CI: 0.70–0.93) [7] and a historical cohort study involving 1964 T2DM (mean age 61.7 ± 14.0 y.o.; 49% women) reported that treatment with metformin was protective against risk of fracture even after adjusting for other risk factors (HR 0.70; 95% CI: 0.6–0.96) [17]. Although some observational studies have shown a beneficial effect of metformin on fracture risk, there was a only trial reported a neutral effect of metformin: in a cohort study involving 200,000 Scottish patients with T2DM (mean age 65 y.o.; 47% women) who were followed for 9 years, there was no association between hip fracture and cumulative exposure to metformin [101]. Recently data from the Osteoporotic Fractures in Men (MrOS) study have found that the use of metformin in T2DM men (aged ≥65 y.o.) did not affect the risk of bone fractures [102].

There has been one randomized trial, ADOPT, designed to compare metformin with other treatments on glycaemic control; in particular, 1840 women and 2511 men were randomly assigned to rosiglitazone, metformin, or glyburide [103]. Fractures were identified as adverse events in ADOPT, and it has been reported 200 fractures in 4351 patients followed for a median period of 4 years. In the group treated with metformin (mean age 57 ± 10 y.o.; 44% women), the cumulative incidence of fracture (women and men) was 1.20 per 100 patients years, with a cumulative incidence of fractures (95% CI) of 5.6% (4.1–7.1) at 5 years [104]. Fracture incidence was similar in the group randomized to sulfonylureas (mean age 57 ± 10 y.o.; 42% women).

10.4.2 Sufonylureas

The sulfonylureas cause increased secretion of insulin by binding to an adenosine triphosphate (ATP)-dependent K+ channel on the cell membrane of pancreatic beta cells. This class of drugs increased the risk of hypoglycaemia [105], which is associated with increased fracture risk [106]. However, only a few investigators have examined their biological effects on bone.

10.4.2.1 Preclinical Data

A small number of studies have investigated the effect of these drugs on bone formation and no consistent data have been available about the influence of sulfonylureas on bone resorption. We have only a few preclinical data that seem to not increase the risk of fracture.

10.4.2.2 Clinical Data

There were not many studies that evaluated the effects of this drug on bone metabolism: in most trials, sulfonylureas have been considered as a control group in order to investigate the effects of other anti-diabetic treatments (frequently TZDs). A major limitation of these kind of studies was the lack of distinction between traumatic and fragility fractures. The only randomized trial of sulfonylureas was the ADOPT trial in which were reported fractures on 49 patients (3.4%) that belonged to the glyburide group, with incidence corresponding to 1.15 per 100 patient years, with a cumulative incidence of fractures (95% CI) of 5.7% (3.9–7.6) at 5 years [104]. This was the same incidence of the metformin group in ADOPT (as above). A larger prospective cohort study which involved 84,339 Canadian patients (mean age 59 y.o.; 43% women) has shown that patients treated with sulfonylureas had a lower fracture risk than patients treated with TZDs [107]. Moreover, other observational studies have reported a neutral effect of sulfonylureas on bone. A case–control study involving 1945 Italian patients affected by T2DM who were followed for 4 years has found no significant association between bone fractures and sulfonylurea treatment [108]. Similarly, a population-based study involving 1964 Rochester residents has shown no significant impact of this drug on fracture risk [18]. Recently, data from the MrOS study has been shown that sulfonylurea use may represent a risk factor for non-vertebral fracture in older men with T2DM HR 95% CI 1.66 (1.09, 2.51) [102].

10.4.3 Thiazolidinediones

Thiazolidinediones such as pioglitazone (PIO) and ROSI were introduced in the late 1990s for the treatment of T2DM. They exert their function by activation of peroxisome proliferator-activated receptors (PPARγ) which increase hepatic and peripheral insulin sensitivity. The family of PPARs consists of three isoforms: PPARα, PPARβ/δ, and PPARγ [109]. Activation of PPARγ stimulates adipogenesis and suppresses osteoblastogenesis and so it determines the reduction of the osteoblast pool in bone marrow [110]. Several studies have demonstrated that TZDs negatively affect the bone health, increasing bone resorption and decreasing bone formation. We have a lot of preclinical and clinical data that seem to confirm the association between TZDs use and increased risk of fracture in women. These studies revealed involvement of the central (spine and hip) and peripheral sites and it is likely to be stronger with longer exposure duration in postmenopausal women. There were not clearly data on fracture risk in men.

10.4.3.1 Preclinical Data

Several studies have demonstrated that TZDs have an adverse effect on bone, increasing bone resorption and decreasing bone formation. It has not yet been fully elucidated how the TZDs decrease bone formation. BMPCs are able to differentiate into different cell lines (e.g., osteoblasts, myoblasts, chondrocytes, adipocytes). PPARγ stimulated differentiation into adipocytes, regardless of BMPCs transdifferentiation towards the osteoblast line [110]. This imbalance between adipocyte and osteoblast formation [111, 112] has been the main cause of TZD-induced impairment of bone metabolism. TZDs also interact with the canonical wingless-type MMTV integration site family (Wnt) that is an important regulatory pathway in the osteogenic differentiation of BMPC. In fact, its activation results in enhancement of bone formation. Studies in vitro and in humans have shown that ROSI increased Dickkopf-1 protein (DKK1), an inhibitor of canonical Wnt signalling

[113]. Other studies in osteocytes from a murine cell line have demonstrated that both ROSI and PIO determined osteocyte apoptosis [114, 115], sclerostin up-regulation [114] and enhanced expression of sclerostin in the absence of oestrogen [115]. It has been demonstrated that GH/IGF axis plays a prominent regulatory role in skeletal development and mineral acquisition [116]. Some studies suggest that TZDs may affect bone formation by decreasing the concentration of IGF-1 [117]. TZDs increase bone resorption rate (potentially via enhancement of osteoclast differentiation) [118] and osteoclast number [119], and decrease expression of OPG in a murine model [120] and in human BMPC [121]. The increased resorption rate was associated with significant reductions in BMD, BMC [120], and mechanical strength in mice [119]. Moreover, there was evidence to suggest a link between TZD and oestrogenic metabolism. In fact, in adipose stromal cells, PPARγ ligands inhibit aromatase expression [122, 123]. Studies have shown that in ovarian granulosa cells, TZD inhibits oestrogen synthesis by interfering with binding of androgen to aromatase [123].

10.4.3.2 Clinical Data

A number of observational studies have underlined the reduction in BMD associated with TZD treatment. In particular, the Health, Aging and Body Composition cohort reported a decrease in BMD (total, lumbar spine and trochanteric) among women but not men treated with TZDs after 4 years of follow-up [124]. The detrimental effects of TZDs have been particularly evident in women [107, 125–127] but a small number of studies also suggested the presence of negative effects in men [128–131]. Indeed, in a meta-analysis which included 10 randomized controlled trial (total 13,715 participants) and two observational studies (31,679 participants), it has been shown that there was no significant association between TZD therapy and fragility fracture in men, while both ROSI and PIO treatment increased fracture risk in women compared to control therapy. Regarding the site of fractures, these studies have demonstrated involvement of the vertebrae [126, 129, 131, 132] and hip [128, 129, 131, 132], but have also documented bone damage at peripheral sites such as ankle and foot [107, 127, 131, 133, 134]. The fracture risk was similar both with ROSI than PIO [129–131, 134, 135] and it was likely to be stronger with longer exposure duration of treatment [131, 132].

10.4.3.3 Rosiglitazone

In healthy [136, 137] postmenopausal women with T2DM [138] and in men affected by T2DM, treatment with ROSI has been associated with a significant reduction in BMD [139], specially at the femoral neck and total hip [140]. The same study has shown that there was not further bone loss after cessation of ROSI administration, and that bone loss at the total hip was reduced when treatment was switched from ROSI to metformin [140]. The treatment with ROSI is associated with an increased risk of fracture specially in women >60 years of age. The lower and upper limbs were the sites most commonly affected [104]. Instead, in men, studies have seemed to show a neutral effect of ROSI treatment, on the risk of fractures [104, 141].

10.4.3.4 Pioglitazone

Studies have shown that treatment with PIO induces a significant reduction in BMD at the lumbar spine and femoral neck and radius but not at the lumbar spine in women and men with T2DM [142, 143]. As regards the fracture risk the treatment with PIO, as the ROSI, is associated with an increase of fracture. The fracture rate was higher in older women and risk raised only after the first year of treatment. No increase in fracture risk was found in men [144].

10.4.4 Incretin System

Incretins are a group of gastrointestinal hormones that causes a decrease in blood glucose levels by inhibiting glucagon release, reducing gastric emptying and food intake and potentially raising the amount of insulin released from the beta cells. Exendin-4 is a peptide agonist of the GLP receptor. Both GLP-1 and GIP are rapidly inactivated by the enzyme dipeptidyl peptidase-4 (DPP-4) [145]. Incretins may regulate bone system, due to the regulation of cellular proliferation of progenitor bone forming mesenchymal cells [146]. Several preclinical studies have showed positive effects of the incretin system on bone: they determine an increase in bone formation and a decrease in bone resorption otherwise, recent studies have demonstrated no significant clinical effect of this system on skeletal tissues.

10.4.4.1 Preclinical Data of GLP-1

Some studies, which have investigated the effects of GLP analogues on bone tissue have demonstrated rate in response to these agents. Receptors for GLP-1, GLP-2, and GIP are present on human osteoblastic cells at different stages of differentiation, and this may be the link between GLP1 and bone formation [146]. Probably, exendin-4, a GLP-1 analogue, interacts with the WNT pathway to rise bone formation; indeed, the treatment with exendin-4 is associated with a reduction in sclerostin in murine osteocytes and, in vivo, in diabetic rats [147]. Both GLP-1 and exendin-4 interact with bone resorption: increasing the OPG/RANKL ratio [65, 148, 149] and increased expression of calcitonin [150].

10.4.4.2 Preclinical Data of DPP-4 Inhibitors

The studies that evaluated the effects of DPP-4 inhibitors on bone formation have shown contradictory results. Anyway, no strong evidence is available about the relationship between DPP-4 inhibitors and bone resorption.

10.4.4.3 Clinical Data

There are contrasting data about BMD change and treatment with GLP analogues. Recently, Su et al. have reported a different fracture risk based on the different GLP-1 analogues treatment. In particular, liraglutide was correlated with a significant reduced risk of fractures (MH-OR = 0.38, 95% CI: 0.17–0.87), instead exenatide was associated with increased fracture rate (MH-OR = 2.09, 95% CI: 1.03–4.21) [151]. DPP-4 inhibitor therapy was associated with reduced risk of fracture (OR

0.60; 95% CI: 0.37–0.99) even after the exclusion of comparisons with TZDs or sulfonylureas [152]. The main limitations of the study were that fractures were reported as adverse events and not as primary or secondary end points, and that the mean duration of the trials was only 35 weeks.

10.4.5 SGLT2 Inhibitors

Sodium glucose co-transporters 2 (SGLT2) allow the reabsorption of glucose in the proximal tubule of the kidney. SGLT2 inhibitors decrease plasma glucose by lowering the renal threshold for glucose and increasing urinary glucose excretion. The mechanism of action of these agents has raised concerns about bone safety but, currently, only a few studies have focused on the relationship between SGLT2 inhibitors and fragility fractures. Canagliflozin seems to negatively affect bone.

10.4.5.1 Clinical Data

It has been shown that Canagliflozin was associated with a slight decrease in total hip BMD but not at other sites measured and no meaningful changes in bone strength were observed [153]. Watts and colleagues have confirmed the impairment of bone health related to the use of canaglifozin [154]. Indeed, in CANVAS trial a significant increase in fractures was recorded with canagliflozin versus placebo that was balanced between upper and lower limbs [154]. Although there is poor evidence that has investigated the relation between bone system and dapaglifozin, it seems to have a neutral effect on bone. There are only two studies in which effects of dapagliflozin on bone-related primary or secondary endpoints have been examined and no BMD and/or fracture risk changes have been reported [155, 156].

10.5 Bone Biomarkers in Diabetes Mellitus

Several studies have investigated bone biomarkers in patients affected by DM aiming to understand how DM affects bone formation and bone resorption.

In children affected by *T1D*, both formation markers (OC, TRAP and P1NP) [157, 158] and resorption marker (CTX) [157] seem to be lower at onset [157], even if they tend to get normalized over the time.

In adults T1D, contrasting evidences have been reported. Some authors have found no differences in bone biomarkers between patients with T1D compared to control [159], whereas in other study it has been revealed a reduction of bone formation markers OC and BAP in T1D patients compared to control [160]; these evidences suggest a reduced bone metabolism in T1DM. Moreover, a reduced level of IGF-1 was recorded in patients with T1DM compared to T2DM [161].

Although in *T2D* evidences have not been univocal, newer evidences seem to suggest a reduction in both formation and resorption markers [162].

Recently, it has been reported that sclerostin, an inhibitor of WNT-signaling, was increased in patients affected by T2DM compared to T1DM and control subjects

[163, 164]. It has also been found a positive correlation with BMD [165]. These data suggested a potential pathogenic role of sclerostin in bone metabolism of T2DM patients.

Several studies investigated the relationship between bone biomarkers and vertebral fractures in T2DM and all evidences seem to point out a decreased bone turnover sustained by a reduction in IGF-1 [31] and OC [166] levels and by an increase in sclerostin levels [31, 167]. This observation was also supported by Jiajue and colleagues who have found an association between low P1NP levels and high CTX levels with bone fractures in patients with T2DM [168].

Finally, a recent meta-analysis which included 22 studies has shown that OC and CTX were usually decreased in patients affected with DM; in particular, in T1D there was a significant reduction in OC levels compared to controls whereas a borderline significance was reported in T2D. It has been also found a significant increase in ALP values in subjects with DM compared to control subjects [169].

Furthermore, P1NP, PTH, calcium, BAP, CICP, and DPD were also evaluated, but no differences were found between subjects with diabetes and controls.

10.6 How to Estimate the Fracture Risk in Diabetes

10.6.1 Bone Mineral Density

It is well known that fracture risk is increased in patients affected by DM, both type1 and type2, but this observation is not sustained by the same trend in BMD values.

In a meta-analysis, reduced BMD *Z*-score was found at the spine and at the hip in patients affected by *T1DM*, with an average decrease of 22% in spine BMD and of −37% at hip *Z*-score when T1DM patients were compared with age and gender matched controls [5]. Instead, increased BMD at the spine and at the hip were found in T2DM patients [5].

Moreover, in T1D subjects, several studies have reported a significant decrease in BMD at either the spine, hip or total [170–172], although few studies have reported no reduction in BMD values [173].

When T1DM onset was reported in childhood before the peak of bone mass, BMD was 0.5–1.0 SD lower [174], but seems only be transiently reduced, with an increase during the puberty [175]. However, the majority of the studies reported a decreased BMD with longstanding T1DM [170, 176]. Furthermore, diabetic complications and poor glycaemic control seem to have a detrimental effect on BMD in T1DM patients as most of the studies reported [174, 177].

Instead, *T2DM* has characterized by an increased risk of fractures despite normal to high BMD at both the hip and spine [178]. In a meta-analysis, Vestergaard et al. have reported 4–5% higher BMD in T2DM patients compared to controls [5].

No significant differences were reported between men and women [178] and across different ethnic groups as Mexican American, white, and black [179]. Fewer studies have been conducted among Asian populations and results have shown a less marked association between T2DM and increased BMD [180].

It is controversial the relationship between BMD and BMI. In several studies BMI is strongly positive associated with BMD [133, 178], although higher values of BMD persist in T2DM patients after adjusting for BMI [179].

However, despite the relatively higher BMD, it has been well documented an increased rate of bone loss among patients affected by T2DM. Several studies such as the Study of Osteoporotic Fractures [181], the Fracture Intervention Trial [182] and the Study of Women Across the Nation [183] have documented an increased BMD loss, especially at the hip, in T2DM women compared with matched controls without diabetes. Only in the multiracial Health, Ageing, and Body Composition Study these findings have been reported only in white women and not in black women and men with diabetes [184].

10.6.2 Bone Quality

In the recent years, bone quality has raised as a relevant element to understand the detrimental impact of DM on bone. Different procedures have been used to assess bone quality in subjects affected by T1D or T2DM.

High-resolution peripheral quantitative CT (HR-pQCT) is a non-invasive method used to assess bone microarchitecture in vivo. In *T1DM* patients affected by retinopathy, bone volume of the proximal tibia was lower compared with control subjects [185]. Furthermore, lower trabecular volumetric BMD at the ultradistal radius and tibia and lower cortical thickness at the tibia have been reported in T1DM patients compared to healthy subjects. HR-pQCT impairments were more severe in patients with microvascular complications [186].

In *T2DM* it has been reported a deficit in cortical bone represented by cortical porosity and lower cortical density. In particular, for the first time, Burghardt et al. have reported a deficit in cortical bone among postmenopausal women with T2DM, whereas trabecular bone microarchitecture was similar to control subjects [187]. This pattern was also reported in postmenopausal African-American women with T2DM [188] and in postmenopausal women with T2DM and fragility fractures [189].

In the recent years it has been developed the *microindentation*, a new technique able to test the bone material properties in vivo, producing microindents over the midshaft of the anterior tibia, which provides a measure of bone resistance using the "bone material strength index" or BMSi (24123088). Farr and colleagues have found a significant BMSi reduction in T2D patients compared to control healthy subjects [190].

Trabecular bone score (TBS) is another recent method to assess bone quality in patients with osteoporosis and it is related to textural parameter correlated with bone microarchitecture, expression of trabecular number and disposition. A low value of TBS reflects a weak bone architecture that can lead to an increased risk of fracture.

In two different cohorts of patients with T2DM, TBS was lower in women [191, 192] and men [192], despite higher values of BMD. Interestingly, in these studies TBS was negatively correlated with glycaemic control. Finally, in a large retrospective analysis of postmenopausal women, after adjustment for possible confounding factors, women with diabetes showed reduced values of lumbar TBS but not impaired BMD values [193].

Only one study was conducted among patients with T1DM and it has been found lower TBS values among patients with T1DM with previous history of bone fractures [194].

References

1. Hough S, Pierroz D, Cooper C, Ferrari S. Mechanisms in endocrinology: mechanisms and evaluation of bone fragility in type 1 diabetes mellitus. Eur J Endocrinol. 2016;174(4):R127–38. https://doi.org/10.1530/EJE-15-0820.
2. Nicodemus KK, Folsom AR, Iowa Women's Health Study. Type 1 and type 2 diabetes and incident hip fractures in postmenopausal women. Diabetes Care. 2001;24:1192–7. https://doi.org/10.2337/diacare.24.7.1192.
3. Ahmed LA, Joakimsen RM, Berntsen GK, Fønnebø V, Schirmer H. Diabetes mellitus and the risk of non-vertebral fractures: the Tromsø study. Osteoporos Int. 2006;17:495–500. https://doi.org/10.1007/s00198-005-0013-x.
4. Miao J, Brismar K, Nyrén O, Ugarph-Morawski A, Ye W. Elevated hip fracture risk in type 1 diabetic patients: a population-based cohort study in Sweden. Diabetes Care. 2005;28:2850–5. https://doi.org/10.2337/diacare.28.12.2850.
5. Vestergaard P. Discrepancies in bone mineral density and fracture risk in patients with type 1 and type 2 diabetesDOUBLEHYPHENa meta-analysis. Osteoporos Int. 2007;18:427–44. https://doi.org/10.1007/s00198-006-0253-4.
6. Janghorbani M, Van Dam RM, Willett WC, Hu FB. Systematic review of type 1 and type 2 diabetes mellitus and risk of fracture. Am J Epidemiol. 2007;166:495–505. https://doi.org/10.1093/aje/kwm106.
7. Vestergaard P, Rejnmark L, Mosekilde L. Relative fracture risk in patients with diabetes mellitus, and the impact of insulin and oral antidiabetic medication on relative fracture risk. Diabetologia. 2005;48:1292–9. https://doi.org/10.1007/s00125-005-1786-3.
8. Zhukouskaya VV, Eller-Vainicher C, Vadzianava VV, Shepelkevich AP, Zhurava IV, Korolenko GG, et al. Prevalence of morphometric vertebral fractures in patients with type 1 diabetes. Diabetes Care. 2013;36:427–44. https://doi.org/10.2337/dc12-1355.
9. Shah VN, Shah CS, Snell-Bergeon JK. Type 1 diabetes and risk of fracture: meta-analysis and review of the literature. Diabet Med. 2015;32:1134–42. https://doi.org/10.1111/dme.12734.
10. Weber DR, Haynes K, Leonard MB, Willi SM, Denburg MR. Type 1 diabetes is associated with an increased risk of fracture across the life span: a population-based cohort study using The Health Improvement Network (THIN). Diabetes Care. 2015;38:1913–20. https://doi.org/10.2337/dc15-0783.
11. Shanbhogue VV, Mitchell DM, Rosen CJ, Bouxsein ML, Leslie W, Rubin M, et al. Type 2 diabetes and the skeleton: new insights into sweet bones. Lancet Diabetes Endocrinol. 2016;4:159–73. https://doi.org/10.1016/S2213-8587(15)00283-1.
12. Strotmeyer ES, Cauley JA, Schwartz AV, Nevitt MC, Resnick HE, Bauer DC, et al. Nontraumatic fracture risk with diabetes mellitus and impaired fasting glucose in older white and black adults: the health, aging, and body composition study. Arch Intern Med. 2005;165:1612–7. https://doi.org/10.1001/archinte.165.14.1612.
13. Bonds DE, Larson JC, Schwartz AV, Strotmeyer ES, Robbins J, Rodriguez BL, et al. Risk of fracture in women with type 2 diabetes: the women's health initiative observational study. J Clin Endocrinol Metab. 2006;91:3404–10. https://doi.org/10.1210/jc.2006-0614.
14. Koh W-P, Wang R, Ang L-W, Heng D, Yuan J-M, Yu MC, et al. Diabetes and risk of hip fracture in the Singapore Chinese health study. Diabetes Care. 2010;33:213–5. https://doi.org/10.2337/dc10-0067.

15. Looker AC, Eberhardt MS, Saydah SH, Janghorbani M, Van Dam RM, Willett WC, et al. Diabetes and fracture risk in older U.S. adults. Bone. 2007;82:9–15. https://doi.org/10.1016/j.bone.2014.12.008.
16. Holmberg AH, Johnell O, Nilsson PM, Nilsson J, Berglund G, Akesson K. Risk factors for fragility fracture in middle age. A prospective population-based study of 33,000 men and women. Osteoporos Int. 2006;17:1065–77. https://doi.org/10.1007/s00198-006-0137-7.
17. Melton LJ, Leibson CL, Achenbach SJ, Therneau TM, Khosla S. Fracture risk in type 2 diabetes: update of a population-based study. J Bone Miner Res. 2008;23:1334–42. https://doi.org/10.1359/jbmr.080323.
18. Schwartz AV, Sellmeyer DE, Ensrud KE, Cauley JA, Tabor HK, Schreiner PJ, et al. Older women with diabetes have an increased risk of fracture: a prospective study. J Clin Endocrinol Metab. 2001;86:32–8. https://doi.org/10.1210/jcem.86.1.7139.
19. Pun KK, Lau P, Ho PW. The characterization, regulation, and function of insulin receptors on osteoblast-like clonal osteosarcoma cell line. J Bone Miner Res. 1989;4:853–62. https://doi.org/10.1002/jbmr.5650040610.
20. Cornish J, Callon KE, Reid IR. Insulin increases histomorphometric indices of bone formation in vivo. Calcif Tissue Int. 1996;59:492–5.
21. Ogata N, Chikazu D, Kubota N, Terauchi Y, Tobe K, Azuma Y, et al. Insulin receptor substrate-1 in osteoblast is indispensable for maintaining bone turnover. J Clin Invest. 2000;105:935–43. https://doi.org/10.1172/JCI9017.
22. Hie M, Tsukamoto I. Increased expression of the receptor for activation of NF-kappaB and decreased runt-related transcription factor 2 expression in bone of rats with streptozotocin-induced diabetes. Int J Mol Med. 2010;26:611–8.
23. Campos Pastor MM, López-Ibarra PJ, Escobar-Jiménez F, Serrano Pardo MD, García-Cervigón AG. Intensive insulin therapy and bone mineral density in type 1 diabetes mellitus: a prospective study. Osteoporos Int. 2000;11:455–9.
24. Xiang G, Sun H, Zhao L. Changes of osteoprotegerin before and after insulin therapy in type 1 diabetic patients. Diabetes Res Clin Pract. 2007;76:199–206. https://doi.org/10.1016/j.diabres.2006.09.008.
25. Hsu C-N, Chang C-H, Lin Y-S, Lin J-W, Caffrey JL. Association of serum C-peptide concentrations with cancer mortality risk in pre-diabetes or undiagnosed diabetes. PLoS One. 2013;8:e55625. https://doi.org/10.1371/journal.pone.0055625.
26. Montalcini T, Gallotti P, Coppola A, Zambianchi V, Fodaro M, Galliera E, et al. Association between low C-peptide and low lumbar bone mineral density in postmenopausal women without diabetes. Osteoporos Int. 2015;26:1639–46. https://doi.org/10.1007/s00198-015-3040-2.
27. Yamaguchi T, Kanazawa I, Yamamoto M, Kurioka S, Yamauchi M, Yano S, et al. Associations between components of the metabolic syndrome versus bone mineral density and vertebral fractures in patients with type 2 diabetes. Bone. 2009;45:174–9. https://doi.org/10.1016/j.bone.2009.05.003.
28. Moyer-Mileur LJ, Slater H, Jordan KC, Murray MA. IGF-1 and IGF-binding proteins and bone mass, geometry, and strength: relation to metabolic control in adolescent girls with type 1 diabetes. J Bone Miner Res. 2008;23:1884–91. https://doi.org/10.1359/jbmr.080713.
29. Fulzele K, DiGirolamo DJ, Liu Z, Xu J, Messina JL, Clemens TL. Disruption of the insulin-like growth factor type 1 receptor in osteoblasts enhances insulin signaling and action. J Biol Chem. 2007;282:25649–58. https://doi.org/10.1074/jbc.M700651200.
30. Lee YH, White MF. Insulin receptor substrate proteins and diabetes. Arch Pharm Res. 2004;27:361–70.
31. Ardawi MS, Akhbar DH, Alshaikh A, Ahmed MM, Qari MH, Rouzi AA, et al. Increased serum sclerostin and decreased serum IGF-1 are associated with vertebral fractures among post-menopausal women with type-2 diabetes. Bone. 2013;56:355–62. https://doi.org/10.1016/j.bone.2013.06.029.
32. Barrett-Connor E, Kritz-Silverstein D. Does hyperinsulinemia preserve bone? Diabetes Care. 1996;19:1388–92.

33. Stolk RP, Van Daele PL, Pols HA, Burger H, Hofman A, Birkenhäger JC, et al. Hyperinsulinemia and bone mineral density in an elderly population: the Rotterdam study. Bone. 1996;18:545–9.
34. Choi YJ, Kim DJ, Lee Y, Chung Y-S. Insulin is inversely associated with bone mass, especially in the insulin-resistant population: the Korea and US national health and nutrition examination surveys. J Clin Endocrinol Metab. 2014;99:1433–41. https://doi.org/10.1210/jc.2013-3346.
35. Fulzele K, Riddle RC, DiGirolamo DJ, Cao X, Wan C, Chen D, et al. Insulin receptor signaling in osteoblasts regulates postnatal bone acquisition and body composition. Cell. 2010;142:309–19. https://doi.org/10.1016/j.cell.2010.06.002.
36. Abrahamsen B, Rohold A, Henriksen JE, Beck-Nielsen H. Correlations between insulin sensitivity and bone mineral density in non-diabetic men. Diabet Med. 2000;17:124–9.
37. Shin D, Kim S, Kim KH, Lee K, Park SM. Association between insulin resistance and bone mass in men. J Clin Endocrinol Metab. 2014;99:988–95. https://doi.org/10.1210/jc.2013-3338.
38. Hie M, Iitsuka N, Otsuka T, Tsukamoto I. Insulin-dependent diabetes mellitus decreases osteoblastogenesis associated with the inhibition of Wnt signaling through increased expression of Sost and Dkk1 and inhibition of Akt activation. Int J Mol Med. 2011;28:455–62. https://doi.org/10.3892/ijmm.2011.697.
39. Okazaki K, Yamaguchi T, Tanaka K-I, Notsu M, Ogawa N, Yano S, et al. Advanced glycation end products (AGEs), but not high glucose, inhibit the osteoblastic differentiation of mouse stromal ST2 cells through the suppression of osterix expression, and inhibit cell growth and increasing cell apoptosis. Calcif Tissue Int. 2012;91:286–96. https://doi.org/10.1007/s00223-012-9641-2.
40. Kim JH, Kim Y-Y, Kim S-J. High glucose inhibits gene expression of tyrosyl-tRNA synthetase in osteoblast cells. Methods Find Exp Clin Pharmacol. 2009;31:639–44. https://doi.org/10.1358/mf.2009.31.10.1441114.
41. Villarino ME, Sánchez LM, Bozal CB, Ubios AM. Influence of short-term diabetes on osteocytic lacunae of alveolar bone. A histomorphometric study. Acta Odontológica Latinoam AOL. 2006;19:23–8.
42. Gennari L, Merlotti D, Valenti R, Ceccarelli E, Ruvio M, Pietrini MG, et al. Circulating sclerostin levels and bone turnover in type 1 and type 2 diabetes. J Clin Endocrinol Metab. 2012;97:1737–44. https://doi.org/10.1210/jc.2011-2958.
43. Neumann T, Hofbauer LC, Rauner M, Lodes S, Kästner B, Franke S, et al. Clinical and endocrine correlates of circulating sclerostin levels in patients with type 1 diabetes mellitus. Clin Endocrinol. 2014;80:649–55. https://doi.org/10.1111/cen.12364.
44. Wittrant Y, Gorin Y, Woodruff K, Horn D, Abboud HE, Mohan S, et al. High d(+)glucose concentration inhibits RANKL-induced osteoclastogenesis. Bone. 2008;42:1122–30. https://doi.org/10.1016/j.bone.2008.02.006.
45. Hie M, Shimono M, Fujii K, Tsukamoto I. Increased cathepsin K and tartrate-resistant acid phosphatase expression in bone of streptozotocin-induced diabetic rats. Bone. 2007;41:1045–50. https://doi.org/10.1016/j.bone.2007.08.030.
46. Saito M, Soshi S, Tanaka T, Fujii K. Intensity-related differences in collagen post-translational modification in MC3T3-E1 osteoblasts after exposure to low- and high-intensity pulsed ultrasound. Bone. 2004;35:644–55. https://doi.org/10.1016/j.bone.2004.04.024.
47. Saito M, Marumo K. Bone quality in diabetes. Front Endocrinol (Lausanne). 2013;4:72. https://doi.org/10.3389/fendo.2013.00072.
48. Turecek C, Fratzl-Zelman N, Rumpler M, Buchinger B, Spitzer S, Zoehrer R, et al. Collagen cross-linking influences osteoblastic differentiation. Calcif Tissue Int. 2008;82:392–400. https://doi.org/10.1007/s00223-008-9136-3.
49. Raposo B, Rodríguez C, Martínez-González J, Badimon L. High levels of homocysteine inhibit lysyl oxidase (LOX) and downregulate LOX expression in vascular endothelial cells. Atherosclerosis. 2004;177:1–8. https://doi.org/10.1016/j.atherosclerosis.2004.06.015.

50. Leslie WD, Rubin MR, Schwartz AV, Kanis JA. Type 2 diabetes and bone. J Bone Miner Res. 2012;27:2231–7. https://doi.org/10.1002/jbmr.1759.
51. Cui S, Xiong F, Hong Y, Jung J-U, Li X-S, Liu J-Z, et al. APPswe/Aβ regulation of osteoclast activation and RAGE expression in an age-dependent manner. J Bone Miner Res. 2011;26:1084–98. https://doi.org/10.1002/jbmr.299.
52. Zhou Z, Han J-Y, Xi C-X, Xie J-X, Feng X, Wang C-Y, et al. HMGB1 regulates RANKL-induced osteoclastogenesis in a manner dependent on RAGE. J Bone Miner Res. 2008;23:1084–96. https://doi.org/10.1359/jbmr.080234.
53. Saito M, Fujii K, Mori Y, Marumo K. Role of collagen enzymatic and glycation induced cross-links as a determinant of bone quality in spontaneously diabetic WBN/Kob rats. Osteoporos Int. 2006;17:1514–23. https://doi.org/10.1007/s00198-006-0155-5.
54. Silva MJ, Brodt MD, Lynch MA, McKenzie JA, Tanouye KM, Nyman JS, et al. Type 1 diabetes in young rats leads to progressive trabecular bone loss, cessation of cortical bone growth, and diminished whole bone strength and fatigue life. J Bone Miner Res. 2009;24:1618–27. https://doi.org/10.1359/jbmr.090316.
55. Okazaki R, Totsuka Y, Hamano K, Ajima M, Miura M, Hirota Y, et al. Metabolic improvement of poorly controlled noninsulin-dependent diabetes mellitus decreases bone turnover. J Clin Endocrinol Metab. 1997;82:2915–20. https://doi.org/10.1210/jcem.82.9.4258.
56. Yamamoto M, Yamaguchi T, Yamauchi M, Yano S, Sugimoto T. Serum pentosidine levels are positively associated with the presence of vertebral fractures in postmenopausal women with type 2 diabetes. J Clin Endocrinol Metab. 2008;93:1013–9. https://doi.org/10.1210/jc.2007-1270.
57. Dorrian CA, Cathcart S, Clausen J, Shapiro D, Dominiczak MH. Factors in human serum interfere with the measurement of advanced glycation endproducts. Cell Mol Biol (Noisy-le-Grand). 1998;44:1069–79.
58. Baggio LL, Drucker DJ. Biology of incretins: GLP-1 and GIP. Gastroenterology. 2007;132:2131–57. https://doi.org/10.1053/j.gastro.2007.03.054.
59. Zhong Q, Itokawa T, Sridhar S, Ding K-H, Xie D, Kang B, et al. Effects of glucose-dependent insulinotropic peptide on osteoclast function. Am J Physiol Endocrinol Metab. 2007;292:E543–8. https://doi.org/10.1152/ajpendo.00364.2006.
60. Nissen A, Christensen M, Knop FK, Vilsbøll T, Holst JJ, Hartmann B. Glucose-dependent insulinotropic polypeptide inhibits bone resorption in humans. J Clin Endocrinol Metab. 2014;99:E2325–9. https://doi.org/10.1210/jc.2014-2547.
61. Faienza MF, Luce V, Ventura A, Colaianni G, Colucci S, Cavallo L, et al. Skeleton and glucose metabolism: a bone-pancreas loop. Int J Endocrinol. 2015;2015:758148. https://doi.org/10.1155/2015/758148.
62. Nuche-Berenguer B, Portal-Núñez S, Moreno P, González N, Acitores A, López-Herradón A, et al. Presence of a functional receptor for GLP-1 in osteoblastic cells, independent of the cAMP-linked GLP-1 receptor. J Cell Physiol. 2010;225:585–92. https://doi.org/10.1002/jcp.22243.
63. Jeon YK, Bae MJ, Kim JI, Kim JH, Choi SJ, Kwon SK, et al. Expression of glucagon-like peptide 1 receptor during Osteogenic differentiation of adipose-derived stem cells. Endocrinol Metab (Seoul). 2014;29:567–73. https://doi.org/10.3803/EnM.2014.29.4.567.
64. Gilbert MP, Pratley RE. The impact of diabetes and diabetes medications on bone health. Endocr Rev. 2015;36:194–213. https://doi.org/10.1210/er.2012-1042.
65. Nuche-Berenguer B, Moreno P, Esbrit P, Dapía S, Caeiro JR, Cancelas J, et al. Effect of GLP-1 treatment on bone turnover in normal, type 2 diabetic, and insulin-resistant states. Calcif Tissue Int. 2009;84:453–61. https://doi.org/10.1007/s00223-009-9220-3.
66. Mansur SA, Mieczkowska A, Bouvard B, Flatt PR, Chappard D, Irwin N, et al. Stable incretin mimetics counter rapid deterioration of bone quality in type 1 diabetes mellitus. J Cell Physiol. 2015;230:3009–18. https://doi.org/10.1002/jcp.25033.
67. Zhao Y, Kachroo S, Kawabata H, Colilla S, Mukherjee J, Fonseca V, et al. Association between hypoglycemia and fall-related fractures and health care utilization in older veterans with type 2 diabetes. Endocr Pract. 2016;22:196–204. https://doi.org/10.4158/EP15640.OR.

68. Khan TS, Fraser L-A. Type 1 diabetes and osteoporosis: from molecular pathways to bone phenotype. J Osteoporos. 2015;2015:174186. https://doi.org/10.1155/2015/174186.
69. Formiga F, Chivite D, Ruiz D, Navarro M, Perez Castejon JM, Duaso E, et al. Clinical evidence of diabetes mellitus end-organ damage as risk factor for falls complicated by hip fracture: a multi-center study of 1225 patients. Diabetes Res Clin Pract. 2015;109:233–7. https://doi.org/10.1016/j.diabres.2015.05.050.
70. Shanbhogue VV, Hansen S, Frost M, Jørgensen NR, Hermann AP, Henriksen JE, et al. Compromised cortical bone compartment in type 2 diabetes mellitus patients with microvascular disease. Eur J Endocrinol. 2015;174:115–24. https://doi.org/10.1530/EJE-15-0860.
71. Jules J, Feng X. In vitro investigation of the roles of the proinflammatory cytokines tumor necrosis factor-α and interleukin-1 in murine osteoclastogenesis. Methods Mol Biol. 2014;1155:109–23. https://doi.org/10.1007/978-1-4939-0669-7_10.
72. Diarra D, Stolina M, Polzer K, Zwerina J, Ominsky MS, Dwyer D, et al. Dickkopf-1 is a master regulator of joint remodeling. Nat Med. 2007;13:156–63. https://doi.org/10.1038/nm1538.
73. Roggia C, Gao Y, Cenci S, Weitzmann MN, Toraldo G, Isaia G, et al. Up-regulation of TNF-producing T cells in the bone marrow: a key mechanism by which estrogen deficiency induces bone loss in vivo. Proc Natl Acad Sci U S A. 2001;98:13960–5. https://doi.org/10.1073/pnas.251534698.
74. Kristiansen OP, Mandrup-Poulsen T. Interleukin-6 and diabetes: the good, the bad, or the indifferent? Diabetes. 2005;54(Suppl 2):S114–24.
75. Park JH, Park KH, Cho S, Choi YS, Seo SK, Lee BS, et al. Concomitant increase in muscle strength and bone mineral density with decreasing IL-6 levels after combination therapy with alendronate and calcitriol in postmenopausal women. Menopause. 2013;20:747–53. https://doi.org/10.1097/GME.0b013e31827cabca.
76. Taguchi Y, Yamamoto M, Yamate T, Lin SC, Mocharla H, DeTogni P, et al. Interleukin-6-type cytokines stimulate mesenchymal progenitor differentiation toward the osteoblastic lineage. Proc Assoc Am Physicians. 1998;110:559–74.
77. Nouh MR, Eid AF. Magnetic resonance imaging of the spinal marrow: basic understanding of the normal marrow pattern and its variant. World J Radiol. 2015;7:448–58. https://doi.org/10.4329/wjr.v7.i12.448.
78. Patsch JM, Li X, Baum T, Yap SP, Karampinos DC, Schwartz AV, et al. Bone marrow fat composition as a novel imaging biomarker in postmenopausal women with prevalent fragility fractures. J Bone Miner Res. 2013;28:1721–8. https://doi.org/10.1002/jbmr.1950.
79. Piccinin MA, Khan ZA. Pathophysiological role of enhanced bone marrow adipogenesis in diabetic complications. Adipocytes. 2014;3:263–72. https://doi.org/10.4161/adip.32215.
80. Krause MP, Riddell MC, Gordon CS, Imam SA, Cafarelli E, Hawke TJ. Diabetic myopathy differs between Ins2Akita+/– and streptozotocin-induced type 1 diabetic models. J Appl Physiol. 2009;106:1650–9. https://doi.org/10.1152/japplphysiol.91565.2008.
81. Jerković R, Bosnar A, Jurisić-Erzen D, Azman J, Starcević-Klasan G, Peharec S, et al. The effects of long-term experimental diabetes mellitus type I on skeletal muscle regeneration capacity. Coll Antropol. 2009;33:1115–9.
82. Kim TN, Park MS, Yang SJ, Yoo HJ, Kang HJ, Song W, et al. Prevalence and determinant factors of sarcopenia in patients with type 2 diabetes: the Korean sarcopenic obesity study (KSOS). Diabetes Care. 2010;33:1497–9. https://doi.org/10.2337/dc09-2310.
83. Umegaki H. Sarcopenia and diabetes: Hyperglycemia is a risk factor for age-associated muscle mass and functional reduction. J Diabetes Investig. 2015;6:623–4. https://doi.org/10.1111/jdi.12365.
84. Macgilchrist C, Paul L, Ellis BM, Howe TE, Kennon B, Godwin J. Lower-limb risk factors for falls in people with diabetes mellitus. Diabet Med. 2010;27:162–8. https://doi.org/10.1111/j.1464-5491.2009.02914.x.
85. Palermo A, Strollo R, Maddaloni E, Tuccinardi D, D'Onofrio L, Briganti SI, et al. Irisin is associated with osteoporotic fractures independently of bone mineral density, body composition or daily physical activity. Clin Endocrinol. 2015;82(4):615–9. https://doi.org/10.1111/cen.12672.

86. Choi Y-K, Kim M-K, Bae KH, Seo H-A, Jeong J-Y, Lee W-K, et al. Serum irisin levels in new-onset type 2 diabetes. Diabetes Res Clin Pract. 2013;100:96–101. https://doi.org/10.1016/j.diabres.2013.01.007.
87. Kanazawa I, Yamaguchi T, Yano S, et al. Metformin enhances the differentiation and mineralization of osteoblastic MC3T3-E1 cells via AMP kinase activation as well as eNOS and BMP-2 expression. Biochem Biophys Res Commun. 2008;375:414–9. https://doi.org/10.1016/j.bbrc.2008.08.034.
88. Jang WG, Kim EJ, Bae I-H, et al. Metformin induces osteoblast differentiation via orphan nuclear receptor SHP-mediated transactivation of Runx2. Bone. 2011;48:885–93. https://doi.org/10.1016/j.bone.2010.12.003.
89. Zhen D, Chen Y, Tang X. Metformin reverses the deleterious effects of high glucose on osteoblast function. J Diabetes Complicat. 2010;24:334–44. https://doi.org/10.1016/j.jdiacomp.2009.05.002.
90. Molinuevo MS, Schurman L, McCarthy AD, et al. Effect of metformin on bone marrow progenitor cell differentiation: in vivo and in vitro studies. J Bone Miner Res. 2010;25:211–21. https://doi.org/10.1359/jbmr.090732.
91. Gao Y, Li Y, Xue J, et al. Effect of the anti-diabetic drug metformin on bone mass in ovariectomized rats. Eur J Pharmacol. 2010;635:231–6. https://doi.org/10.1016/j.ejphar.2010.02.051.
92. Sedlinsky C, Molinuevo MS, Cortizo AM, et al. Metformin prevents anti-osteogenic in vivo and ex vivo effects of rosiglitazone in rats. Eur J Pharmacol. 2011;668:477–85. https://doi.org/10.1016/j.ejphar.2011.07.033.
93. Tolosa MJ, Chuguransky SR, Sedlinsky C, et al. Insulin-deficient diabetes-induced bone microarchitecture alterations are associated with a decrease in the osteogenic potential of bone marrow progenitor cells: preventive effects of metformin. Diabetes Res Clin Pract. 2013;101:177–86. https://doi.org/10.1016/j.diabres.2013.05.016.
94. Kasai T, Bandow K, Suzuki H, et al. Osteoblast differentiation is functionally associated with decreased AMP kinase activity. J Cell Physiol. 2009;221:740–9. https://doi.org/10.1002/jcp.21917.
95. Salai M, Somjen D, Gigi R, et al. Effects of commonly used medications on bone tissue mineralisation in SaOS-2 human bone cell line: an in vitro study. Bone Joint J. 2013;95-B:1575–80. https://doi.org/10.1302/0301-620X.95B11.31158.
96. Mai Q-G, Zhang Z-M, Xu S, et al. Metformin stimulates osteoprotegerin and reduces RANKL expression in osteoblasts and ovariectomized rats. J Cell Biochem. 2011;112:2902–9. https://doi.org/10.1002/jcb.23206.
97. Liu L, Zhang C, Hu Y, Peng B. Protective effect of metformin on periapical lesions in rats by decreasing the ratio of receptor activator of nuclear factor kappa B ligand/osteoprotegerin. J Endod. 2012;38:943–7. https://doi.org/10.1016/j.joen.2012.03.010.
98. Wu W, Ye Z, Zhou Y, Tan W-S. AICAR, a small chemical molecule, primes osteogenic differentiation of adult mesenchymal stem cells. Int J Artif Organs. 2011;34:1128–36. https://doi.org/10.5301/ijao.5000007.
99. Patel JJ, Butters OR, Arnett TR. PPAR agonists stimulate adipogenesis at the expense of osteoblast differentiation while inhibiting osteoclast formation and activity. Cell Biochem Funct. 2014;32(4):368–77. https://doi.org/10.1002/cbf.3025.
100. Jeyabalan J, Viollet B, Smitham P, et al. The anti-diabetic drug metformin does not affect bone mass in vivo or fracture healing. Osteoporos Int. 2013;24:2659–70. https://doi.org/10.1007/s00198-013-2371-0.
101. Colhoun HM, Livingstone SJ, Looker HC, et al. Hospitalised hip fracture risk with rosiglitazone and pioglitazone use compared with other glucose-lowering drugs. Diabetologia. 2012;55:2929–37. https://doi.org/10.1007/s00125-012-2668-0.
102. Napoli N, Strotmeyer ES, Ensrud KE, et al. Fracture risk in diabetic elderly men: the MrOS study. Diabetologia. 2014;57:2057–65. https://doi.org/10.1007/s00125-014-3289-6.

103. Kahn SE, Haffner SM, Heise MA, et al. Glycemic durability of rosiglitazone, metformin, or glyburide monotherapy. N Engl J Med. 2006;355:2427–43. https://doi.org/10.1056/NEJMoa066224.
104. Kahn SE, Zinman B, Lachin JM, et al. Rosiglitazone-associated fractures in type 2 diabetes: an Analysis from A Diabetes Outcome Progression Trial (ADOPT). Diabetes Care. 2008;31:845–51. https://doi.org/10.2337/dc07-2270.
105. Monami M, Dicembrini I, Kundisova L, et al. A meta-analysis of the hypoglycemic risk in randomized controlled trials with sulphonylureas in patients with type 2 diabetes. Diabetes Obes Metab. 2014;16(9):833–40. https://doi.org/10.1111/dom.12287.
106. Johnston SS, Conner C, Aagren M, et al. Association between hypoglycaemic events and fall-related fractures in Medicare-covered patients with type 2 diabetes. Diabetes Obes Metab. 2012;14:634–43. https://doi.org/10.1111/j.1463-1326.2012.01583.x.
107. Dormuth CR, Carney G, Carleton B, et al. Thiazolidinediones and fractures in men and women. Arch Intern Med. 2009;169:1395–402. https://doi.org/10.1001/archinternmed.2009.214.
108. Monami M, Cresci B, Colombini A, et al. Bone fractures and hypoglycemic treatment in type 2 diabetic patients: a case-control study. Diabetes Care. 2008;31:199–203. https://doi.org/10.2337/dc07-1736.
109. Michalik L, Auwerx J, Berger JP, et al. International Union of Pharmacology. LXI. Peroxisome proliferator-activated receptors. Pharmacol Rev. 2006;58:726–41. https://doi.org/10.1124/pr.58.4.5.
110. Ahmadian M, Suh JM, Hah N, et al. PPARγ signaling and metabolism: the good, the bad and the future. Nat Med. 2013;19:557–66. https://doi.org/10.1038/nm.3159.
111. Shockley KR, Lazarenko OP, Czernik PJ, et al. PPARgamma2 nuclear receptor controls multiple regulatory pathways of osteoblast differentiation from marrow mesenchymal stem cells. J Cell Biochem. 2009;106:232–46. https://doi.org/10.1002/jcb.21994.
112. Johnson TE, Vogel R, Rutledge SJ, et al. Thiazolidinedione effects on glucocorticoid receptor-mediated gene transcription and differentiation in osteoblastic cells. Endocrinology. 1999;140:3245–54. https://doi.org/10.1210/endo.140.7.6797.
113. Gustafson B, Eliasson B, Smith U. Thiazolidinediones increase the wingless-type MMTV integration site family (WNT) inhibitor Dickkopf-1 in adipocytes: a link with osteogenesis. Diabetologia. 2010;53:536–40. https://doi.org/10.1007/s00125-009-1615-1.
114. Mieczkowska A, Baslé MF, Chappard D, Mabilleau G. Thiazolidinediones induce osteocyte apoptosis by a G protein-coupled receptor 40-dependent mechanism. J Biol Chem. 2012;287:23517–26. https://doi.org/10.1074/jbc.M111.324814.
115. Mabilleau G, Mieczkowska A, Edmonds ME. Thiazolidinediones induce osteocyte apoptosis and increase sclerostin expression. Diabet Med. 2010;27:925–32. https://doi.org/10.1111/j.1464-5491.2010.03048.x.
116. Yakar S, Courtland H-W, Clemmons D. IGF-1 and bone: new discoveries from mouse models. J Bone Miner Res. 2010;25:2543–52. https://doi.org/10.1002/jbmr.234.
117. Lecka-Czernik B, Ackert-Bicknell C, Adamo ML, et al. Activation of peroxisome proliferator-activated receptor gamma (PPARgamma) by rosiglitazone suppresses components of the insulin-like growth factor regulatory system in vitro and in vivo. Endocrinology. 2007;148:903–11. https://doi.org/10.1210/en.2006-1121.
118. Wan Y, Chong L-W, Evans RM. PPAR-gamma regulates osteoclastogenesis in mice. Nat Med. 2007;13:1496–503. https://doi.org/10.1038/nm1672.
119. Sottile V, Seuwen K, Kneissel M. Enhanced marrow adipogenesis and bone resorption in estrogen-deprived rats treated with the PPARgamma agonist BRL49653 (rosiglitazone). Calcif Tissue Int. 2004;75:329–37. https://doi.org/10.1007/s00223-004-0224-8.
120. Syversen U, Stunes AK, Gustafsson BI, et al. Different skeletal effects of the peroxisome proliferator activated receptor (PPAR)alpha agonist fenofibrate and the PPARgamma agonist pioglitazone. BMC Endocr Disord. 2009;9:10. https://doi.org/10.1186/1472-6823-9-10.

121. Krause U, Harris S, Green A, et al. Pharmaceutical modulation of canonical Wnt signaling in multipotent stromal cells for improved osteoinductive therapy. Proc Natl Acad Sci U S A. 2010;107:4147–52. https://doi.org/10.1073/pnas.0914360107.
122. Seto-Young D, Paliou M, Schlosser J, et al. Direct thiazolidinedione action in the human ovary: insulin-independent and insulin-sensitizing effects on steroidogenesis and insulin-like growth factor binding protein-1 production. J Clin Endocrinol Metab. 2005;90:6099–105. https://doi.org/10.1210/jc.2005-0469.
123. Seto-Young D, Avtanski D, Parikh G, et al. Rosiglitazone and pioglitazone inhibit estrogen synthesis in human granulosa cells by interfering with androgen binding to aromatase. Horm Metab Res. 2011;43:250–6. https://doi.org/10.1055/s-0030-1270525.
124. Schwartz AV, Sellmeyer DE, Vittinghoff E, et al. Thiazolidinedione (TZD) use and bone loss in older diabetic adults. J Clin Endocrinol Metab. 2006;91:3349–54.
125. Solomon DH, Cadarette SM, Choudhry NK, et al. A cohort study of thiazolidinediones and fractures in older adults with diabetes. J Clin Endocrinol Metab. 2009;94:2792–8. https://doi.org/10.1210/jc.2008-2157.
126. Kanazawa I, Yamaguchi T, Yamamoto M, Sugimoto T. Relationship between treatments with insulin and oral hypoglycemic agents versus the presence of vertebral fractures in type 2 diabetes mellitus. J Bone Miner Metab. 2010;28:554–60. https://doi.org/10.1007/s00774-010-0160-9.
127. Habib ZA, Havstad SL, Wells K, et al. Thiazolidinedione use and the longitudinal risk of fractures in patients with type 2 diabetes mellitus. J Clin Endocrinol Metab. 2010;95:592–600. https://doi.org/10.1210/jc.2009-1385.
128. Douglas IJ, Evans SJ, Pocock S, Smeeth L. The risk of fractures associated with thiazolidinediones: a self-controlled case-series study. PLoS Med. 2009;6:e1000154. https://doi.org/10.1371/journal.pmed.100015.
129. Meier C, Kraenzlin ME, Bodmer M, et al. Use of thiazolidinediones and fracture risk. Arch Intern Med. 2008;168:820–5. https://doi.org/10.1001/archinte.168.8.820.
130. Aubert RE, Herrera V, Chen W, et al. Rosiglitazone and pioglitazone increase fracture risk in women and men with type 2 diabetes. Diabetes Obes Metab. 2010;12:716–21. https://doi.org/10.1111/j.1463-1326.2010.01225.x.
131. Bilik D, McEwen LN, Brown MB, et al. Thiazolidinediones and fractures: evidence from translating research into action for diabetes. J Clin Endocrinol Metab. 2010;95:4560–5. https://doi.org/10.1210/jc.2009-2638.
132. Hsiao F-Y, Mullins CD. The association between thiazolidinediones and hospitalisation for fracture in type 2 diabetic patients: a Taiwanese population-based nested case-control study. Diabetologia. 2010;53:489–96. https://doi.org/10.1007/s00125-009-1609-z.
133. Bazelier MT, Vestergaard P, Gallagher AM, van Staa T-P, Cooper C, Leufkens HGM, et al. Risk of fracture with thiazolidinediones: disease or drugs? Calcif Tissue Int. 2012;90:450–7. https://doi.org/10.1007/s00223-012-9591-8.
134. Jones SG, Momin SR, Good MW, et al. Distal upper and lower limb fractures associated with thiazolidinedione use. Am J Manag Care. 2009;15:491–6.
135. Zhu Z-N, Jiang Y-F, Ding T. Risk of fracture with thiazolidinediones: an updated meta-analysis of randomized clinical trials. Bone. 2014;68:115–23. https://doi.org/10.1016/j.bone.2014.08.010.
136. Grey A, Bolland M, Gamble G, et al. The peroxisome proliferator-activated receptor-gamma agonist rosiglitazone decreases bone formation and bone mineral density in healthy postmenopausal women: a randomized, controlled trial. J Clin Endocrinol Metab. 2007;92:1305–10. https://doi.org/10.1210/jc.2006-2646.
137. Harsløf T, Wamberg L, Møller L, et al. Rosiglitazone decreases bone mass and bone marrow fat. J Clin Endocrinol Metab. 2011;96:1541–8. https://doi.org/10.1210/jc.2010-2077.
138. Berberoglu Z, Yazici AC, Demirag NG. Effects of rosiglitazone on bone mineral density and remodelling parameters in Postmenopausal diabetic women: a 2-year follow-up study. Clin Endocrinol. 2010;73:305–12. https://doi.org/10.1111/j.1365-2265.2010.03784.x.

139. Yaturu S, Bryant B, Jain SK. Thiazolidinedione treatment decreases bone mineral density in type 2 diabetic men. Diabetes Care. 2007;30:1574–6. https://doi.org/10.2337/dc06-2606.
140. Bilezikian JP, Josse RG, Eastell R, et al. Rosiglitazone decreases bone mineral density and increases bone turnover in postmenopausal women with type 2 diabetes mellitus. J Clin Endocrinol Metab. 2013;98:1519–28. https://doi.org/10.1210/jc.2012-4018.
141. Home PD, Pocock SJ, Beck-Nielsen H, et al. Rosiglitazone evaluated for cardiovascular outcomes in oral agent combination therapy for type 2 diabetes (RECORD): a multicentre, randomised, open-label trial. Lancet. 2009;373:2125–35. https://doi.org/10.1016/S0140-6736(09)60953-3.
142. Kanazawa I, Yamaguchi T, Yano S, et al. Baseline atherosclerosis parameter could assess the risk of bone loss during pioglitazone treatment in type 2 diabetes mellitus. Osteoporos Int. 2010;21:2013–8. https://doi.org/10.1007/s00198-009-1161-1.
143. Grey A, Bolland M, Fenwick S, et al. The skeletal effects of pioglitazone in type 2 diabetes or impaired glucose tolerance: a randomized controlled trial. Eur J Endocrinol. 2014;170:255–62. https://doi.org/10.1530/EJE-13-0793.
144. Dormandy J, Bhattacharya M, van Troostenburg de Bruyn A-R. Safety and tolerability of pioglitazone in high-risk patients with type 2 diabetes: an overview of data from PROactive. Drug Saf. 2009;32:187–202.
145. Drucker DJ, Nauck MA. The incretin system: glucagon-like peptide-1 receptor agonists and dipeptidyl peptidase-4 inhibitors in type 2 diabetes. Lancet. 2006;368:1696–705. https://doi.org/10.1016/S0140-6736(06)69705-5.
146. Pacheco-Pantoja EL, Ranganath LR, Gallagher JA, et al. Receptors and effects of gut hormones in three osteoblastic cell lines. BMC Physiol. 2011;11:12. https://doi.org/10.1186/1472-6793-11-12.
147. Kim J-Y, Lee S-K, Jo K-J, et al. Exendin-4 increases bone mineral density in type 2 diabetic OLETF rats potentially through the down-regulation of SOST/sclerostin in osteocytes. Life Sci. 2013;92:533–40. https://doi.org/10.1016/j.lfs.2013.01.001.
148. Nuche-Berenguer B, Lozano D, Gutiérrez-Rojas I, et al. GLP-1 and exendin-4 can reverse hyperlipidic-related osteopenia. J Endocrinol. 2011;209:203–10. https://doi.org/10.1530/JOE-11-0015.
149. Ma X, Meng J, Jia M, et al. Exendin-4, a glucagon-like peptide-1 receptor agonist, prevents osteopenia by promoting bone formation and suppressing bone resorption in aged ovariectomized rats. J Bone Miner Res. 2013;28:1641–52. https://doi.org/10.1002/jbmr.1898.
150. Yamada C, Yamada Y, Tsukiyama K, et al. The murine glucagon-like peptide-1 receptor is essential for control of bone resorption. Endocrinology. 2008;149:574–9. https://doi.org/10.1210/en.2007-1292.
151. Su B, Sheng H, Zhang M, et al. Risk of bone fractures associated with glucagon-like peptide-1 receptor agonists' treatment: a meta-analysis of randomized controlled trials. Endocrine. 2014;48(1):107–15. https://doi.org/10.1007/s12020-014-0361-4.
152. Monami M, Dicembrini I, Antenore A, Mannucci E. Dipeptidyl peptidase-4 inhibitors and bone fractures: a meta-analysis of randomized clinical trials. Diabetes Care. 2011;34:2474–6. https://doi.org/10.2337/dc11-1099.
153. Bilezikian JP, Watts NB, Usiskin K, et al. Evaluation of bone mineral density and bone biomarkers in patients with type 2 diabetes treated with canagliflozin. J Clin Endocrinol Metab. 2016;101(1):44–51. https://doi.org/10.1210/jc.2015-1860.
154. Watts NB, Bilezikian JP, Usiskin K, et al. Effects of canagliflozin on fracture risk in patients with type 2 diabetes mellitus. J Clin Endocrinol Metab. 2016;101(1):157–66. https://doi.org/10.1210/jc.2015-3167.
155. Ljunggren Ö, Bolinder J, Johansson L, et al. Dapagliflozin has no effect on markers of bone formation and resorption or bone mineral density in patients with inadequately controlled type 2 diabetes mellitus on metformin. Diabetes Obes Metab. 2012;14:990–9. https://doi.org/10.1111/j.1463-1326.2012.01630.x.

156. Bolinder J, Ljunggren O, Johansson L, et al. Dapagliflozin maintains glycaemic control while reducing weight and body fat mass over 2 years in patients with type 2 diabetes mellitus inadequately controlled on metformin. Diabetes Obes Metab. 2013;16(2):159–69. https://doi.org/10.1111/dom.12189.
157. Pater A, Sypniewska G, Pilecki O. Biochemical markers of bone cell activity in children with type 1 diabetes mellitus. J Pediatr Endocrinol Metab. 2010;23:81–6.
158. Karagüzel G, Akçurin S, Ozdem S, Boz A, Bircan I. Bone mineral density and alterations of bone metabolism in children and adolescents with type 1 diabetes mellitus. J Pediatr Endocrinol Metab. 2006;19:805–14.
159. Alexopoulou O, Jamart J, Devogelaer JP, Brichard S, de Nayer PBM. Bone density and markers of bone remodeling in type 1 male diabetic patients. Diabetes Metab. 2006;32:453–8.
160. Lumachi F, Camozzi V, Tombolan V, Luisetto G. Bone mineral density, osteocalcin, and bone-specific alkaline phosphatase in patients with insulin-dependent diabetes mellitus. Ann N Y Acad Sci. 2009;1173:E64–7. https://doi.org/10.1111/j.1749-6632.2009.04955.x.
161. Jehle PM, Jehle DR, Mohan S, Böhm BO. Serum levels of insulin-like growth factor system components and relationship to bone metabolism in Type 1 and Type 2 diabetes mellitus patients. J Endocrinol. 1998;159:297–306.
162. Starup-Linde J, Vestergaard P, Vestergaard P, Giangregorio LM, Leslie WD, Lix LM, et al. Biochemical bone turnover markers in diabetes mellitus — a systematic review. Bone. 2015;82:69–78. https://doi.org/10.1016/j.bone.2015.02.019.
163. Gaudio A, Privitera F, Battaglia K, Torrisi V, Sidoti MH, Pulvirenti I, et al. Sclerostin levels associated with inhibition of the Wnt/β-catenin signaling and reduced bone turnover in type 2 diabetes mellitus. J Clin Endocrinol Metab. 2012;97:3744–50. https://doi.org/10.1210/jc.2012-1901.
164. Catalano A, Pintaudi B, Morabito N, Di Vieste G, Giunta L, Bruno ML, et al. Gender differences in sclerostin and clinical characteristics in type 1 diabetes mellitus. Eur J Endocrinol. 2014;171:293–300. https://doi.org/10.1530/EJE-14-0106.
165. Register TC, Hruska KA, Divers J, Bowden DW, Palmer ND, Carr JJ, et al. Sclerostin is positively associated with bone mineral density in men and women and negatively associated with carotid calcified atherosclerotic plaque in men from the African American-diabetes heart study. J Clin Endocrinol Metab. 2014;99:315–21. https://doi.org/10.1210/jc.2013-3168.
166. Kanazawa I, Yamaguchi T, Sugimoto T. Serum insulin-like growth factor-I is a marker for assessing the severity of vertebral fractures in postmenopausal women with type 2 diabetes mellitus. Osteoporos Int. 2011;22:1191–8. https://doi.org/10.1007/s00198-010-1310-6.
167. Yamamoto M, Yamauchi M, Sugimoto T. Elevated sclerostin levels are associated with vertebral fractures in patients with type 2 diabetes mellitus. J Clin Endocrinol Metab. 2013;98:4030–7. https://doi.org/10.1210/jc.2013-2143.
168. Jiajue R, Jiang Y, Wang O, Li M, Xing X, Cui L, et al. Suppressed bone turnover was associated with increased osteoporotic fracture risks in non-obese postmenopausal Chinese women with type 2 diabetes mellitus. Osteoporos Int. 2014;25:1999–2005. https://doi.org/10.1007/s00198-014-2714-5.
169. Starup-Linde J, Eriksen SA, Lykkeboe S, Handberg A, Vestergaard P. Biochemical markers of bone turnover in diabetes patientsDOUBLEHYPHENa meta-analysis, and a methodological study on the effects of glucose on bone markers. Osteoporos Int. 2014;25:1697–708. https://doi.org/10.1007/s00198-014-2676-7.
170. Hampson G, Evans C, Petitt RJ, Evans WD, Woodhead SJ, Peters JR, et al. Bone mineral density, collagen type 1 alpha 1 genotypes and bone turnover in premenopausal women with diabetes mellitus. Diabetologia. 1998;41:1314–20.
171. Eller-Vainicher C, Zhukouskaya VV, Tolkachev YV, Koritko SS, Cairoli E, Grossi E, et al. Low bone mineral density and its predictors in type 1 diabetic patients evaluated by the classic statistics and artificial neural network analysis. Diabetes Care. 2011;34:2186–91. https://doi.org/10.2337/dc11-0764.
172. Joshi A, Varthakavi P, Chadha M, Bhagwat N. A study of bone mineral density and its determinants in type 1 diabetes mellitus. J Osteoporos. 2013;2013:397814. https://doi.org/10.1155/2013/397814.

173. Bridges MJ, Moochhala SH, Barbour J, Kelly CA. Influence of diabetes on peripheral bone mineral density in men: a controlled study. Acta Diabetol. 2005;42:82–6. https://doi.org/10.1007/s00592-005-0183-1.
174. Hofbauer LC, Brueck CC, Singh SK, Dobnig H. Osteoporosis in patients with diabetes mellitus. J Bone Miner Res. 2007;22:1317–28. https://doi.org/10.1359/jbmr.070510.
175. Bechtold S, Putzker S, Bonfig W, Fuchs O, Dirlenbach I, Schwarz HP. Bone size normalizes with age in children and adolescents with type 1 diabetes. Diabetes Care. 2007;30:2046–50. https://doi.org/10.2337/dc07-0142.
176. Mastrandrea LD, Wactawski-Wende J, Donahue RP, Hovey KM, Clark A, Quattrin T. Young women with type 1 diabetes have lower bone mineral density that persists over time. Diabetes Care. 2008;31:1729–35. https://doi.org/10.2337/dc07-2426.
177. Sellmeyer DE, Civitelli R, Hofbauer LC, Khosla S, Lecka-Czernik B, Schwartz AV. Skeletal metabolism, fracture risk, and fracture outcomes in type 1 and type 2 diabetes. Diabetes. 2016;65:1757–66. https://doi.org/10.2337/db16-0063.
178. Ma L, Oei L, Jiang L, Estrada K, Chen H, Wang Z, et al. Association between bone mineral density and type 2 diabetes mellitus: a meta-analysis of observational studies. Eur J Epidemiol. 2012;27:319–32. https://doi.org/10.1007/s10654-012-9674-x.
179. Strotmeyer ES, Cauley JA, Schwartz AV, Nevitt MC, Resnick HE, Zmuda JM, et al. Diabetes is associated independently of body composition with BMD and bone volume in older white and black men and women: the health, aging, and body composition study. J Bone Miner Res. 2004;19:1084–91. https://doi.org/10.1359/JBMR.040311.
180. Shan PF, Wu XP, Zhang H, Cao XZ, Yuan LQ, Liao EY. Age-related bone mineral density, osteoporosis rate and risk of vertebral fracture in mainland Chinese women with type 2 diabetes mellitus. J Endocrinol Investig. 2011;34:190–6. https://doi.org/10.1007/BF03347065.
181. Schwartz AV, Ewing SK, Porzig AM, McCulloch CE, Resnick HE, Hillier TA, et al. Diabetes and change in bone mineral density at the hip, calcaneus, spine, and radius in older women. Front Endocrinol (Lausanne). 2013;4:62. https://doi.org/10.3389/fendo.2013.00062.
182. Keegan THM, Schwartz AV, Bauer DC, Sellmeyer DE, Kelsey JL, Fracture Intervention Trial. Effect of alendronate on bone mineral density and biochemical markers of bone turnover in type 2 diabetic women: the fracture intervention trial. Diabetes Care. 2004;27:1547–53.
183. Khalil N, Sutton-Tyrrell K, Strotmeyer ES, Greendale GA, Vuga M, Selzer F, et al. Menopausal bone changes and incident fractures in diabetic women: a cohort study. Osteoporos Int. 2011;22:1367–76. https://doi.org/10.1007/s00198-010-1357-4.
184. Schwartz AV, Sellmeyer DE, Strotmeyer ES, Tylavsky FA, Feingold KR, Resnick HE, et al. Diabetes and bone loss at the hip in older black and white adults. J Bone Miner Res. 2005;20:596–603. https://doi.org/10.1359/JBMR.041219.
185. Abdalrahaman N, McComb C, Foster JE, McLean J, Lindsay RS, McClure J, et al. Deficits in trabecular bone microarchitecture in young women with type 1 diabetes mellitus. J Bone Miner Res. 2015;30:1386–93. https://doi.org/10.1002/jbmr.2465.
186. Shanbhogue VV, Hansen S, Frost M, Jørgensen NR, Hermann AP, Henriksen JE, et al. Bone geometry, volumetric density, microarchitecture, and estimated bone strength assessed by HR-pQCT in adult patients with type 1 diabetes mellitus. J Bone Miner Res. 2015;30:2188–99. https://doi.org/10.1002/jbmr.2573.
187. Burghardt AJ, Issever AS, Schwartz AV, Davis KA, Masharani U, Majumdar S, et al. High-resolution peripheral quantitative computed tomographic imaging of cortical and trabecular bone microarchitecture in patients with type 2 diabetes mellitus. J Clin Endocrinol Metab. 2010;95:5045–55. https://doi.org/10.1210/jc.2010-0226.
188. Yu EW, Putman MS, Derrico N, Abrishamanian-Garcia G, Finkelstein JS, Bouxsein ML. Defects in cortical microarchitecture among African-American women with type 2 diabetes. Osteoporos Int. 2015;26:673–9. https://doi.org/10.1007/s00198-014-2927-7.
189. Patsch JM, Burghardt AJ, Yap SP, Baum T, Schwartz AV, Joseph GB, et al. Increased cortical porosity in type 2 diabetic postmenopausal women with fragility fractures. J Bone Miner Res. 2013;28:313–24. https://doi.org/10.1002/jbmr.1763.

190. Farr JN, Drake MT, Amin S, Melton LJ, McCready LK, Khosla S. In vivo assessment of bone quality in postmenopausal women with type 2 diabetes. J Bone Miner Res. 2014;29:787–95. https://doi.org/10.1002/jbmr.2106.
191. Dhaliwal R, Cibula D, Ghosh C, Weinstock RS, Moses AM. Bone quality assessment in type 2 diabetes mellitus. Osteoporos Int. 2014;25(7):1969–73. https://doi.org/10.1007/s00198-014-2704-7.
192. Kim JH, Choi HJ, Ku EJ, Kim KM, Kim SW, Cho NH, et al. Trabecular bone score as an indicator for skeletal deterioration in diabetes. J Clin Endocrinol Metab. 2015;100(2):475–82. https://doi.org/10.1210/jc.2014-2047.
193. Leslie WD, Aubry-Rozier B, Lamy O, Hans D, Manitoba Bone Density Program. TBS (trabecular bone score) and diabetes-related fracture risk. J Clin Endocrinol Metab. 2013;98:602–9. https://doi.org/10.1210/jc.2012-3118.
194. Neumann T, Lodes S, Kästner B, Lehmann T, Hans D, Lamy O, et al. Trabecular bone score in type 1 diabetesDOUBLEHYPHENa cross-sectional study. Osteoporos Int. 2016;27:127–33. https://doi.org/10.1007/s00198-015-3222-y.

11 Renal Diseases and Skeletal Health

Sandro Mazzaferro, Silverio Rotondi, Lida Tartaglione, Natalia De Martino, Cristiana Leonangeli, and Marzia Pasquali

11.1 Renal Disease and Mineral and Bone Disease

According to the international KDIGO guidelines, the diagnosis of chronic kidney damage (CKD) or of decreased kidney function (chronic renal failure, CRF) is defined by the evidence, for 3 or more months, of any pathologic abnormality of the kidney. Abnormalities can be evidenced by urinary sediment, renal biopsy, or imaging studies. First thing to notice is that these abnormalities may occur in the presence of normal or decreased glomerular filtration rate. Glomerular filtration rate (GFR), the most widely employed method to assess renal function, is commonly referred to as creatinine clearance; however, in recent years, different formulas have been provided that allow to estimate GFR (eGFR). The esteem can be obtained with few anthropometric parameters and/or biochemicals and, importantly, serum creatinine. Following their diffusion, these formulas have been applied also to the general population, and it has become evident that the reduction of GFR is more common than expected, in particular in elderly people. It is now appreciated that CRF prevalence in the general population averages 9% in Europe but has been reported to reach 13% in countries outside Europe. The condition of reduced GFR cannot be regarded as a nephrologic problem, since it is commonly recognized that CRF carries a significant increase in the overall and cardiovascular risk of mortality. A seminal publication by Levey et al. [1] has clearly evidenced that it is not only the reduction of GFR (which could arise from aging or from vascular diseases like hypertension) but also the degree of proteinuria (which is expected to arise from glomerular or tubular damage) that contributes to increase the cardiovascular burden of renal insufficiency [1]. CRF is thus divided into five different grades of

S. Mazzaferro (✉) · S. Rotondi · L. Tartaglione · N. D. Martino · C. Leonangeli · M. Pasquali
Unit of Nephrology, Dipartimento di Scienze Cardiovascolari Respiratorie Nefrologiche Anestesiologiche e Geriatriche, Azienda Policlinico Umberto I, Sapienza Università di Roma, Rome, Italy
e-mail: sandro.mazzaferro@uniroma1.it

A. Lenzi, S. Migliaccio (eds.), *Multidisciplinary Approach to Osteoporosis*, https://doi.org/10.1007/978-3-319-75110-8_11

reduction (G, 1–5) and three levels of albuminuria (A, 1–3). The resulting GA classification of the individual patient is relevant for the prognostic value in terms of both progression of renal disease and cardiovascular risk. Accordingly, any physician should know and apply this classification to their patients.

Another cultural achievement in the field of nephrology has been the recognition that also the disturbances in mineral and bone metabolism may play a role in the increment of morbidity and mortality that goes along with progression of CRF. Until recently, the attention on bone disease in CRF was focused on the more severe and advanced stages of the disease, in patients receiving dialysis. In these patients, the disease of the bone was severe with deformities and/or non-healing fractures which were mostly referred to secondary hyperparathyroidism (SHP) and hypovitaminosis D. In more recent years, the attention has moved to the early stages of CRF which involve a much larger number of subjects. The biochemical derangements of SHP (hypocalcemia, hyperphosphatemia, hyperparathyroidism, and hypovitaminosis D) have been enriched by the discovery of specific receptors for serum Ca and vitamin D (which are expressed in most of the cells in the organism) and of the FGF23/Klotho system. This last system can be regarded as responsible for the dialogue between the bone and kidney. Bone cells synthesize FGF23 which is determinant for the regulation of renal phosphate excretion and balance and for the fine-tuning of vitamin D synthesis; renal tubular cells, on the other side, produce klotho, a coreceptor that renders the selective action of FGF23 at renal and extrarenal sites. Also, other bone proteins (e.g., osteocalcin, sclerostin, DKK1, the SIBLINGS family, etc.) have gained attention because of their potential role in extra-skeletal calcification which is now regarded as essential for the cardiovascular morbidity and mortality specifically carried by CRF.

As a result, renal osteodystrophy, the disease of bone that affects patients with CRF, is now re-comprised in a larger clinical entity named CKD-MBD which includes the biochemical derangements of divalent ions of renal patients, the presence of bone disease, and the presence of vascular and ectopic calcifications. All of these derangements are considered to occur together and in variable degrees as a consequence of CRF and to be responsible, at least in part, of the cardiovascular risk now appreciated in renal patients. For this reason, numerous research efforts are under way to try to discover the precise pathomechanisms of these derangements with the aim of discovering new, more successful, therapeutic strategies.

11.2 Pathogenesis of Bone Disease in Renal Patients

The pathophysiology of bone disease in chronic kidney disease (CKD) is complex. The kidney is essential for regulation of mineral metabolism, and it has been known for many years that renal patients are affected with bone disease as a result of significant derangements in divalent ions. Kidneys are involved in divalent ion homeostasis not only by renal handling of ions but also because of the synthesis of hormones affecting mineral metabolism and bone cell activity.

As a consequence, mineral abnormalities can be secondary to either a defect of some specific renal tubular cell activity (generally associated with normal glomerular filtration rate) or a generalized involvement of the organ affecting both glomerular and tubular structures (mostly resulting in variable degrees of renal failure).

Different renal diseases may produce different bone diseases as a reflection of the resulting metabolic alteration [2], and the presence or not of renal insufficiency is always essential for the final clinical picture. Accordingly, we can consider that bone disease may be secondary to CKD with or without reduced glomerular filtration rate (or chronic renal failure).

11.2.1 Bone Disease in Chronic Kidney Disease Without Chronic Renal Failure

Calcium and phosphate are divalent ions essential for skeletal health. Kidneys play a central role in the handling of these ions, through processes of glomerular filtration and tubular reabsorption and/or secretion. Under physiologic conditions, the balance of calcium and phosphate is maintained by tiny adjustments of urinary excretion that guarantee neutral balance. Renal tubular disorders that lead to calcium and/or phosphorus imbalance result in bone disease.

In particular, tubular defects of calcium handling are responsible for calcium leak, negative calcium balance, and osteoporosis [3]. Interestingly hypercalciuria can be secondary to genetic disorders [4] referable to single or multiple transport protein defects. For example, genetic disorders of the voltage-dependent chloride transporter, CLC-5, have been reported in four different hereditary hypercalciuric syndromes with nephrolithiasis: Dent's disease, X-linked recessive nephrolithiasis (XRN), X-linked recessive hypophosphatemic rickets (XLRH), and Japanese idiopathic low molecular weight proteinuria (JILMWP). The first and the third of these syndromes are also characterized by bone involvement [5]. In these syndromes, defects in tubular endocytosis and/or protein trafficking, resulting in defective reabsorption of the vitamin D-binding protein-25-hydroxyvitamin D complex and in defective activation of vitamin D [6], are claimed to explain the presence of rickets.

Genetic mutations of phosphate transport proteins also result in bone disease. For example, hereditary hypophosphatemic rickets with hypercalciuria (HHRH) is a rare autosomal recessive disorder characterized by hypophosphatemia secondary to renal phosphate wasting, muscle weakness, bone pain, limb deformities, and rickets. HHRH is distinct from other forms of hypophosphatemic rickets since it results from a loss-of-function mutation in sodium/phosphate cotransporter 2c (Na/P 2c) [7] leading to hypophosphatemia, low FGF23 levels, increased 1,25-dihydroxyvitamin D synthesis, increased intestinal absorption of calcium, and finally, hypercalciuria.

Renal tubular acidosis, a group of renal transport defects of bicarbonate reabsorption or of hydrogen excretion, also affects bone mineral composition. In fact, acidosis favors ion exchange between H+ and Ca++ [8] and stimulates the buffer function of bone by directly dissolving the mineral component. Further, chronic acidosis affects bone cell activity through induction of PGE2 [9] and RANK-L production [10], which result in disturbed collagen synthesis and increased osteoclast differentiation [11]. Also, acidosis inhibits expression of selective calcium transport channels in renal tubular cells, thus inducing urinary calcium excretion and negative calcium balance [12]. Further possible links between acidosis and bone can be guessed from the recent experimental evidence of proton-sensing receptors [13] and of acid-sensing ion channels in bone cells [14]. The typical clinical manifestations of bone involvement in acidosis are osteomalacia, osteopenia, and/or osteoporosis resulting from either defective mineralization, increased osteoclastic activity, or urinary calcium leak.

Multiple defects in tubular transportation are also possible in Fanconi syndrome which leads to hypophosphatemia, hypercalciuria, aminoaciduria, glycosuria, acidosis, vitamin D deficit, and then, osteomalacia or rickets (Table 11.1) [15].

Table 11.1 Bone involvement in kidney diseases

Bone disease	Kidney disease	Biochemical derangement
Osteoporosis	RTA1, RTA2 (tubular disorders with metabolic acidosis)	Low pH Normal anion gap High serum Cl
	Idiopathic hypercalciuria – X-linked recessive nephrolithiasis (XRN) – Japanese idiopathic low molecular weight proteinuria (JILMWP)	High urinary Ca Renal failure High urinary Ca Proteinuria
Osteomalacia rickets	– Dent's disease – X-linked recessive hypophosphatemic rickets (XLRH)	Renal failure High urinary Ca High urinary PO_4 Proteinuria
	Hereditary hypophosphatemic rickets with hypercalciuria (HHRH)	Low serum PO_4 High serum 1,25D High urinary Ca High urinary PO_4 Multiple renal tubular defects
	Fanconi syndrome	Multiple renal tubular defects
Renal osteodystrophy	Chronic kidney failure	High PTH Low serum 1,25D Low serum Ca High serum PO_4 High/normal BALP Low pH Low Klotho High FGF23

RTA renal tubular acidosis, *1,25D* calcitriol, *PTH* parathyroid hormone, *FGF23* fibroblast growth factor 23, *Ca* calcium, PO_4 phosphate, *BALP* bone-specific alkaline phosphatase, *Cl* chloride

11.2.2 Bone Disease in Chronic Kidney Disease with Chronic Renal Failure

The presence of reduced GFR changes completely the clinical spectrum of bone disease secondary to CKD. In fact, besides the classical derangement in divalent ions and the associated SHP, new pathomechanisms have been recently discovered. Further, in particular in the more advanced stages of renal disease, CRF carries the metabolic abnormalities of uremia, responsible for very specific clinical pictures.

11.2.2.1 Calcium, Phosphate, PTH, and the Vitamin D/FGF23/Klotho System

Chronic renal failure typically associates with a complex endocrinopathy whose pathomechanisms are still incompletely understood. A major aspect of this endocrinopathy involves divalent ions and bone metabolism. It is interesting to note that until recently, the disorders of calcium, phosphate, parathyroid hormone, and vitamin D have been regarded as the culprits of renal bone disease, generically recapitulated in the term ROD.

However, the discovery of new actors like the FGF23/Klotho system and the Wnt pathway (see later) which are deeply intertwined with bone function has changed the picture. In fact, it is now possible to envisage that the diseased bone of renal patients is itself responsible of or involved with the systemic manifestations of CRF including left ventricle hypertrophy (LVH) and vascular calcification.

Typical disturbances of mineral metabolism in chronic renal failure are hyperphosphatemia, hypocalcemia, low vitamin D, and high PTH. Divalent ions are regulated by kidney filtration, resorption, and excretion. Abnormal levels of these ions are detectable only late in the course of renal failure, when glomerular filtration rate (GFR) is less than 30 ml/min. In fact, in the early phases of CRF, the initial loss of nephrons associates with increased fractional excretion in the intact nephrons aiming at maintaining normal levels of phosphate. Two hormones are essential to drive this adaptation: parathyroid hormone (PTH) and fibroblast growth factor 23 (FGF23). Both are responsible for internalization and degradation of the sodium-dependent phosphate cotransporter 2a (Na/P 2a) in the proximal tubule [16]. Hyperphosphatemia increases PTH and FGF23 secretion [17, 18], thus rising phosphate excretion. However, this system becomes insufficient when the residual number of functional nephrons cannot face the dietary load of phosphate. Kidney resistance to phosphaturic hormones secondary to reduced tubular expression of Klotho may also play a role. Klotho is a transmembrane protein primarily expressed in the distal tubular cells [19] where it acts as an obligate coreceptor for the bone-derived protein fibroblast growth factor 23 (FGF23). Clinical data in CKD evidence early reduction of circulating renal Klotho expression [20, 21], which is considered a hallmark of tubular cell resistance to FGF23, whose levels eventually increase. As a result, circulating levels of calcitriol (1,25D) decrease [22] since FGF23 is a potent inhibitor of vitamin D metabolism, both by inhibiting its synthesis (through inhibition of the enzyme 25-hydroxyvitamin D-1-alpha-hydroxylase) and by increasing its degradation (through activation of the enzyme 24-hydroxylase) [23]. 1,25D declines progressively also as a consequence of tubular damage leading to reduced ability to synthesize 1,25D. Calcitriol deficiency in turn decreases intestinal absorption of phosphate. However, also intestinal absorption of calcium is reduced and is responsible for hypocalcemia.

Reduction in 1,25D, hypocalcemia, and hyperphosphatemia is all capable of stimulating parathyroid gland secretion and cell proliferation. 1,25D normally suppresses PTH by several mechanisms: PTH gene transcription inhibition [24], antiproliferative action on parathyroid cells, and upregulation of calcium-sensing receptor expression (CaSR), which sensitizes parathyroid cells to the inhibitory effect of calcium [25]. Hypocalcemia stimulates PTH secretion directly by increasing PTH gene expression and indirectly by exerting an antiproliferative role on parathyroid gland [26]. Hyperphosphatemia contributes to secondary hyperparathyroidism through direct effects on PTH synthesis (stabilization of PTH mRNA) and cell proliferation [27].

As a whole, these biochemical alterations combine to produce the clinical picture of secondary hyperparathyroidism of uremia, including the complex and specific bone disease known as renal osteodystrophy (ROD). In fact, the alterations of mineral metabolism lead to defective skeletal mineralization, while the chronic excess in circulating PTH, according to its catabolic action [28], leads to both high bone formation and resorption rates and accumulation of unmineralized osteoid.

11.2.2.2 The Canonical Wnt/Beta-Catenin Pathway

The canonical Wnt/beta-catenin signaling pathway has been recognized in the last decade as a major player in bone formation and resorption. In particular the canonical Wnt pathway is activated when any of several ligands interact with a complex receptor formed by the transmembrane Frizzled (Frz) receptor and the low-density lipoprotein coreceptor-related proteins (LRP) 5/6. When stimulated, the key function of the canonical Wnt pathway is to increase bone mass through a number of mechanisms including renewal of stem cells, stimulation of preosteoblast replication, induction of osteoblastogenesis, and inhibition of osteoblast and osteocyte apoptosis [29].

The Wnt pathway is tightly regulated by several receptor inhibitors, including Dickkopf-related protein 1 (DKK1), sclerostin, and secreted frizzled-related protein 4 (sFRP4). Wnt receptor inhibition reduces osteoblastogenesis and promotes osteoblast and osteocyte apoptosis, thus exerting a powerful anti-anabolic effect.

Alterations in Wnt signaling or of Wnt inhibitor levels are present in patients with CKD. In particular, recent evidences suggest that Wnt pathway inhibition could be an early event in the pathogenesis of ROD. An increase in circulating blood levels of Wnt inhibitors (DKK1 and sclerostin) can be observed in CKD patients since the early stages [30, 31]. Indeed, CKD mice showed increased expression of Wnt antagonists (sclerostin and sFRP4) [32] associated with progressive increment of osteoclast activity. Similarly, bone expression of sclerostin increased in CKD patients starting from stage 2 [33], and most of the patients in this study showed a low bone turnover, despite progressive increments in PTH levels [33]. Finally, sclerostin has been shown to correlate negatively with osteoblast number and bone turnover in hemodialysis patients [34]. According to these evidences, it has been suggested that the inhibition of Wnt pathway, in the early stages of CKD, could be determinant for the development of the frequently observed low turnover ROD [35].

In addition to Wnt inhibitors, other osteocyte-derived factors are involved in the regulation of bone metabolism and turnover in CKD. In particular, FGF23 and dentin matrix protein 1 (DMP1) are both upregulated in all stages of CKD, as compared to normal controls [33, 36]. DMP1, a member of the small integrin-binding ligand, N-linked glycoprotein (SIBLING) family proteins, is a powerful suppressor of bone FGF23 expression [37]. However, its osteocytic expression increases early in CKD despite high osteocytic FGF23 synthesis [33, 36], and the expression of both proteins is inversely related to osteoid accumulation [36] suggesting a role in bone mineralization. The increase in bone FGF23 and DMP1 expression suggests that osteocyte function is altered early in the course of CKD. Importantly, the mechanism by which these proteins regulate the process of calcification in bone could be exactly the same as that of ectopic vascular calcification. No surprise then that they are the subject of significant research investment for the potential therapeutic implication.

11.2.2.3 Metabolic Acidosis

In normal conditions acid-base balance is maintained by renal excretion of the daily acid load. Elimination of this acid load is achieved by the urinary excretion of hydrogen ions, both as titratable acidity and as ammonium. Along with the decline of functioning nephrons, acid excretion is initially maintained by increasing the fractional excretion of ammonium, but later retention of hydrogen ions is unavoidable and responsible for metabolic acidosis. A diminished excretion of titratable acidity (primarily as phosphoric acid) also plays a role. Since bone is a powerful buffer reservoir, chronic acidosis affects bone metabolism and in particular increases bone resorption (through stimulation of osteoclast activity) and inhibits mineralization, thus producing osteomalacia, as already mentioned.

11.2.2.4 Abnormal Endocrine Hormones

In general, chronic renal insufficiency is associated with variable degrees of uremic toxicity which is responsible for a systemic disturbance of metabolism eventually leading to a generalized organ dysfunction. With the contribution of inflammation and malnutrition that plagues renal patients, almost all of the endocrine organs become dysfunctional and associated with some bone involvement. The most frequently claimed endocrine derangements in renal patients are those of the hypothalamic-pituitary axis and of the sexual and thyroid hormones. A common finding along with GFR reduction is an increment in serum prolactin associated with hypogonadism, infertility, and bone loss. In advanced CKD, women suffer from oligomenorrhea or amenorrhea and low estrogen levels [38], whereas men are hypogonadal with low concentrations of total and free testosterone [39]. These alterations of sex steroids can be referred to either primary or secondary hypogonadism [39]. Uremic toxins, comorbid conditions, and medications all contribute to sex hormone derangements in CRF [38]. Abnormalities of gonadal hormones contribute to bone disease because both androgens and estrogens modulate bone cell activity [40, 41]. In particular, the frequently observed hypogonadism of uremia is considered to contribute to the development of osteoporosis. The most frequent disturbance in thyroid function in uremia is hypothyroidism which is mainly prevalent in elderly people and potentially associated with osteoporosis.

11.2.2.5 Uremic Toxins

Several uremic toxins accumulate in the blood of patients with severely impaired renal function. Among them, indoxyl sulfate (IS), which is produced from the metabolism of dietary tryptophan, has recently gained attention and may have bone effects [42]. In osteoblast cultures IS, internalized via organic anion transporter-3 (OAT-3), impairs osteoblast function and downregulates expression of parathyroid/parathyroid hormone-related peptide receptor (PTHR) [43]. Further, IS inhibits osteoclast differentiation and bone resorption activity [44]. In experimental renal failure, IS reduces bone formation through downregulation of alkaline phosphatase, osteocalcin, and PTHR expression. Administration of an oral charcoal adsorbent inhibited IS accumulation in blood and ameliorated bone formation [45]. These findings strongly suggest that it is at least one of the factors responsible for the skeletal resistance to PTH described in uremia and considered responsible for low bone turnover.

11.2.3 Types of Bone Disease in Chronic Renal Failure Patients

The term "renal osteodystrophy" has been commonly attributed to every disturbance in mineral metabolism and skeletal health occurring in CKD, most frequently linked to secondary hyperparathyroidism. More recently, the new clinical entity of CKD-MBD (chronic kidney disease-mineral and bone disorder) has been established aiming at encompassing the complex endocrine disturbance of mineral metabolism, bone and the pathologic calcification processes associated with CKD [46]. CKD-MBD includes:

- *Laboratory findings*: abnormal values of mineral metabolism biomarkers like calcium, phosphate, parathormone, and vitamin D
- *Renal osteodystrophy*: every morphologic alteration of bone occurring in chronic renal failure
- *Ectopic calcifications*: in particular those involving soft tissues and blood vessels

The reason to include this triad in a common disorder arises from the acknowledgment that the underlying individual pathomechanisms are deeply intertwined and responsible for an increased morbidity that is not limited to bones but involves the cardiovascular system. The laboratory findings are those classically linked with SHP; however, new molecules have been discovered in recent years (e.g., FGF23 and sclerostin) which are produced by bone cells and potentially involved with cardiovascular disease. Renal osteodystrophy refers to the multiple bone changes ranging from high to low turnover, with or without mineralization defects that are described in CKD [47]. Low turnover lesions with defective mineralization (caused by vitamin D deficiency) characterize *osteomalacia*. If associated with normal mineralization, low turnover is typically identified as *adynamic bone disease*, recently thought to be the earliest bone adaptation to mineral derangements in CKD. High turnover bone is usually related to secondary hyperparathyroidism occurring in advanced CKD; when severe it leads to *osteitis fibrosa*, evidenced by the presence of marrow fibrosis. Further, also *mild* or *mixed* forms of ROD can be observed.

This histopathologic classification is based on morphologic changes of bone and has some pathophysiologic value but is not ideal for routine clinical evaluation due to the variability in the methods of reporting. Accordingly, a unified classification system, known as TMV classification, has been introduced by the KDIGO guidelines aiming at achieving a homogeneous and simple description of bone changes in CKD. Three essential histomorphometry-derived parameters are taken into account:

- *Turnover*, as a measure of skeletal remodeling rate, which can be low, normal, or high
- *Mineralization*, evaluating the matrix calcification process that can be either normal or low
- *Volume*, reflecting the amount of bone (bone matrix, both mineralized and not) in respect to the entire bone tissue (including marrow, nerves, and vessels)

The two classifications are clearly different and can be compared only tentatively, as illustrated in Table 11.2. Whatever the underlying lesion, skeletal health is severely compromised in renal patients who suffer a remarkably increased risk of bone fractures impacting life quality and expectancy.

Table 11.2 ROD: histopathologic vs TMV classification

Morphologic classification	Features	KDIGO new classification		
		Turnover	Mineralization	Volume
Osteomalacia	Defective mineralization of bone organic matrix	Low	Abnormal	Normal/low
Adynamic bone disease	Low bone formation with normal osteoid	Low	Normal/abnormal	Normal/low
Osteitis fibrosa	Accelerated mineral apposition and bone formation	High	Abnormal	High/normal/low
Mixed uremic osteodystrophy	Coexistence of changes typical of osteitis fibrosa and osteomalacia	High/normal	Abnormal	Normal/low

11.2.4 Diagnosis of Bone Disease in Renal Patients

Given the variety of bone lesions in CKD, the gold standard technique for the diagnosis of renal osteodystrophy still remains the invasive bone biopsy. Less invasively, skeletal status can be investigated by using blood or urinary circulating biomarkers or by imaging findings obtained with radiologic equipment.

11.2.4.1 Bone Biomarkers

Biomarkers are defined as easily identifiable and quantifiable molecules detectable in biological fluids, whose levels express specific pathophysiological processes, identify patients at risk, or highlight the response to therapeutic treatments. On practical ground, no single biomarker is available to identify a specific type of bone disease [48]. Rather, it is necessary to evaluate several biomarkers together, and more than a single evaluation, their temporal trend is most useful to guess the underlying bone lesion. Widely employed biomarkers are serum calcium and phosphate, PTH, alkaline phosphatase, and vitamin D. More speculative and limited to research purpose are recently discovered biomarkers like FGF23, klotho, sclerostin, DKK1, etc. We will briefly go through the diagnostic value of the principal biomarkers currently employed (Table 11.3).

Table 11.3 Biomarkers involved in ROD

Biomarkers	Production site	Target	Actions on bone	Levels in CKD	Diagnostic role
25D	Hepatocytes			Reduced	Vitamin D deficiency
1,25D	Kidney tubular cells	Intestinal cell	Increase calcium and phosphate absorption	Reduced	Markers of: – Inappropriate kidney function – Initial bone involvement
		Osteoblast	Induction of osteoblastic and osteoclastic differentiation		
		Parathyroid cell	Inhibition of PTH production		
		Kidney tubular cell	1α-Hydroxylase inhibition 24-Hydroxilase stimulation		
PTH	Parathyroid gland	Osteoblast	Increase osteoid formation	Increased	Indicative of SHP
		Kidney tubular cell	Increase 1,25D synthesis Increase calcium resorption Decrease phosphorus resorption		

Table 11.3 (continued)

Biomarkers	Production site	Target	Actions on bone	Levels in CKD	Diagnostic role
BALP	Osteoblast (during bone formation)	Bone tissue	Inactivation of pyrophosphate, an inhibitor of mineralization	Reduced or increased	Indicative of bone turnover
TRAP-5b	Osteoclast	Osteopontin, bone sialoproteins and collagen 1	Active in bone resorption		Marker of osteoclast activity
OPG	Osteoblast, T and B cells, endothelial and VSMC, kidney, spleen, lung, liver, and skin	Osteoclast	Inhibition of osteoclastogenesis	Increased	Not a marker of bone histology in CKD
PINP	Osteoblast		Produced during bone formation	Increased	Indicative of bone collagen synthesis
CTX	Osteoblast		Produced during bone resorption	Increased (highly dependent on kidney function)	Limited use in CKD
FGF23	Osteocyte	Kidney tubular cell	Decrease phosphorus resorption Decrease 1,25D synthesis Increase 24,25D synthesis	Increased	Limited to research
		Parathyroid gland	Decrease PTH synthesis		
Klotho	Kidney tubular cells	Kidney tubular cell	FGF23 coreceptor Decrease phosphorus resorption Increase calcium resorption	Reduced	No diagnostic role in bone disease
Sclerostin	Osteocyte	Osteoblast Osteoclast	Reduction of osteoblastogenesis Induction of osteoblast and osteoclast apoptosis Stimulation of osteoclastogenesis	Increased	Diagnostic role in bone disease still unsettled
SIBLINGs	Bone cells	Paracrine actions	Inhibition of mineralization and renal/intestinal phosphate uptake		Potentially involved with CKD-MBD

25D 25OH-vitamin D, *1,25D* calcitriol, *PTH* parathyroid hormone, *BALP* bone-specific alkaline phosphatase, *TRAP-5b* tartrate-resistant acid phosphatase, *OPG* osteoprotegerin, *PINP* procollagen type I peptide, *CTX* C-terminal cross-linking telopeptide, *FGF23* fibroblast growth factor 23, *SHP* secondary hyperparathyroidism, *CKD* chronic kidney disease, *MBD* mineral and bone disorder

- *Serum Calcium*
  Renal patients usually develop hypocalcemia which promotes parathyroid gland secretion and hypertrophy up to adenoma formation and autonomous hypersecretion with hypercalcemia. Therefore, serum calcium can be low, normal, or high in CRF. The best method for serum calcium measurement is ionized calcium which is not widely and routinely used. Total serum calcium can be misleading in renal patients because of possible changes in serum albumin. Accordingly, it is advisable to correct total calcium concentration for serum albumin concentration or to measure the ionized fraction.
- *Serum Phosphate*
  Serum phosphate levels inexorably increase in advanced CKD. However, in early stages of CKD, dietary phosphate load may be determinant for the development of SHP even in the presence of normal serum levels. The early stimulation of PTH in these stages can also result in mild hypophosphatemia. Also, hypophosphatemia can be observed in malnourished patients. Therefore, hypo-, normal, and hyperphosphatemia are possible in renal patients. Their diagnostic value for bone disease requires a careful clinical evaluation.
- *pH*
  Because of its role in skeletal mineralization, acidosis, the most frequent abnormality in CRF, should be considered as a possible cause of osteomalacia. Metabolic alkalosis is also possible, secondary to volume depletion or drugs or dietary excess. Alkalosis is considered a risk condition for ectopic calcifications.
- *Vitamin D*
  In renal patients, 25OH vitamin D deficiency is very common and is a recognized cause of SHP. Moreover, severe insufficiency (<10 ng/ml) associates with osteomalacia. The reduction of circulating calcitriol, the active hormonal form of vitamin D, is one of the earliest markers of inappropriate kidney function, indicative of initial bone involvement. However, intracellular or local tissue levels are more important than the circulating ones. Accordingly, its assay is not widely employed.
- *PTH*
  Plasma PTH concentration is strictly linked to parathyroid secretion, thus making the hormone a validated marker of hyperparathyroidism. However, due to biological complexity and variability and to technical laboratory aspects, there is a weak correspondence between serum values and bone histology findings [49]. In fact, PTH increment in CKD is influenced by reduced renal function; circulating levels include active, less active, and possibly antagonistic fragments; and preanalytic pitfalls are not rare.
  For this reason, on practical ground it is recommended to evaluate multiple values over time and balance them with other biomarkers of bone, e.g., alkaline phosphatase. In general, extremely high PTH levels correlate best with high turnover and increased resorption aspects; moderate increments overlap widely with bone lesions, and low values indicate low turnover.

- *Alkaline Phosphatase*
  Total serum ALP is usually considered indicative of bone turnover in CKD patients. Its serum concentration includes tissue-specific and tissue non-specific enzymes (accounting for 95% of the entire value) and is represented by similar percentages of liver and bone isoenzymes [50]. The bone specific alkaline phosphatase (BALP) is more sensitive and specific of osteoblast activity and bone turnover and has strong correlation with histologic findings. Moreover, its stability, hepatic excretion, limited biologic variation, and easily comparable assays would favor its use as the first choice bone disease biomarker, if it was not for the costs. Intriguingly, recent clinical observations indicate AP as a biomarker of cardiovascular risk [51].
- *TRAP*
  Tartrate-resistant acid phosphatase, particularly its isoform TRAP-5b produced by osteoclasts, is a good marker of bone resorption, correlated with bone histomorphometric parameters. Its circulating levels are not influenced by renal function [52] and are representative of the underlying osteoclast activity [53]. Its wider use is limited by high costs.
- *Osteocalcin (OC) and Osteoprotegerin (OPG)*
  For many years OC has been recognized as a biomarker of renal osteodystrophy involved in matrix mineralization and positively correlated with bone remodeling [54]. More recent experimental data suggest that its under-carboxylated metabolite, produced along with bone resorption, may have systemic metabolic effects through modulation of insulin sensitivity.
  OPG serum levels are not a good marker of bone histology in CKD. However, in the absence of renal insufficiency, its ratio with RANK ligand is measured, estimating the degree of bone cell coupling activity.
- *Bone Collagen-Derived Peptides*
  PINP (procollagen type I N-terminal peptide) is a marker of bone collagen synthesis whose levels correlate positively with bone resorption markers and negatively with BMD [55]. Its concentration is not affected by GFR, but it is not widely used in CKD, and thus its clinical value is underappreciated.
  CTX (C-terminal cross-linking telopeptide) can be detected in blood and urine as a biomarker of bone resorption [56]. Increments have been associated with higher risk of osteoporotic fractures, but due to renal elimination, its value in ROD is limited.
- *FGF 23/Klotho*
  Recently, the bone-released FGF23 has been proposed as the earliest and most reliable biomarker of mineral imbalance in CKD. Its serum levels increase since the first stages of CKD and definitively reflect CKD-MBD pathophysiology. However, despite its bone specificity, FGF23 is not a marker of bone turnover or disease. Instead, FGF23 levels associate best with cardiac hypertrophy and cardiovascular disease [57]. Its assay is still limited to research laboratories. Reduction of both transmembrane and soluble Klotho can be observed since early stages of CKD. S-Klotho concentration in blood and urine is directly proportional to calcemia but negatively related to phosphoremia and FGF23 levels

[58]. Moreover, low s-Klotho seems to associate with worse cardiovascular prognosis. Produced by the kidney, Klotho is determinant of some tissue-specific effects of FGF23, but no diagnostic role is evident for bone disease.

- *Sclerostin and the SIBLINGs*
  Sclerostin levels may increase in the earliest stages of CKD as a reflection of increased bone production [30, 31]. Given the inhibitory effect on osteoblast, its increment correlates with the development of adynamic bone. Importantly, sclerostin synthesis could be involved with the processes of ectopic vascular calcification and cardiovascular mortality. Its diagnostic role for bone disease is still unsettled.
  SIBLINGs proteins (MEPE, DMP1, OPN, DSPP, BSP) are a family of bone-synthetized proteins involved with local regulation of bone cell activity [48]. As such, they are potentially involved in the pathogenesis of CKD-MBD and could be novel biomarkers of bone disease.

11.2.5 Details of Bone Histology in ROD

Though invasive and expensive, bone biopsy still remains the only method to diagnose renal osteodystrophy properly. It represents the single available tool that definitely identifies the various bone lesions underlying skeletal fragility of patients with CKD and that informs us about bone quality in terms of turnover, mineralization, volume, microarchitecture, remodeling, fibrosis, and matrix composition. For this reason, it remains the reference gold standard to assess renal bone disease. Unfortunately, because of practical limitations, bone biopsy is an exceptional procedure and clinical and pathological expertise is becoming rare. On the contrary, recent evidence shows that its use should be encouraged because of its diagnostic and prognostic value and in order to set up the most appropriate therapeutic interventions [35, 59]. According to current guidelines, bone biopsy in CKD is indicated in a limited and generic number of clinical conditions like unexplained fractures or bone pain, unexplained hypercalcemia or hypophosphatemia, discordance between serum biomarkers, unexplained radiologic abnormalities, and suspected toxicity of heavy or rare metals, prior to parathyroidectomy or to exclude low bone turnover before initiating antiresorptive drugs [60].

Bone biopsy technique should be performed according to standard methods: iliac bone sampling, either by vertical or, preferably, horizontal approach; no decalcification of the sample; toluidine blue, Masson-Goldner trichrome, and aluminum staining; chemical tests for metals; and last but not least, histomorphometric analysis. The main parameters to evaluate are bone volume, mineralization, and turnover (the latter by measuring the double tetracycline labeling in fluorescence microscopy of unstained sections). Thus, appropriate tetracycline administration is necessary before biopsy procedure. The most frequent schedule of labeling is with demeclocycline 150 mg or tetracycline hydrochloride 250 mg four times per day; the same schedule is then repeated after 14 days; then the biopsy is performed after 3–5 days. However, different protocols are employed, and it is mandatory to take a record of the exact days of administration to allow proper evaluation of the dynamic parameters. After sampling, the bone specimen is embedded in methacrylate to allow its cutting with the microtome. Stained slices are viewed at the optical microscope for description. In this way, calcified and non-calcified areas, trabeculae, osteoblast, and osteoclast (either active or inactive) are evaluated to recognize the standard histologic types of ROD.

11.2.5.1 Types of ROD

The different types of ROD can be distinguished by taking into account the main morphologic and histomorphometric aspects, as shown in Table 11.4. Indeed, *osteomalacia* is characterized by increased osteoid volume and prolonged mineralization lag time (Mlt) with low bone turnover and normal volume; *adynamic bone* disease is

Table 11.4 Main parameters in bone histomorphometry

	Acronym	Explanation	Definition note
Structural parameters	BV/TV	Bone volume/ tissue volume	Quantity of BV (mineralized and non-mineralized) as percentage of TV (bone matrix, cells, nerves marrow)
	Tb. N Tb. Th Tb. Sp	Trabecular number Trabecular thickness Trabecular separation	Number, width, and distance between trabeculae
Static remodeling parameters	OV/BV OS/BS O. Th	Osteoid volume/ bone volume Osteoid surface/ bone surface Osteoid thickness	Non-mineralized bone matrix vs BV or BS, indicative of mineralization state
	Ob. S/BS	Osteoblastic surface/bone surface	Area occupied by Ob. as percentage of BS indicative of active formation processes
	ES/BS Oc. S/BS	Eroded surface/ bone surface Osteoclastic surface/bone surface	Area occupied by Oc. indicative of bone resorption
Dynamic remodeling parameters	dLS/BS sLS/BS	Double-labeled/ BS Single-labeled/BS	Types, extension, and distance between the fluorescent signals of tetracyclines deposited on the mineralization front. Measure of new bone apposition
	MS/BS	Mineralizing surface/BS	Measure of the extension of surface active in mineralization
	MAR	Mineral apposition rate	Indicative of the quantity of newly mineralized bone
	Aj. AR	Adjusted apposition rate	Estimate of osteoid deposition per time unit (Aj.AR = MAR*MS/OS)
	BFR	Bone formation rate	Estimate of bone turnover (BFR = MS/ BS*MAR)
	Mlt	Mineralization lag time	Estimated time elapsed between matrix deposition and mineralization (Mlt = O. Th/ Aj. AR)

represented by low bone formation rate (BFR) evidenced by single tetracycline labeling, with low or normal volume and normal Mlt. On the other hand, *severe SHP* is presented with high turnover, accelerated mineralization, and increased bone volume; a *mild SH* is also possible when these lesions are of limited entity; finally *mixed uremic osteodystrophy* presents with both aspects of osteomalacia and of SHP [60].

Osteomalacia is secondary to defective mineralization. Mlt is extremely prolonged, and osteoid surface is wide but not associated with increased number of active osteoblasts; trabeculae can be completely substituted by non-mineralized matrix. Bone turnover is low, as indicated by limited eroded surfaces and osteoclast number. Similar aspects are observed in the presence of aluminum toxicity.

Reduced bone remodeling with low BFR is a peculiar adynamic bone. Bone volume can be reduced because of the loss of osteoblastic activity, and trabecular thickness is extremely low. Active cells and mineralizing and eroded surfaces are sporadic.

Severe SHP is characterized by increased bone turnover of both formation and resorption, with endosteal fibrosis. Mineralization is also increased but may be insufficient for the increased rate of bone formation. Wide eroded surfaces with numerous active osteoclasts and increased osteoid surface with activated osteoblasts can be seen. However, matrix deposition occurs irregularly and leads to the dysfunctional woven bone, whose aspect can be identified by polarized light microscopy. Findings of both high turnover and insufficient mineralization characterize the mixed renal osteopathy. Figure 11.1 shows the four typical histologic aspect of ROD, compared with a normal bone.

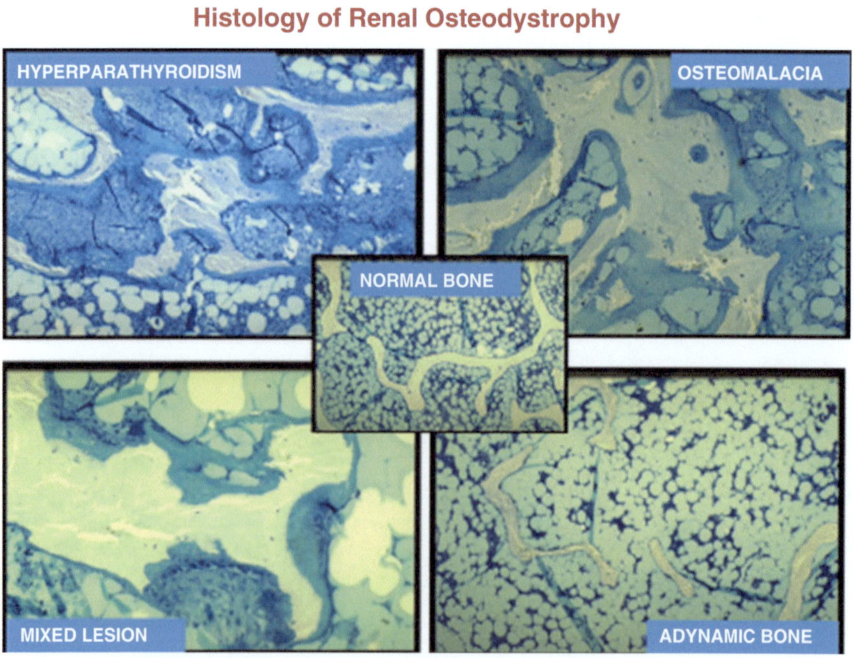

Fig. 11.1 Morphology of the four typical lesions of ROD, as compared with normal histology

11.3 Imaging

Imaging may represent a useful tool to estimate bone disease in CKD.

Conventional X-ray examination of bone in CKD may reveal significant signs of disease, like generalized demineralization (detected when bone loss reaches about −30%); subperiosteal, intracortical, trabecular, and subchondral resorption; loss of cortical definition and corticomedullary differentiation; and "pseudo-widening" of joint spaces. Trabecular resorption is typically revealed by "salt and pepper" skull, a "ground-glass" appearance due to spotty deossification, and loss of distinction between inner and outer tables. Brown tumors are possible and described as cyst-like, well-delimited, lytic lesions affecting the jaw, pelvis, and metaphyses of long bones, typically lacking of associated reactive bone formation. Osteosclerosis is seen in SHP in the axial skeleton, where excessive accumulation of osteoid results in the classic "rugger-jersey" aspect of the spine, with sclerotic endplates of vertebral bodies alternating to radiolucent bands.

Bowing deformities, sometimes with Looser-Milkman zones consisting in linear radiolucent bands perpendicular to the long axis of the bone located at their concave (compressive) side, can frequently be noted in osteomalacia and found in pubic and ischial rami, medial femoral necks, ribs, scapulae, and weight-bearing long bones. Conventional lateral X-ray of the spine is useful to recognize the presence of vertebral fractures which are asymptomatic but frequent in CKD. Vertebral fractures are best examined with a morphometric method according to the visual approach first suggested by Genant. Alternatively, vertebral morphometry can be obtained automatically with dedicated softwares applied to computerized radiologic or DXA images. Importantly, lateral X-ray of the spine is very useful to measure vascular and soft tissue calcifications that are now included in the CKD-MBD syndrome (Fig. 11.2). In fact, vascular calcification is now considered part of the bone disease in CKD, directly linked to cardiovascular risk.

Dual energy X-ray absorptiometry (DXA) allows to calculate bone mineral density (BMD), the most diffuse parameter employed to diagnose osteoporosis. In the general population without CKD, BMD, which is representative mainly of the bone volume, is able to predict fracture risk. In CKD patients, the risk of fractures is high [61, 62], and fractures impact morbidity and mortality with both clinical and social consequences. Therefore, diagnosis, prevention, and treatment represent critical points for these patients [46]. However, the role of DXA in predicting fracture risk in patients with CKD has been controversial until recently. The Kidney Disease Improving Global Outcomes (KDIGO) guidelines suggested to measure DXA for fracture risk evaluation only in early CKD stages (stages 1–3) [47]. In fact, in older individuals DXA BMD indicates the risk of fracture also in renal patients with an estimated GFR >60 ml/min per 1.73 m^2 [63]. In more advanced stages, other factors in addition to bone mass become determinant for bone strength: turnover, mineralization, microarchitecture, and matrix. Further, DXA does not differentiate cortical from trabecular bone, does not recognize the types of ROD, and, when applied on the lumbar vertebrae, measurements may be imprecise for the presence of aortic calcification and/or deformities. For these reasons, BMD measurement has been considered inadequate

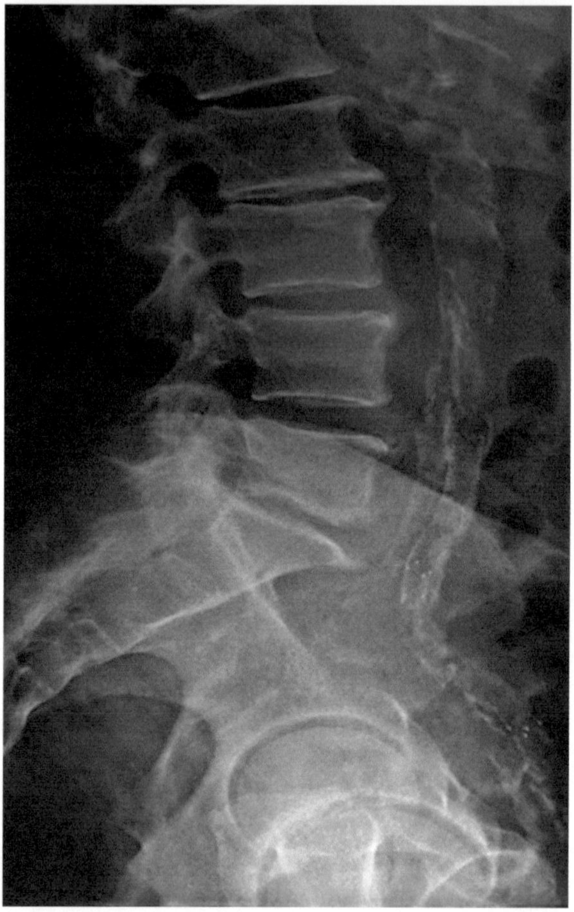

Fig. 11.2 X-ray of the lumbosacral spine with almost complete aortic and iliac artery vascular calcification in a hemodialysis female patient

and discouraged in advanced renal failure (stage 4 and 5 CKD) for the theoretical risk of underestimating the fracture risk [64–66]. However, recent observational studies have documented that low BMD predicts incident fractures also in patients with CKD 3a–5D [67, 68]. Accordingly, the updated KDIGO guidelines suggest to perform BMD measurement even in patients with advanced CKD in order to recognize those at increased risk of fracture deserving therapeutic attention.

BMD can also be measured by quantitative computed tomography (QCT) which, at variance with DXA, differentiates cortical and trabecular bone and is more accurate in assessing spinal volumetric BMD. Further, high-resolution radiologic techniques (HR-QCT) analyze cortical porosity [69] and trabecular microarchitecture [70] and provide detailed 3-D images. Recently, these sophisticated tools have been used in ESRD patients to determine the relationship with bone histomorphometry [71]. Interestingly, not only bone volume could be assessed but also mineralization and some parameters of bone quality. The limitations of this technique include increased radiation dose, limited availability, high costs, and space requirements.

11.3.1 Osteoporosis and Renal Osteodystrophy

Osteoporosis, is a common disease in aging people, responsible for reduction of bone strength and, consequently, of increased fracture risk. Bone strength is determined by both bone quantity and bone quality [72]. The first component can be easily estimated by measuring BMD with a DXA or a QCT equipment. The second main component of bone strength, bone quality, is determined by bone matrix composition, mineralization, remodeling, and architecture. Defects of bone quality can be evidenced with bone histomorphometry. In osteoporosis the peculiar histologic finding is bone volume reduction due to prevalence of bone resorption over formation; turnover can be either high or low, while mineralization, matrix composition, and microarchitecture are mostly regular. In the absence of CKD, the most common way to assess fracture risk is represented by FRAX®, an algorithm provided by the WHO [73] which takes into account the following factors: age, sex, body mass index, ethnicity, family history, peak bone mass, hormone deficiency, falls, previous fractures, smoking, alcohol use, glucocorticoids, and diseases like rheumatoid arthritis, diabetes, osteogenesis imperfecta, long-standing hyperthyroidism, hypogonadism, premature menopause, chronic malnutrition, or malabsorption syndromes. Notably, no mention is made for CRF or CKD. This is because renal patients have always been recognized to be affected with any type of ROD [46, 47] but not with OP. However, coexistence and relationships between OP and ROD warrant investigation because of the rising number of elderly population that typically suffer both osteoporosis and variable degrees of kidney failure [74]. Indeed, aging people may have OP before developing renal insufficiency or vice versa. In any case, given that both diseases negatively affect bone quality and are responsible for an increased risk of fractures, more than giving the exact name to the disease, it seems relevant to develop efficacious diagnostic and therapeutic strategies. On the clinical daily practice, it is possible that BMD performed in aging people will indicate some degree of OP which can be associated or not with some type of ROD. The description of morphology and biochemistry of ROD claims for its substantial difference with OP, and it is difficult to imagine that the therapy could be the same. Also, the new concept of bone as an endocrine gland possibly linked with cardiovascular disease suggests that therapies affecting bone cell (endocrine) activity may impact the cardiovascular system. Accordingly, it would be wise to distinguish the two disorders. Regrettably, there is still no agreement on how to recognize OP in CKD [75]. Early alterations in Klotho and FGF23 are now regarded as the earliest disturbance of the bone-kidney cross talk [2] and thus of the ensuing of ROD. Also, higher FGF23 quartiles have been reported to predict incident fractures specifically in patients with CKD from 3A to 5D stages and not in the population as a whole [76]. Thus, considering that the recognized eGFR threshold for Klotho reduction and FGF23 increments is set at <60 ml/min, this value of eGFR could be reasonably adopted to separate patients with CKD and initial ROD from non-CKD pure OP patients.

Recent evidence shows that BMD and FRAX risk assessment are relevant in patients with CKD [77, 78]. In particular, a significant reduction in BMD (diagnostic for OP) identifies CKD patients at increased risk of fracture [63, 79, 80], with proportional rise of morbidity and mortality along with the development of major fractures [61, 81–85]. Recently the KDIGO committee recommended BMD assessment in renal patients to highlight the fracture risk and individualize clinical management [86]. Importantly, in recent years new drugs have been developed for the treatment of OP. These drugs specifically modify the activity of bone cells and could therefore have a role in the treatment of the different types of ROD. Unfortunately, CKD patients have been excluded from clinical trials evaluating pharmacotherapies for OP. Some authors suggest that ROD should be regarded as a secondary cause of OP, and the term "CKD-induced osteoporosis" has been coined [87]. While the debate is open, the single physician is faced with significant therapeutic choices.

11.4 Available Therapies for ROD

Therapy of ROD is focused mostly on the control of SHP. For this purpose, therapeutic efforts are directed toward improvement of the biochemical derangements that characterize it. The most important drugs available and employed in renal patients are schematically illustrated in Table 11.5. We will briefly analyze the rationale for their use.

First of all, hyperphosphatemia, which manifests in the late stages of the disease, is tentatively corrected through dietary restriction of proteins (down to 0.6 g/kg/day) which are the major source of phosphate. If insufficient, phosphate binders are available to reduce intestinal absorption. The most common and ancient phosphate binder is calcium carbonate that, administered during foods, binds phosphate and provides calcium for absorption. In this way, besides reducing serum phosphate, there is also an increment of serum calcium which could be desirable in the presence of hypocalcemia. In fact, improvement of hypocalcemia or even the induction of hypercalcemia is expected to reduce serum levels of PTH. However, since the recognition of the importance of vascular calcification, hypercalcemia is an untoward effect. For this reason, a number of calcium-free phosphate binders have been developed. First it was sevelamer, a synthetic resin that binds dietary phosphate without calcium release. Further, sevelamer improves serum lipid levels and could theoretically improve cardiovascular outcome. However, prospective randomized trials have not been able to demonstrate a significant effect on mortality. Another non-calcium-based phosphate binder is lanthanum carbonate which is more potent than sevelamer and requires less pills to improve hyperphosphatemia but, again, without evidence of improved cardiovascular survival. Recently, also iron-based phosphate binders are made available. Control of hyperphosphatemia is an issue in advanced stages of renal disease, in particular in dialysis patients, in whom substitutive therapy is not capable of correcting it. But in recent years the attention has been directed also toward the phosphate load in the early stages of the disease, when serum levels are still normal. There is a debate on the opportunity of administering phosphate binders early in renal patients (stages 3–4), even in the absence of

Table 11.5 Available therapies for ROD

	Indications	Mechanism	Bone effects	Dosing
Cholecalciferol	Vitamin D deficiency Treatment of SHP Osteomalacia	Vitamin D storage	Increased 25-hydroxyvitamin D levels with possible PTH reduction and secondary improvement of bone disease Improvement of mineralization	200–1000 IU/die to max 4000 IU/d or 5000–10,000 IU/weekly or 25,000–50,000 IU/monthly
VDR activators				
Calcitriol	Treatment of SHP	Activation of VDR	Modulation of osteoblastogenesis and skeletal anabolism; osteoclast activation Reduction in PTH with secondary improvement of bone disease	0.5–1 mcg/d
Paricalcitol	Treatment of SHP	Activation of VDR (mostly on parathyroid gland)	Reduction in PTH and fewer hypercalcemic episodes; improvement of biochemical markers of bone disease	CRF stages 3–4: 1 mcg–2 mcg/d CRF stage 5: max 32 mcg/week
Calcimimetic *cinacalcet*	Treatment of SHP	Allosteric modulation of CaSR	Reduction of PTH levels with secondary improvement of bone disease	30–120 mg/d
Phosphate binders	Treatment of hyperphosphoremia and SHP	Phosphate binding in the gastrointestinal tract	Reduction in phosphatemia and of PTH levels with secondary improvement of bone disease	*Calcium based*: Calcium carbonate 500 mg–2000 mg die *Calcium free*: sevelamer carbonate or hydrochloride 800 mg–4800 mg/die Lanthanum carbonate 1000–3000 mg/die

(continued)

Table 11.5 (continued)

	Indications	Mechanism	Bone effects	Dosing
Teriparatide	Adynamic bone disease	Activation of PTH1R on osteoblasts	Anabolic effects on bone	Intermittent: 20 or 40 mcg/daily Weekly: 56.5 mcg
Denosumab	OP	Inhibition by binding of the Ocl activator RANKL	Inhibition of resorption	60 mg every 6 m

ROD Renal osteodystrophy, *SHP* secondary hyperthyroidism, *VDR* vitamin D receptor, *CaSR* calcium-sensing receptor, *PTH1R* PTH/PTH-related protein receptor, *RANKL* receptor activator of nuclear factor kappa-B ligand

hyperphosphatemia, with the aim of preventing the bone adaptive response in terms of increased FGF23 synthesis [46, 86].

Another way to improve SHP, given the evidence of vitamin D deficiency in renal patients, is by administering vitamin D compounds [88]. Cholecalciferol, the oldest of available drugs, has been used at high dosages to correct hypocalcemia. In this way serum levels of PTH dropped a little, but long-lasting hypercalcemia could develop. For this reason, cholecalciferol was substituted for calcitriol, the active hormonal form of vitamin D. Given the direct action on VDR expressed on parathyroid glands, calcitriol is definitely more active than cholecalciferol to reduce PTH. Also, in renal patients, the step of renal hydroxylation is skipped. However, high doses may be necessary with the untoward effect of hypercalcemia secondary to the contemporary stimulation of VRD in the intestine [89]. As already indicated, hypercalcemia, once tolerated, is now forbidden. Therefore, vitamin D analogues, more selective on parathyroid tissue and less active on intestinal receptors, have been developed. Paricalcitol is the most widely used vitamin D analogue in Europe and has a lower calcemic effect than calcitriol, with powerful suppression of PTH [90]. Importantly, none of the claimed pleiotropic effects of vitamin D and/or of analogues (e.g., improvement of left ventricle hypertrophy, of hypertension, of endothelial function, etc.) that, beyond control of SHP, could ameliorate patients' prognosis have been demonstrated in randomized clinical trials. These days the use of vitamin D in renal patients is a subject of controversies. In general, there is renewed attention on the use of cholecalciferol since the early stages of the disease, at doses capable of avoiding deficiency and with the aim of avoiding the amount of SHP that could be referred to vitamin D insufficiency. The more active metabolites are used in the presence of significant elevations of PTH levels or when/if cholecalciferol seems insufficient. In any case, high doses should be avoided since hypercalcemia is considered worse than mild hypocalcemia [86].

The discovery of calcium-sensing receptor prompted the research for drugs capable of stimulating it. Cinacalcet is the first calcium-sensing receptor activator made available for clinical use. Many patients with end-stage renal disease have been and are treated with cinacalcet to control SHP. Indeed, the drug increases the sensitivity of the receptor toward circulating calcium levels, thus inhibiting PTH secretion and proliferation. Therefore, cinacalcet can be employed for prevention and treatment of severe SHP in renal patients [91]. Claimed positive clinical effects on calcification and survival are less evident, as for vitamin D.

All of the above drugs, even though with possible untoward effects, are capable of suppressing SHP in most of the cases. Evidence for this powerful efficacy comes from the modification of the prevalence of the different types of ROD evidenced in recent years. In fact, the most frequently described bone lesion in renal patients these days seems to be adynamic bone disease, i.e., a possible consequence of excessive PTH suppression. Adynamic bone is also described in patients who received parathyroid surgery and developed hypoparathyroidism. For these cases, the theoretical possibility exists to employ teriparatide, the synthetic biological drug reproducing the 1–34 fragment of the human PTH molecule [92]. Teriparatide is now indicated for some types of OP with normal renal function, and its use could be indicated in the presence of adynamic bone. However, the presence of renal insufficiency may change the pharmacodynamic profile and the biological effect of the drug, and for this reason, its use in CKD is limited to single, episodic, or case series experience [74].

More recently, another biological drug, denosumab, a monoclonal antibody directed against the RANKL, has been successfully employed in OP. Positive results in terms of reduced fracture rate incidence have been reported also in subpopulations with mild renal insufficiency [93]. Theoretically, this drug specifically inhibits osteoclast recruitment and bone resorption leaving space for osteoblastic bone building activity. Further, at variance with bisphosphonates that are excreted by the kidney, its pharmacodynamic is not influenced by renal function. Therefore, its application could be useful in renal patients with high bone turnover but seems less suitable in case of adynamic bone. A diagnostic bone biopsy seems mandatory before use in single cases, and randomized trials are warranted to define the potential utility of denosumab in renal patients [74].

In summary, therapy of ROD has been mostly focused on the control of SHP, but this seems insufficient to reduce the burden of skeletal fractures in renal disease. Drugs employed for OP should be considered in renal patients with the target of fractures and not simply of the biochemical control of SHP.

References

1. Levey AS, de Jong PE, Coresh J, et al. The definition, classification, and prognosis of chronic kidney disease: a KDIGO Controversies Conference report. Kidney Int. 2011;80:17–28.
2. Mazzaferro S, Pasquali M, Pirrò G, Rotondi S, Tartaglione L. The bone and the kidney. Arch Biochem Biophys. 2010;503:95–102.
3. Heilberg IP, Weisinger JR. Bone disease in idiopathic hypercalciuria. Curr Opin Nephrol Hypertens. 2006;15:394–402.
4. Vezzoli G, Soldato L, Gambaro G. Hypercalciuria revisited: one or many conditions? Pediatr Nephrol. 2008;23:503–606.
5. Thakker RV. Pathogenesis of Dent's disease and related syndromes of X-linked nephrolithiasis. Kidney Int. 2000;57:787–93.
6. Devuyst O, Pirson Y. Genetics of hypercalciuric stone forming disease. Kidney Int. 2007;72:1065–72.

7. Bergwitz C, Roslin NM, Tieder M, et al. SCL34A3 mutations in patient with hereditary hypophosphatemic rickets with hypercalciuria predict key role for the sodium-phosphate cotransporter NaPi-IIc in maintaining phosphate homeostasis. Am J Hum Genet. 2006;78:179–92.
8. Bushinsky DA, Goldring JM, Coe FL. Cellular contribution to pH-mediated calcium flux in neonatal mouse calvariae. Am J Physiol. 1985;248:F785–9.
9. Krieger NS, Parker WR, Alexander KM, Bushinsky DA. Prostaglandins regulate acid-induced cell-mediated bone resorption. Am J Physiol Renal Physiol. 2000;279:F1077–82.
10. Frick KK, Bushinsky DA. Metabolic acidosis stimulates RANKL RNA expression in bone through a cyclo-oxygenase-dependent mechanism. J Bone Miner Res. 2003;18:1317–25.
11. Bushinsky DA. Stimulated osteoclastic and suppressed osteoblastic activity in metabolic but not respiratory acidosis. Am J Physiol. 1995;268:C80–8.
12. Nijenhuis T, Renkema KY, Hoenderop JG, Bindels RY. Acid-base status determines the renal expression of Ca2+ and Mg2+ transport proteins. J Am Soc Nephrol. 2006;17:617–26.
13. Ludwig MG, Vanek M, Guerini D, et al. Proton sensing G-protein–coupled receptors. Nature. 2003;425:93–8.
14. Jahr H, van Driel M, van Osch GJ, Weinans H, van Leeuwen JP. Identification of acid-sensing ion channels in bone. Biochem Biophys Res Commun. 2005;337:349–54.
15. Clarke BL, Wynne AG, Wilson DM, Fitzpatrick LA. Osteomalacia associated with adult Fanconi's syndrome: clinical and diagnostic features. Clin Endocrinol. 1995;43:479–90.
16. Shimada T, Urakawa I, Yamazaki Y, et al. FGF-23 transgenic mice demonstrate hypophosphatemic rickets with reduced expression of sodium phosphate cotransporter type IIa. Biochem Biophys Res Commun. 2004;312:409–14.
17. Slatopolsky E, Caglar S, Pennell JP, et al. On the pathogenesis of hyperparathyroidism in chronic experimental renal insufficiency in the dog. J Clin Invest. 1971;50:492–9.
18. Slatopolsky E, Finch J, Denda M, et al. Phosphorus restriction prevents parathyroid gland growth. High phosphorus directly stimulates PTH secretion in vitro. J Clin Invest. 1996;97:2534–40.
19. Mian IS. Sequence, structural, functional, and phylogenetic analyses of three glycosidase families. Blood Cells Mol Dis. 1998;2:83–100.
20. Rotondi S, Pasquali M, Tartaglione L, et al. Soluble α-Klotho serum levels in chronic kidney disease. Int J Endocrinol. 2015;2015:1–8.
21. Yu J, Deng M, Zhao J, Huang L. Decreased expression of klotho gene in uremic atherosclerosis in apolipoprotein E deficient mice. Biochem Biophys Res Comm. 2010;391:261–6.
22. Levin A, Bakris GL, Molitch M, et al. Prevalence of abnormal serum vitamin D, PTH, calcium, and phosphorus in patients with chronic kidney disease: results of the study to evaluate early kidney disease. Kidney Int. 2007;71:31–8.
23. Shimada T, Hasegawa H, Yamazaki Y, et al. FGF23 is a potent regulator of vitamin D metabolism and phosphate homeostasis. J Bone Miner Res. 2004;19:429–35.
24. Silver J, Naveh-Many T. FGF23 and the parathyroid glands. Pediatr Nephrol. 2010;25:2241–5.
25. Canaff L, Hendy GN. Human calcium-sensing receptor gene. Vitamin D response elements in promoters P1 and P2 confer transcriptional responsiveness to 1,25-dihydroxyvitamin D. J Biol Chem. 2002;277:30337–50.
26. Tfelt-Hansen J, Brown EM. The calcium-sensing receptor in normal physiology and pathophysiology: a review. Crit Rev Clin Lab Sci. 2005;42:35–70.
27. Dusso A, Arcidiacono MV, Yang J, Tokumoto M. Vitamin D inhibition of TACE and prevention of renal osteodystrophy and cardiovascular mortality. J Steroid Biochem Mol Biol. 2010;121:193–8.
28. Silverberg SJ, Shane E, de la Cruz L, et al. Skeletal disease in primary hyperparathyroidism. J Bone Miner Res. 1989;4:283–91.
29. Rodda SJ, McMahon AP. Distinct role for Hedgehog and canonical Wnt signaling in specification, differentiation and maintenance of osteoblast progenitors. Development. 2006;133:3231–44.
30. Fang Y, Ginsberg C, Seifert M, et al. CKD-induced wingless/integration1 inhibitors and phosphorus cause the CKD-mineral and bone disorder. J Am Soc Nephrol. 2014;25:1760–73.

31. Pelletier S, Dubourg L, Carlier MC, Hadj-Aissa A, Fouque D. The relation between renal function and serum sclerostin in adult patients with CKD. Clin J Am Soc Nephrol. 2013;8:819–23.
32. Sabbagh Y, Graciolli FG, O'Brien S, et al. Repression of osteocyte Wnt/beta-catenin signaling is an early event in the progression of renal osteodystrophy. J Bone Miner Res. 2012;27:1757–72.
33. Graciolli FG, Naves KR, Barreto F, et al. The complexity of chronic kidney disease-mineral bone disorder across stages of chronic kidney disease. Kidney Int. 2017;91:1436–46.
34. Cejka D, Herberth J, Branscum AJ, et al. Sclerostin and dickkopf-1 in renal osteodystrophy. Clin J Am Soc Nephrol. 2011;6:877–82.
35. Drueke TB, Massy ZA. Changing bone patterns with progression of chronic kidney disease. Kidney Int. 2016;89:289–302.
36. Pereira RC, Valta H, Tumber N, et al. Altered osteocyte-specific protein expression in bone after childhood solid organ transplantation. PLoS One. 2015;10:1–12.
37. Martin A, David V, Li H, et al. Overexpression of the DMP1 C-terminal fragment stimulates FGF23 and exacerbates the hypophosphatemic rickets phenotype in Hyp mice. Mol Endocrinol. 2012;26:1883–95.
38. Gomez F, de la Cueva R, Wauters JP, Lemarchand-Beraud T. Endocrine abnormalities in patients undergoing longterm hemodialysis: the role of prolactin. Am J Med. 1980;68:522–30.
39. Handelsman DJ, Dong Q. Hypothalamo-pituitary gonadal axis in chronic renal failure. Endocrinol Metab Clin North Am. 1993;22:145–61.
40. Kousteni S, Bellido T, Plotkin LI, et al. Non genotropic, sex-non specific signaling through the estrogen or androgen receptors: dissociation from transcriptional activity. Cell. 2001;104:719–30.
41. Pederson L, Kremer M, Judd J, et al. Androgens regulate bone resorption activity of isolated osteoclasts in vitro. Proc Natl Acad Sci U S A. 1999;96:505–10.
42. Niwa T, Takeda N, Tatematsu A, et al. Accumulation of indoxyl sulfate, an inhibitor of drug-binding, in uremic serum as demonstrated by internal-surface reversed-phase liquid chromatography. Clin Chem. 1988;34:2264–7.
43. Nii-Kono T, Iwasaki Y, Uchida M, et al. Indoxyl sulfate induces skeletal resistance to parathyroid hormone in cultured osteoblastic cells. Kidney Int. 2007;71:738–43.
44. Mozar A, Louvet L, Godin C, et al. Indoxyl sulphate inhibits osteoclast differentiation and function. Nephrol Dial Transplant. 2012;27:2176–81.
45. Iwasaki Y, Yamato H, Nii-Kono T, et al. Administration of oral charcoal adsorbent (AST-120) suppresses low-turnover bone progression in uraemic rats. Nephrol Dial Transplant. 2006;21:2768–74.
46. Moe S, Drüeke T, Block GA, et al. KDIGO clinical practice guideline for the diagnosis, evaluation, prevention, and treatment of Chronic Kidney Disease-Mineral and Bone Disorder (CKD-MBD). Kidney Int. 2009;76:S3–S130.
47. Moe S, Drüeke T, Cunningham J, et al. Definition, evaluation, and classification of renal osteodystrophy: a position statement from Kidney Disease: Improving Global Outcomes (KDIGO). Kidney Int. 2006;69:1945–53.
48. Mazzaferro S, Tartaglione L, Rotondi S, Bover J, Goldsmith D, Pasquali M. News on biomarkers in CKD-MBD. Semin Nephrol. 2014;34:598–611.
49. Garrett G, Sardiwal S, Lamb EJ, Goldsmith DJ. PTH--a particularly tricky hormone: why measure it at all in kidney patients? Clin J Am Soc Nephrol. 2013;8:299–312.
50. Ureña P, Hruby M, Ferreira A, Ang KS, de Vernejoul MC. Plasma total versus bone alkaline phosphatase as markers of bone turnover in hemodialysis patients. J Am Soc Nephrol. 1996;7:506–12.
51. Drechsler C, Verduijn M, Pilz S, Krediet RT, et al. Bone alkaline phosphatase and mortality in dialysis patients. Clin J Am Soc Nephrol. 2011;6:1752–9.
52. Yamada S, Inaba M, Kurajoh M, Shidara K, Imanishi Y, Ishimura E, et al. Utility of serum tartrate-resistant acid phosphatase (TRAP5b) as a bone resorption marker inpatients with chronic kidney disease: independence from renal dysfunction. Clin Endocrinol. 2008;69:189–96.

53. Henriksen K, Tanko LB, Qvist P, Delmas PD, Christiansen C, Karsdal MA. Assessment of osteoclast number and function: application in the development of new and improved treatment modalities for bone diseases. Osteoporos Int. 2007;18(5):681.
54. Coen G, Mazzaferro S, Bonucci E, Taggi F, Ballanti P, Bianchi AR, et al. Bone GLA protein in predialysis chronic renal failure. Effects of 1,25(OH)2D3 administration in a long term follow-up. Kidney Int. 1985;28:783–90.
55. Vasikaran S, Eastell R, Bruyere O, et al. Markers of bone turnover for the prediction of fracture risk and monitoring of osteoporosis treatment: a need for international reference standards. Osteoporos Int. 2011;22:391–420.
56. Johnell O, Oden A, De Laet C, et al. Biochemical indices of bone turnover and the assessment of fracture probability. Osteoporos Int. 2002;13:523–6.
57. Grabner A, Mazzaferro S, Cianciolo G, et al. Fibroblast growth factor 23: mineral metabolism and beyond. Contrib Nephrol. 2017;190:83–95.
58. Marçais C, Maucort-Boulch D, Drai J, et al. Circulating Klotho associates with cardiovascular morbidity and mortality during hemodialysis. J Clin Endocrinol Metab. 2017;102(9):3154–61. [Epub ahead of print].
59. Evenepoel P, D'Haese P, Bacchetta J, et al. Bone biopsy practice patterns across Europe: the European renal osteodystrophy initiative-a position paper. Nephrol Dial Transplant. 2017;32(10):1608–13. [Epub ahead of print].
60. Torres PU, Bover J, Mazzaferro S. When, how, and why a bone biopsy should be performed in patients with chronic kidney disease. Semin Nephrol. 2014;34:612–25.
61. Alem AM, Sherrard DJ, Gillen DL, et al. Increased risk of hip fracture among patients with end-stage renal disease. Kidney Int. 2000;58:396–9.
62. Wakasugi M, Kazama JJ, Taniguchi M, et al. Increased risk of hip fracture among Japanese hemodialysis patients. J Bone Miner Metab. 2013;31:315–21.
63. Yenchek RH, Ix JH, Shlipak MG, Bauer DC, Rianon NJ, Kritchevsky SB, Harris TB, Newman AB, Cauley JA, Fried LF, Health, Aging, and Body Composition Study. Bone mineral density and fracture risk in older individuals with CKD. Clin J Am Soc Nephrol. 2012;7:1130–6.
64. Jamal SA, West SL, Miller PD. Fracture risk assessment in patients with chronic kidney disease. Osteoporos Int. 2012;23:1191–8.
65. Jamal SA, West SL, Miller PD. Bone and kidney disease: diagnostic and therapeutic implications. Curr Rheumatol Rep. 2012;14:217–23.
66. Ott SM. When bone mass fails to predict bone failure. Calcif Tissue Int. 1993;53(Suppl. 1):S7–13.
67. Jamal SA, Hayden JA, Beyene J. Low bone mineral density and fractures in long term hemodialysis patients: a meta-analysis. Am J Kidney Dis. 2007;49:674–81.
68. Jamal SA, Cheung AM, West S, Lok C. Bone mineral density by DXA and HR pQCT can discriminate fracture status in men and women with stages 3 to 5 chronic kidney disease. Osteoporos Int. 2012;23:2805–13.
69. Nishiyama KK, Macdonald HM, Buie HR, Hanley DA, Boyd SK. Postmenopausal women with osteopenia have higher cortical porosity and thinner cortices at the distal radius and tibia than women with normal aBMD: an in vivo HR-pQCT study. J Bone Miner Res. 2010;25:882–90.
70. Liu XS, Stein EM, Zhou B, et al. Individual trabecula segmentation (ITS)-based morphological analyses and microfinite element analysis of HRpQCT images discriminate postmenopausal fragility fractures independent of DXA measurements. J Bone Miner Res. 2012;27:263–72.
71. Pereira RC, Bischoff DS, Yamaguchi D, Salusky IB, Wesseling-Perry K. Micro-CT in the assessment of pediatric renal osteodystrophy by bone histomorphometry. Clin J Am Soc Nephrol. 2016;11:481–7.
72. NIH Consensus Development Panel on Osteoporosis Prevention, Diagnosis, and Therapy. Osteoporosis prevention, diagnosis, and therapy. JAMA. 2010;285:785–95.
73. Kanis JA, on behalf of the World Health Organization Scientific Group. Assessment of osteoporosis at the primary health-care level. Technical report. Sheffield: World Health Organization Collaborating Centre for Metabolic Bone Diseases, University of Sheffield; 2007. Printed by the University of Sheffield.

74. Tartaglione L, Pasquali M, Rotondi S, Muci ML, Covic A, Mazzaferro S. Positioning novel biologicals in CKD mineral and bone disorders. J Nephrol. 2017;30(5):689–99. [Epub ahead of print].
75. Miller PD. Diagnosis and treatment of osteoporosis in chronic renal disease. Semin Nephrol. 2009;29:144–55.
76. Lane NE, Parimi N, Corr M, et al. Association of serum fibroblast growth factor 23 (FGF23) and incident fractures in older men: the Osteoporotic Fractures in Men (MrOS) study. J Bone Miner Res. 2013;28:2325–32.
77. Jamal SA, West SL, Nickolas TL. The clinical utility of FRAX to discriminate fracture status in men and women with chronic kidney disease. Osteoporos Int. 2014;25(1):71–6.
78. Naylor KL, Leslie WD, Hodsman AB, Rush DN, Garg AX. FRAX predicts fracture risk in kidney transplant recipients. Transplantation. 2014;97:940–5.
79. West SL, Lok CE, Langsetmo L, Cheung AM, Szabo E, Pearce D, et al. Bone mineral density predicts fractures in chronic kidney disease. J Bone Miner Res. 2015;30:913–919 8.
80. Nickolas TL, Cremers S, Zhang A, et al. Discriminants of prevalent fractures in chronic kidney disease. J Am Soc Nephrol. 2011;22:1560–72.
81. Naylor KL, Garg AX, Zou G, et al. Comparison of fracture risk prediction among individuals with reduced and normal kidney function. Clin J Am Soc Nephrol. 2015;10:646–53.
82. Fried LF, Biggs ML, Shlipak MG, et al. Association of kidney function with incident hip fracture in older adults. J Am Soc Nephrol. 2007;18:282–6.
83. Coco M, Rush H. Increased incidence of hip fractures in dialysis patients with low serum parathyroid hormone. Am J Kidney Dis. 2000;36:1115–21.
84. Beaubrun AC, Kilpatrick RD, Freburger JK, Bradbury BD, Wang L, Brookhart MA. Temporal trends in fracture rates and postdischarge outcomes among hemodialysis patients. J Am Soc Nephrol. 2013;24(9):1461.
85. Naylor K, McArthur E, Leslie W, et al. Three three-year incidence of fracture in chronic kidney disease. Kidney Int. 2014;86:810–8.
86. Ketteler M, Block GA, Evenepoel P, et al. Executive summary of the 2017 KDIGO Chronic Kidney Disease-Mineral and Bone Disorder (CKD-MBD) Guideline Update: what's changed and why it matters. Kidney Int. 2017;92:23–36.
87. Moe SM. Renal osteodystrophy or kidney-induced osteoporosis? Curr Osteoporos Rep. 2017;15:194–7.
88. Mazzaferro S, Goldsmith D, Larsson TE, Massy ZA, Cozzolino M. Vitamin D metabolites and/or analogs: which D for which patient? Curr Vasc Pharmacol. 2014;12:339–49.
89. Andress DL, Keith MD, Norris C, et al. Intravenous calcitriol in the treatment of refractory osteitis fibrosa of chronic renal failure. N Engl J Med. 1989;321:274–9.
90. Bover J, Cozzolino M. Mineral and bone disorders in chronic kidney disease and end-stage renal disease patients: new insights into vitamin D receptor activation. Kidney Int Suppl. 2011;1:122–9.
91. Behets GJ, Spasovski G, Sterling LR, et al. Bone histomorphometry before and after long-term treatment with cinacalcet in dialysis patients with secondary hyperparathyroidism. Kidney Int. 2015;87:846–56.
92. Sumida K, Ubara Y, Hoshino J, Mise K, Hayami N, Suwabe T, et al. Once-weekly teriparatide in hemodialysis patients with hypoparathyroidism and low bone mass: a prospective study. Osteoporos Int. 2016;27:1441–50.
93. Chen CL, Chen NC, Hsu CY, et al. An open-label, prospective pilot clinical study of denosumab for severe hyperparathyroidism in patients with ow bone mass undergoing dialysis. J Clin Endocrinol Metab. 2014;99:2426–32.

Osteoporosis and Cardiovascular Risk 12

Giancarlo Isaia, Lorenzo Marchese, Margherita Marchetti, and Mario Bo

12.1 Introduction

Osteoporosis and cardiovascular diseases are two of the major public health problems: both are associated with high morbidity and mortality, increased recourse to hospital services, loss of independence, increased risk of institutionalization and high health-related costs. The socio-economic consequences of both these diseases are very important bearing in mind the facts that OP is the second highest world health problem after CVD, and this number will increase with the growth of the elderly population over the next decades.

Prevalence and incidence of either cardiovascular disease (CVD) and osteoporosis (OP) increase with advancing age. Traditionally these two conditions were considered unrelated and their coexistence has been attributed to ageing-associated independent processes. Indeed, CVD and OP involve different apparatus, have distinct well-defined pathogenetic pathway and are treated with specific therapeutic interventions. However, growing evidence indicates the existence of a correlation between CVD and OP fractures, irrespective of age. Some studies showed that OP fractures are associated with higher risk of cardiovascular event. Moreover, CVD and OP share some common risk factors (estrogens deficiency and many other

G. Isaia (✉)
Unit of Geriatrics and Metabolic Bone Disease, Molinette Hospital and School of Geriatric Medicine, University of Torino, Torino, Italy
e-mail: giancarlo.isaia@unito.it

L. Marchese
Presidio Ausiliatrice, Fondazione Don Carlo Gnocchi, Torino, Italy

M. Marchetti · M. Bo
Department of Geriatrics, Città della Salute e della Scienza - Molinette Hospital, University of Torino, Torino, Italy
e-mail: margherita.marchetti@to.omceo.it; mario.bo@unito.it

A. Lenzi, S. Migliaccio (eds.), *Multidisciplinary Approach to Osteoporosis*,
https://doi.org/10.1007/978-3-319-75110-8_12

factors may be involved either in bone formation or in development of atherosclerosis) and some therapeutic drugs currently used in the treatment of these conditions might not be exclusive for a single system (bone or cardiovascular) but take part both in bone metabolism and atherosclerosis.

Hereafter, we will briefly review the evidence supporting a link between CVD and OP.

12.2 Epidemiology

A growing evidence indicates the existence of an association between CVD and OP fractures, irrespective of age, and some studies suggested a causal relationship between these two conditions.

Winkelmann et al. firstly reported an association between low femoral BMD and atherosclerosis in the elderly, in which severe OP in the hip was not only a risk factor for hip fractures, but also a marker of coronary heart disease [1]. Tanko et al. showed an important increase of cardiovascular risk in patients with bone loss representing the placebo group of Multiple Outcome of Raloxifene Evaluation study [2]: women with vertebral OP fractures had a 3.9 fold greater risk of cardiovascular events (95% CI, 2.0–7.7; $p < 0.001$) compared with those with osteopenia expressed as low bone mineral density (BMD). Moreover, the cardiovascular risk increased proportionally to the number and severity of vertebral fractures at baseline, suggesting a linear relationship between the severity of OP and CVD risk at the time of diagnosis of bone loss. In a large study carried out in the National Health Insurance Research Database in Taiwan, OP vertebral fracture was associated with higher risk of stroke, whereas hip fracture was associated with higher risk of myocardial infarction [3]. At the same time, it has been reported that individuals with CVD may have higher risk of major OP fractures, including hip or vertebral fracture. In a large cohort of community-dwelling patients (Swedish Twin Register), ischemic heart disease was associated with higher risk of hip fracture [4]. Moreover, several studies show that heart failure is also associated with higher risk of hip fracture [5].

12.3 Risk Factors and Pathophysiology

OP and CVD share several common risk factors. Age, smoking, sedentary life-style and physical inactivity, alcohol consumption, menopause, hypertension, inadequate nutrition and chronic use of some medications (for example, glucocorticoids, diuretics and anticoagulants), can promote atherosclerosis, vascular calcification (VC), bone demineralization.

Age represents per se a high risk factor for both these conditions. Progressive bone loss is a physiological event occurring during aging. The slow reduction of osteoblastic activity and survival, typical of the late post-menopause and aging, gradually worsens bone health. Atherosclerosis/arteriosclerosis is also considered a hallmark of aging process, contributing to heart attacks and strokes, significantly enhancing morbidity and mortality in the elderly. Reduced blood flow supply because of atherosclerosis may impair the intraosseous blood circulation. This in turn impairs bone metabolism in the joint resulting in loss of BMD and osteoporosis. In the case of asymmetrical peripheral arterial disease, the hip bone mineral content in the affected limb is lower than that of the contralateral limb. Limited physical activity in patients with cardiovascular disease could be consequently responsible for bone loss [6].

Obesity and *physical inactivity* are well recognized risk factors for CVD and OP, as well as *diabetes*. *Cigarette smoking* is a strong predictor of CVD morbidity and mortality, and it has been associated with an increased risk of bone loss and OP fractures.

Endothelial dysfunction is considered a preclinical marker of atherosclerosis. Some interesting data demonstrated that coronary microvascular endothelial dysfunction is an independent predictor for development of postmenopausal osteoporosis (PMOP). *Arterial stiffness* secondary to VC was also studied in patients affected by OP. Pulse wave velocity (PWV) is considered a reliable surrogate of arterial stiffness, and several studies demonstrated that brachial-ankle PWV (baPWV) correlates well with coronary artery disease (CAD). Hirose et al. observed that baPWV was negatively correlated with BMD. Aortic calcification (AoC) seems to be itself an independent indicator of low BMD and risk of future fractures at the proximal femur: in a recent study, increasing severity of abdominal AoC was associated with prevalent vertebral fractures regardless of age, body mass index (BMI), history of fractures and BMD [7]. Abdominal aortic calcification (AAC) occupies a particular position in this field. Firstly, its assessment is easily available, inexpensive and easy to perform. Most often, AAC is assessed from lateral radiographs of lumbar spine using Kauppila's semi-quantitative 24-point score or using a simplified 8-point semi-quantitative score. These scores estimate AAC severity in the abdominal aorta adjacent to the first four lumbar vertebrae. AAC may be also assessed from lateral spine scan obtained by dual energy X-ray absorptiometry (DXA) (using the above scores) and using quantitative computed tomography.

Secondly, severe AAC is associated with higher cardiovascular mortality and with higher risk of cardiovascular diseases in comparison with individuals without or with milder AAC [8] . This association was found consistently in several large cohorts of men and women as well as confirmed by meta-analyses. Importantly, it remained significant after adjustment for multiple confounders, such as age, weight, negative lifestyle factors (e.g. smoking, sedentary lifestyle), co-morbidities and treatments.

Thirdly, severe AAC is associated with higher risk of osteoporotic fracture. This association was found in cross-sectional and prospective studies. Cross-sectional studies were focused on vertebral fractures. Severe AAC was associated with greater prevalence, higher number and greater severity of vertebral fractures [9]. This association remained significant after adjustment for confounders including bone mineral density (BMD) measured by DXA. Severe AAC and lower BMD were jointly and independently associated with higher number and greater severity of vertebral fractures. In some cohorts, severe AAC was also associated with prior hip fracture [10].

On the other side, some data suggest that OP may be associated with increased risk of CVD. Sumino et al. reported higher arterial stiffness in osteoporotic women compared with healthy controls. Frost et al. demonstrated that decreased BMD is associated with VC and arterial stiffening and proposed a possible role of osteoprotegerin (OPG) as a marker of arterial stiffening, independent of any association with BMD [11]. Furthermore, it was supposed that arterial stiffening is independent of non-calcified atheromatous plaque and BMD, but associated with a calcification process within atherosclerotic plaque distinct from atherosclerosis and due to a natural tendency of vascular wall to calcify. Low BMD appears to be associated with increased prevalence of aortic valve calcification, although the underlying pathophysiologic rationale remains to be elucidated.

Estrogens deficiency occurring in menopause leads to a significant increase of some pro-inflammatory cytokines, such as interleukin-1 (IL-1), interleukin-6 (IL-6), tumor necrosis factor-alpha (TNF-α) and osteoclastic hyperactivity, while osteoprotegerin (OPG) decreases. These phenomena are mostly responsible of bone loss, but seem to be also implicated in the mechanisms of atherogenesis [12].

Moreover, the growing knowledge of bone biology led to recognize that several matrix proteins, such as type 1 collagen, proteoglycan, osteopontin (OPN), osteonectin and also bone morphogenetic proteins (BMPs) and OPG, usually found in bone, are vascular matrix components too. These factors may be involved either in bone formation or in development of vascular calcification (VC) and atherosclerosis [13].

12.3.1 Vascular Calcification and Bone Biology

VC and bone mineralization share several anatomical and pathophysiological common features. In fact the calcification of the arterial wall tissue is not just a simple precipitation or absorption of phosphate and calcium but it is a highly organized process, regulated by mechanisms similar to those involved in bone mineralization [6].

VC is the pathological deposition of calcium and minerals in blood vessels, highly associated with cardiovascular disease mortality: intimal calcification is mainly linked to atherosclerosis, whereas medial calcification is a non-occlusive process which increases vascular stiffness impairing vascular compliance [14]. VC has long been considered simply a passive ageing-related process; however, recent studies showed that vascular calcification is a highly regulated process, involving genetic factors, hormones, cytokines, enzymes involved in the metabolism and transport of calcium and phosphate, and trans-differentiation of vascular smooth muscle cells into osteoblastic cells and other factors.

VC and bone mineralization share some anatomical and pathophysiological common features which could partly explain the link between OP and CVD. VC is an active process, regulated by several factors primarily involved in the osteogenesis process, such as BMPs, OPG, OPN, bone specific-alkaline phosphatase (bALP) and matrix Gla protein (MGP).

Vascular smooth muscle cells (VSMCs) are able to differentiate into osteoblast-like cells under the stimuli of BMPs, RANKL, reactive oxygen species (ROS), inflammation and estrogen deficiency. These osteoblastic cells produce bALP, osteocalcin (OC) and other crucial factors to mineralization.

The unbalance between RANKL and OPG has been indicated as the pivotal mechanism responsible for estrogen deficiency bone loss. RANKL and OPG might play a role in vascular biology: it is known that both RANKL and OPG are present in the plaques and the healthy vessel wall. This data, together with the presence of osteoclasts-like cells in the atherosclerotic plaques, support the hypothesis of a relevant role of this system in controlling vascular biology.

OPG, one of the main regulators of bone resorption mediated by osteoclasts, is another factor found in both vascular and bone tissue. The discovery that mice lacking OPG had severe OP and VC provided the first clue that OPG might be a key molecule linking these vascular and skeletal phenotypes. Elevated level of OPG was also found in patients with CVD, suggesting its abnormal high serum concentration in vivo may be associated with endothelial dysfunction and arterial calcification [15].

It has been suggested that OPG might act as an autocrine/paracrine regulator of vascular calcification and may be useful as a serum marker of vascular disease. OPG is able to prevent VC by blocking the formation of osteoclast-like cells present in calcified arterial walls acting as a decoy receptor of RANKL as in bone. OPG is also able to reduce endothelial and smooth vascular cell apoptosis: the vascular cell's survival mediated by OPG could represent a protective mechanism against atherosclerosis. However, its exact role in vascular calcification is still not completely understood and need further studies [16].

Osteopontin (OPN) is a glycoprotein of extracellular matrix of bone tissue binding to calcium and hydroxyapatite which was also proposed to be a mediator in the pathogenic pathways leading to atherosclerotic vascular disease. Circulating levels of OPN were reported to be independently associated with the severity of coronary atherosclerosis and increased risk for major adverse cardiac events [17].

bALP is an enzyme that catalyzes the hydrolysis of esters, generally located on the osteoblasts surface and used as a marker of bone turnover. Recent evidences show that serum bALP and phosphate may be indicators of VC in chronic kidney disease, ischemic heart disease and stroke [18]. This finding has to be confirmed with studies including large populations.

Several other markers of bone metabolism, including parathyroid hormone (PTH), OC, vitamin K, MGP and other non-collagenous bone proteins take a significant part in the process of calcification. However, their diagnostic role and potential implications in clinical practice need further assessments.

12.3.2 Vitamin D

Vitamin D displays its hormonal effect in the form of its physiological active metabolite 1,25(OH)$_2$D- 1,25 dihydroxyvitamin D$_3$, and Vitamin D receptors (VDR) are present in many different tissues, such as brain, breast, immune cells, muscle tissue, parathyroid glands, cardiomyocytes, vascular endothelial and vascular smooth muscle cells, endothelial cells of colon mucosae, as well as malignant colon cells. Vitamin D has a key role in maintenance of bone quality and reduction of fracture risk. However, low levels of Vitamin D have been associated with muscle weakness, increased risk for cancers, autoimmune disease and infectious [19]. A possible association between low vitamin D levels and metabolic syndrome (MS) has been also proposed, as Vitamin D deficiency may increase the risk of insulin resistance and hypertension, the main components of MS [20]. Clinical studies confirm that Vitamin D deficiency influences the activity of renin in plasma, leading to hypertension. Vitamin D regulation of renin expression is independent of calcium metabolism. Renin transcription has been found being suppressed by a VDR-mediated mechanism. $1.25(OH)_2D_3$ can thus be considered a negative endocrine regulator of the renin-angiotensin system (RAS).

However, these data have yet to be confirmed and the precise role of hypovitaminosis D on metabolic status remains to be clarified.

Observational studies suggest an association of low Vitamin D levels with CVD and atherosclerosis. Data on atherosclerosis of the coronary arteries (CAD) have shown that low 25(OH)D levels are associated both with presence and severity of coronary heart disease, and vitamin D deficiency has been identified as an independent marker for CAD [21]. A variety of anti-atherosclerotic effects seems to be exerted by VDR activation: these involve, amongst others, vitamin D-induced decrease of endothelial adhesion molecules, increase of nitric oxide (NO) production and inhibition of macrophage to foam cell formation. VDR activation can also stimulate insulin secretion, protecting against beta-cell dysfunction, as insulin secretion is a calcium-dependent process. Other suggested anti-diabetic effects include improved peripheral insulin resistance, anti-inflammatory actions, and stimulation of osteocalcin, a bone marker with putative effects on insulin secretion and insulin sensitivity.

Vitamin D deficiency thus directly promote the development of hypertension and, consequently, cardiomyocyte hypertrophy and vascular remodeling, resulting in ventricular hypertrophy and congestive heart failure. Also, this process stimulates the release of cytokines, such as interleukin-10, from smooth muscle vascular cells, that have been identified as having an important role in atherogenesis [22]. Vitamin D analogues have been shown to inhibit the release of several proinflammatory cytokines and adhesion molecules, preventing abnormal changes in smooth muscle cells in vessel walls that lead to vascular calcification. It has been proved that low vitamin D levels are associated with increased risk for development of the coronary arterial calcifications seen in atherosclerosis that, together with increased arterial resistance, results in a significant rise in CVD [23, 24].

Low Vitamin D levels lead to the increased production and release of PTH and, consequently, to secondary hyperparathyroidism, which has negative implications for the cardiovascular system and bone metabolism.

12.3.3 Estrogens

Estrogen physiologically promote bone formation by reducing survival, function and production of osteoclasts, through inhibition of two signaling molecules, receptor activator of nuclear factor κB ligand (RANKL) and colony stimulating factor-1.

Estrogen deficiency occurring with menopause represents the major contributor to gradual bone loss observed in women. Lack of estrogens causes a reduction in bone mineral density and quality, owing to an imbalance between the formation of new bone and removal of old bone (remodeling cycle).

Furthermore, bone and coronary arteries are target organs for estrogens. Woman after the menopause demonstrate accelerated bone loss, but also the beneficial effects of estrogens on the cardiovascular system and atherosclerosis are well established [25].

Menopausal estrogenic deficit is also associated with a significant increase in pro-inflammatory cytokines like tumor necrosis factor (TNF)-α, interleukin (IL-4), IL-10 and IL-12 which enhance bone turnover leading to increased bone loss and greater fracture risk. Specifically, TNF-α, produced by macrophages and granulocytes, contributes to decrease bone mass increasing osteoclastic formation via direct stimulation of pro-osteoclastogenic activity of stromal cells. Moreover, the high levels of follicular stimulating hormone (FSH) during menopause can stimulate osteoclastic differentiation and TNF-α production, both causing bone fragility.

Lots of studies showed that the decline of estrogens, which are considered important natural antioxidants, induces a pro-oxidant state during menopause. Oxidative stress (OxS) might intensify bone resorption, underlying development of post menopausal osteoporosis (PMO). In addition, the majority of studies reported OxS is strongly linked to a variety of pathologies like infections, autoimmune diseases and others, specific to old age: cancer, neurodegenerative and CVD. As OxS is also a risk factor of arteriosclerosis and cardiovascular event, it seems to be an interesting link between low bone quantity/quality, on one hand, and arteriosclerosis, on the other hand [26].

12.3.4 Other Factors

Homocysteine (Hcy) is a factor which may contribute to the high bone remodeling of menopause by its direct and indirect effects on bone metabolism. Hcy can increase osteoclastic activity, decrease osteoblastic function and bind directly to bone extracellular matrix, reducing bone strength. Hyperhomocysteinemia (HHcy) may produce also some mitochondrial abnormalities, which can alter bone properties through generations of ROS. However, the mechanism of HHcy-induced bone loss via the mitochondrial pathway is largely unknown.

Interestingly, Hcy plasma levels can increase in postmenopause, thus enhancing the detrimental effect on the skeleton and on CVD risk. Current reports on whether Hcy affects bone density are still controversal.

Homocysteine is a possible risk factor for atherosclerosis. Homocystinuria is a genetically inherited disease which is characterised by elevated plasma homocysteine concentrations. Its clinical manifestations, apart from skeletal disorders and OP, include a tendency towards premature atherosclerosis and thromboembolism. There is also evidence that postmenopausal woman with a heterozygous mutation in methylenetetrahydrofolate reductase (MTHFR) and, therefore, hyperhomocysteinaemia demonstrate a decrease in BMD. This supports the hypothesis that homocysteine participates in the interaction between oestrogen and bone metabolism [27].

Many studies also found an alteration in bone biomechanical properties in patients affected by vitamin B12 and folate deficiencies, hypothesizing that both could act not only via Hcy-dependent pathways but also via Hcy-independent pathways in determining bone loss. Earlier evidence reported Hcy and vitamin B12, but not folate, was related to BMD in PMO. However, the real impact of lack of folate and vitamin B12 alone or in association with HHcy on bone health has to be better clarified. The relationship between Hcy, folate, and vitamin B12 and BMD in postmenopausal women needs to be further investigated.

Also patients with OP and atherosclerosis exhibit insufficient vitamin K levels. Vitamin K is a cofactor required to convert the amino acid glutamate into gamma-carboxyglutamate, or Gla-proteins. Gla-proteins regulate physiological processes controlled by calcium. These include blood coagulation (clotting) and bone mineralization. Accordingly, Gla-proteins are critical to the formation and replenishment of bone tissue. Unless these proteins are modified by vitamin K, they cannot properly form the matrix in which calcium and phosphorus bind together to make solid, well-mineralized bone. Vitamin K has been shown to stimulate new bone formation and reduce the incidence of vertebral fractures. The Gla-protein osteocalcin, normally present in bone, has been found in calcified atherosclerotic plaque lesions, and production of this protein is pathologically up-regulated in people with atherosclerosis. At the same time, another vitamin K-dependent Gla-protein known as matrix Gla-protein (MGP), normally found in healthy arterial walls, is a strong inhibitor of vascular calcification. In other words, by increasing MGP in the arterial walls, vitamin K protects against the calcification-inducing effects of osteocalcin. Therefore, vitamin K deficiency is also a confounder in the OP/CVD relationship [28].

12.4 Drugs

Some data show that many drugs used for treatment of OP have an interesting impact on cardiovascular system. This evidence could further suggest pathophysiological similarities between bone loss and CVD.

Biphosphonates (BP) are well-known antiresorptive agents used for therapy of post- menopausal osteoporosis (PMO) with proved antifracturative efficacy, mostly due to their ability to increase BMD. Recent studies have supported the hypothesis that BPs may have also some antiatherogenic actions [29]: *ibandronate* (IBN) i.v. produced a significant increase in high-density lipoprotein cholesterol/low-density lipoprotein cholesterol (HDL-C/LDL-C) ratio in 60 postmenopausal osteoporotic women, and *zoledronate* (ZLN) i.v. annually causes a significant reduction of carotid artery intima-media thickness (CA-IMT) and an even more effective reduction of LDL-C compared with that observed with IBN. Fibroblast growth factor 23 and sclerostin—a Wnt/β-catenin signaling antagonist promoting the differentiation of osteoblast precursors towards mature osteoblasts—were proposed to be involved in the mechanism of action of BPs at a vascular level. *Alendronate* (ALN) has been proven effective in reducing CA-IMT and improving lipid profile during 1 year of therapy [30]. ALN seems have also a protective effect from atherosclerosis and abdominal AoC. However, the role of BPs on VC is still conflicting.

Statins lower serum cholesterol by inhibiting 3-hydroxy-3-methylglutaryl coenzyme A (HMG-CoA) reductase in the liver and can decrease LDL cholesterol levels in patients with dyslipidemia, helping prevent the formation of atherosclerotic plaque. Their association with bone miralization is controversial: some reports claim they were associated—alone or in combination with BPs—with an increase in bone mineralization and reduced incidence of fractures in murine and human models, while others seem to deny this hypothesis.

One possible explanation could be that both statins that BP induce inhibition of mevalonate, that leads to the synthesis of both cholesterol and prenylation of proteins which activate the osteoclast cells [31].

Denosumab (Dmab) is a monoclonal antibody that blocks RANKL, inhibiting osteoclast formation and survival, that has been introduced for the therapy of PMO as an effective antiresorptive agent. Its effects in preventing VC in a murine model of glucocorticoid-induced OP have been proven, but data in humans are still lacking. However, patients treated with Dmab do not report effects on progression of AoC or incidence of CVD [32].

Raloxifene (RLX) is a Selective Estrogen Receptor Modulator (SERM). Its protective action from demineralization in women in early postmenopause with normal or low bone mass is well known, and it has proven useful in preventing osteoporosis and fracture risk. It showed a beneficial effect in reducing LDL cholesterol levels, improving vascular endothelial function and reducing risk of coronary heart disease, especially in postmenopausal women.

Recent evidence suggests that *Vitamin D* (Vit D) intakes above current recommendations may be associated with better health outcomes other than reducing the risk of osteopenia and osteoporosis. A daily dose of 700–1000 IU has an anti-inflammatory effect and blocks plaque calcification in arterial blood flow. Its role in blood pressure homeostasis suggests that Vit D analogues could help prevent or ameliorate hypertension. Toxic doses lead to medicalcinosis, which is a reversible process.

The free radical Nitric Oxide (NO), is a powerful vasodilator that helps keep the vascular tone and would inhibit collagen and bone loss. NO could be involved in osteogenesis as knock-out mice show low bone mass, a low BMD and a reduced number of osteoclasts [33]. The endothelial isoform of the synthase (eNOS) is found in high concentrations level in bone where it plays an active role in osteoblast activation and inhibition of bone resorption. Patients treated for 1 year with NO show an increased bone mass. Nitrates (like nitroglycerin) have proven to be useful in enabling osteoclastogenesis and increasing bone mass.

Besides, several data showed some medications, such as bisphosphonates (BPs) and raloxifene (RLX)—mainly used for the treatment of OP and statins, the most important drug for hypercholesterolemia—are effective on both bone loss and CVD risk. These data could indicate that the mechanisms of action of all these medications at cellular level may not be exclusive for a single system (bone or cardiovascular) but take part both in bone metabolism and atherosclerosis.

References

1. Winkelmann BR. American Heart Association scientific sessions. Expert Opin Investig Drugs. 2004;13:435–45.
2. Tanko LB, Christiansen C, Cummings SR. Relationship between osteoporosis and cardiovascular disease in postmenopausal women. J Bone Miner Res. 2005;20:1912–20.
3. Chiang CH, Liu CJ, Chen PJ, Huang CC, Hsu CY, Chen ZY, Chan WL, Huang PH, Chen TJ, Chung CM, Lin SJ, Chen JW, Leu HB. Hip fracture and risk of acute myocardial infarction: a nationwide study. J Bone Miner Res. 2013;28:404–11.
4. Sennerby U, Melhus H, Gedeborg R, Byberg L, Garmo H, Ahlbom A, Pedersen NL, Michaëlsson K. Cardiovascular diseases and risk of hip fracture. JAMA. 2009;302:1666–73.
5. Aluoch AO, Jessee R, Habal H, Garcia-Rosell M, Shah R, Reed G, Carbone L. Heart failure as a risk factor for osteoporosis and fractures. Curr Osteoporos Rep. 2012;10(4):258–69.
6. Sprini D, Rini GB, Di Stefano L, Cianferotti L, Napoli N. Correlation between osteoporosis and cardiovascular disease. Clin Cases Miner Bone Metab. 2014;11(2):117–9.
7. El Maghraoui A, Rezqi A, Mounach A. Vertebral fractures and abdominal aortic calcification in postmenopausal women. A cohort study. Bone. 2013;56:213–9.
8. Bastos Gonçalves F, Voûte MT, Hoeks SE, Chonchol MB, Boersma EE, Stolker RJ, Verhagen HJ. Calcification of the abdominal aorta as an independent predictor of cardiovascular events: a meta-analysis. Heart. 2012;98:988–94.
9. Simon SP, Fodor D, Muntean L, Poanta L, Cristea P, Rednic S. Bone mineral density, vertebral fractures and body mass index in post-menopausal women with abdominal aortic calcification. Endocr Res. 2014;39:1–6.
10. Szulc P. Vascular calcification and fracture risk. Clin Cases Miner Bone Metab. 2015;12(2): 139–41.
11. Frost ML, Grella R, Millasseau SC, Jiang BY, Hampson G, Fogelman I, Chowienczyk PJ. Relationship of calcification of atherosclerotic plaque and arterial stiffness to bone mineral density and osteoprotegerin in postmenopausal women referred for osteoporosis screening. Calcif Tissue Int. 2008;83(2):112–20.
12. Fernández-Murga ML, Vinué Á, Caeiro JR. Impact of estrogens on atherosclerosis and bone in the apolipoprotein E-deficient mouse model. Menopause. 2015;22:428–36.
13. McCarty MF, Di Nicolantonio JJ. The molecular biology and pathophysiology of vascular calcification. Postgrad Med. 2014;126:54–64.
14. Lello S, Capozzi A, Scambia G. Osteoporosis and cardiovascular disease: an update. Gynecol Endocrinol. 2015;31(8):590–4.
15. Lee CJ, Wang JH, Chen ML. Serum osteoprotegerin is associated with arterial stiffness assessed according to the cardio-ankle vascular index in hypertensive patients. J Atheroscler Thromb. 2015;22:304–12.
16. D'Amelio P, Isaia G, Isaia GC. The osteoprotegerin/RANK/RANKL system: a bone key to vascular disease. J Endocrinol Investig. 2009;32(4 Suppl):6–9.
17. Wolak T. Osteopontin – a multi-modal marker and mediator in atherosclerotic vascular disease. Atherosclerosis. 2014;236:327–37.
18. Evrard S, Delanaye P, Kamel S. Vascular calcification: from pathophysiology to biomarkers. Clin Chim Acta. 2014;438C:401–14.
19. Lai YH, Fang TC. The pleiotropic effect of vitamin D. ISRN Nephrol. 2013;2013:898125.
20. Querales MI, Cruces ME, Rojas S. Association between vitamin D deficiency and metabolic syndrome. Rev Med Chil. 2010;138:1312–8.
21. Pilz S, Verheyen N, Grübler MR, Tomaschitz A, März W. Vitamin D and cardiovascular disease prevention. Nat Rev Cardiol. 2016;13(7):404–17.
22. Wang T, Pencina M, Booth S. Vitamin D deficiency and risc of cardiovascular disease. Circulation. 2008;117:503–11.
23. Li YC, Kong J, Wei M, Chen ZF, Liu SQ, Cao LP. 1,25-Dihydroxyvitamin D3 is a negative endocrine regulator of the renin-angiotensin system. J Clin Invest. 2002;110:229–38.

24. Stojanovic OI, Lazovic M, Lazovic M, Vuceljic M. Association between atherosclerosis and osteoporosis, the role of vitamin D. Arch Med Sci. 2011;7(2):179–88.
25. Mendelsohn ME, Karas RH. The protective effects of estrogen on the cardiovascular system. N Engl J Med. 1999;340:1801–11.
26. Cagnacci A, Cannoletta M, Palma F. Relation between oxidative stress and climacteric symptoms in early postmenopausal women. Climacteric. 2015;18(4):1–6.
27. Anagnostis P, Karagiannis A, Kakafika AI, Tziomalos K, Athyros VG, Mikhailidis DP. Atherosclerosis and osteoporosis: age-dependent degenerative processes or related entities? Osteoporos Int. 2009;20:197–207.
28. Shoji S. Vitamin K and vascular calcification. Clin Calcium. 2002;12:1123–8.
29. Igase M, Kohara K, Tabara Y. Change in arterial stiffness associated with monthly bisphosphonate treatment in women with postmenopausal osteoporosis. Menopause. 2014;21:962–6.
30. Celiloglu M, Aydin Y, Balci P, Kolamaz T. The effect of alendronate sodium on carotid artery intima-media thickness and lipid profile in women with postmenopausal osteoporosis. Menopause. 2009;16:689–93.
31. Wu M, Rementer C, Giachelli CM. Vascular calcification: an update on mechanisms and challenges in treatment. Calcif Tissue Int. 2013;93:365–73.
32. Samelson EJ, Miller PD, Christiansen C. RANKL inhibition with denosumab does not influence 3-year progression of aortic calcification or incidence of adverse cardiovascular events in postmenopausal women with osteoporosis and high cardiovascular risk. J Bone Miner Res. 2014;29:450–7.
33. Riancho JA, Salas E, Zarrabeitia MT, Olmos JM, Amado JA, Fernández-Luna JL, González-Macías J. Expression and functional role of nitric oxide synthase in osteoblast-like cells. J Bone Miner Res. 1995;10(3):439–46.

Osteoporosis in Men

13

Elena Nebot Valenzuela and Peter Pietschmann

13.1 Definition of Osteoporosis

Osteoporosis is a skeletal disorder characterized by compromised bone strength predisposing a person to an increased risk of fracture. Bone strength primarily reflects the integration of bone density and bone quality [1]. Bone microarchitecture is an important determinant of bone strength; an example of trabecular alterations in male idiopathic osteoporosis is shown in Fig. 13.1.

13.2 Epidemiology

Due to the essential role of estrogen deficiency in the development of osteoporosis, postmenopausal and elderly women are numerically most affected. However, men are not protected from bone loss and its consequences [2, 3].

E. N. Valenzuela (✉)
Department of Pathophysiology and Allergy Research, Center for Pathophysiology, Infectiology and Immunology, Medical University of Vienna, Vienna, Austria

Department of Physiology, School of Pharmacy and Institute of Nutrition and Food Technology, University of Granada, Granada, Spain
e-mail: enebot@ugr.es

P. Pietschmann
Department of Pathophysiology and Allergy Research, Center for Pathophysiology, Infectiology and Immunology, Medical University of Vienna, Vienna, Austria
e-mail: peter.pietschmann@meduniwien.ac.at

A. Lenzi, S. Migliaccio (eds.), *Multidisciplinary Approach to Osteoporosis*,
https://doi.org/10.1007/978-3-319-75110-8_13

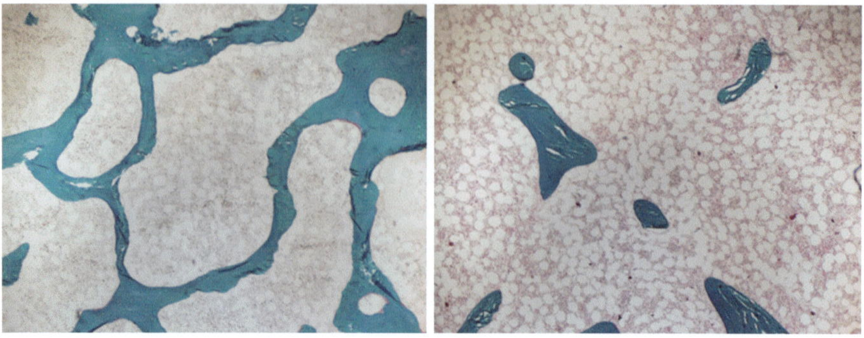

Fig. 13.1 Histologic sections of trabecular bone from iliac crest biopsies of a control subject (left panel) and a man with idiopathic osteoporosis (right panel) [41]. Biopsies were fixed, dehydrated, and embedded in polymethyl methacrylate. Histologic sections were cut from the blocks and stained according to Goldner

Men undergo a relatively slow bone loss with age; bone loss is accelerated from the sixth decade at an average rate of 0.5–1.0% per year and accompanied by a growing incidence of fractures [4]. The most common sites for fragility fractures in men are those of the vertebrae and hip, but also fractures of other sites such as forearm, ribs, pelvis, and clavicle are associated with osteoporosis in men [5].

Osteoporosis affects approximately 10 million subjects in the United States, including 2 million men [6]. It has been estimated that one in five white men will have a fracture related to osteoporosis during his lifetime [7]. In this context, men are estimated to account for 29% of all osteoporotic fractures [8]. The prevalence of the disease in the European Union is estimated at 27.6 million (22.0 million women versus 5.6 million men) [9]. Approximately 6% of men and 21% of women aged 50–84 years are classified as having osteoporosis. The prevalence of osteoporosis in women over the age of 50 years is three to four times greater than in men; this finding is in line with the difference in lifetime risk of an osteoporotic fracture in women and men [9].

Nevertheless, mortality after a hip fracture, (in particular within the first year after the fracture), is higher in men compared to women [10, 11]; the reason for this gender difference has not yet been clarified [12]. For instance, a study by Bass et al. [13] reported that approximately one in three men older than 65 years dies within 1 year after hip fracture.

13.3 Pathophysiology

In osteoporosis, osteoblast and osteoclast activities are unbalanced with decreased bone formation and/or increased bone resorption; this imbalance results in bone loss and increased fracture risk [12].

From a clinical point of view, osteoporosis in men can be classified as primary or secondary [14]. In cases of primary osteoporosis, the condition either is caused by age-related bone loss (senile osteoporosis) or the cause is unknown (idiopathic osteoporosis). The term idiopathic osteoporosis commonly is used only for men less than 70 years old; older men—in the absence of secondary causes—are assumed to suffer from age-related osteoporosis. Nevertheless, in contrast to women, the majority of men with osteoporosis have at least one secondary cause. In secondary osteoporosis, the loss of bone mass is caused by specific lifestyle factors, diseases, or medications.

13.3.1 Primary Osteoporosis

Taking into account that the age-related changes in the male skeleton occur early in adult life and that failure to achieve adequate peak bone mass at a young age is one of the factors leading to osteoporosis, the pathogenesis of the two types of primary male osteoporosis is described together. Quantitative and qualitative alterations of bone are mainly attributed to changes in the concentration of circulating endogenous factors which regulate bone metabolism [15].

13.3.1.1 "Natural" Bone Loss in Men

Adult bone mass is achieved during childhood and particularly during adolescent growth spurt. Interestingly in this period, there is also an increase in fractures, which appears to be due to transient decreases in cortical thickness and increase in cortical porosity [16]. Data obtained by quantitative computer tomography have also demonstrated that trabecular bone mass seems to "peak" in early adult life (although the timing of acquisition of peak bone mass may be different at different sites), with decreases in trabecular bone (evident in both sexes) as early as the third decade. By contrast, in men cortical bone remains stable until later in life, with subsequent decreases [17].

Bone loss generally accelerates after the age of 70 years in men due to a combination of nutritional and hormonal deficiencies [14]. A decrease in intestinal calcium absorption and high prevalence of vitamin D insufficiency both contribute to elevated serum parathyroid hormone (PTH) levels and bone loss [18].

As will be discussed in the next section, rapid bone loss is common in testosterone or estradiol deficiency [19]. Both free or bioavailable testosterone and estradiol levels decline with age due to increased serum sex hormone-binding globulin (SHBG) levels and failure of the hypothalamic-pituitary-testicular axis to compensate [20]. The age-related decrease of insulin-like growth factor 1 (IGF-1) may directly or indirectly decrease bone formation [21].

The pattern of age-related changes in bone structure is an important factor in the pathophysiology of bone loss. As mentioned before, in men, trabecular bone loss starts early in life; this is associated with changes in the IGF-1 regulating system, whereas cortical bone loss occurs later, in association with decreases in testosterone and estrogen and increased bone remodeling [22].

In men, the imbalance of bone resorption relative to formation leads to decreases in bone mineral density (BMD) of about 1% per year, which can begin soon after peak bone mass [22, 23]. As described above, BMD is not the only determinant of fracture risk; bone size, geometry, and microarchitecture are major contributors to bone strength. Men have greater bone size than do women, which confers mechanical advantage. With increasing age, the rate of resorption at the endocortical surface increases. This endocortical resorption is partially compensated by an increase in periosteal circumference, which increases bone size and displaces the cortex outward from the center of the bone (both of which increase bone strength). However, a net decrease in cortical thickness occurs, which reduces bone strength [24]. In addition, microarchitecture deteriorates with aging: cortical porosity increases, endocortical absorption causes trabecularization of cortical bone (Fig. 13.2), and trabecular thickness decreases [25].

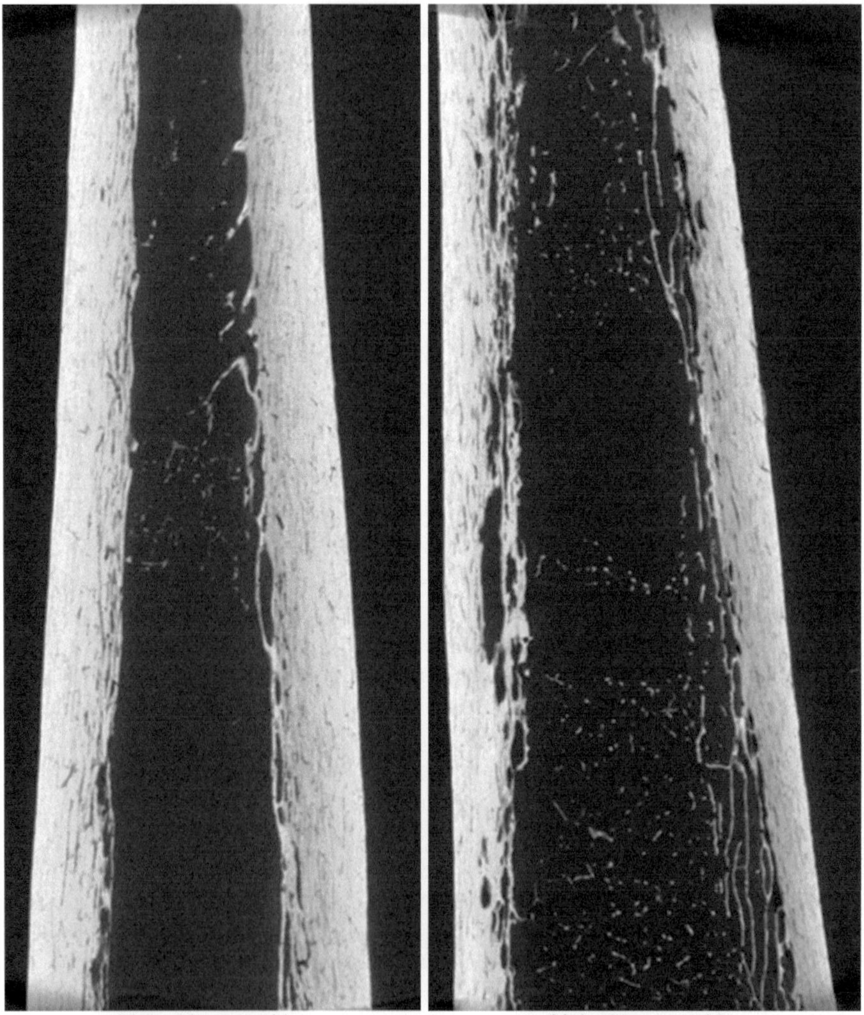

Male, 63 years old

Male, 90 years old

Fig. 13.2 Representative microarchitectural images of middle-age and old human male tibia midshafts, respectively. Tibias were obtained from body donors provided by the Department of Anatomy, Medical University of Vienna, Austria. Analyses of the cortical bone microarchitecture were performed with an X-raying inspection system with a microcomputer tomography scanner (Viscom X-8060-II, Core Facility for Micro-Computed Tomography, University of Vienna, Austria)

13.3.1.2 Hormones and the Male Skeleton

Bone-forming cells contain both androgen and estrogen receptors along with enzymes involved in sex hormone metabolism [15]. It appears that both types of steroids play a role in bone growth. Estrogens, possibly mediated by IGF-1, favor the longitudinal growth of long bones in the epiphyseal plate. Androgens, on the other hand, stimulate periosteal apposition and are responsible for appositional growth which leads to an increase in bone thickness. Moreover, sex hormones play an important role in maintaining bone mass with age: estrogens are regarded to protect both cancellous and cortical bone, whereas androgens predominantly conserve cancellous bone [26].

With aging, in men testosterone and 17β-estradiol levels decline and SHBG levels increase [20, 27, 28]. A study by Orwoll et al. [20] showed that both total and bioavailable testosterone levels are diminished with aging, and a 10% reduction rate per decade was reported. Moreover, there was a strong association between older age and low concentrations of total and bioavailable estradiol. Additionally, low levels of free estradiol were associated with low free testosterone and high SHBG.

It is important to note that independent roles of estrogens and androgens in bone metabolism in healthy men had been demonstrated. A study by Falahati-Nini et al. [29] reported that estrogens were responsible for over 70% of sex hormone-related bone resorption in normal elderly men, while bone formation was equally affected by both types of steroids. However, the study by Leder et al. [30] demonstrated the superiority of androgens in the regulation of bone formation and an independent action of both hormones on bone resorption in healthy young men.

The effect of sex hormones on the male skeleton can also be assessed by the correlation of the hormones with fracture risk [28, 31]. Several studies show that testosterone is not strongly associated with bone loss, while others refer to it as a strong predisposing factor for osteoporotic fractures. A possible explanation is that the hormone affects mostly exoskeletal parameters of fracture risk (e.g., muscle mass), and it appears possible that its aromatization to estrogens could have an effect [32].

The pathogenesis of bone loss in men is closely related to the production and action of estradiol (total, free, or bioavailable). Moreover, the pathogenesis of male osteoporosis is consequently related to quantitative and qualitative changes of aromatase and estrogen receptors which mainly arise from genetic variations of the corresponding genes [33]. Most of the studies using fracture as outcomes have provided support for a key role for estradiol in determining fracture risk in aging men, as well as the presence of a threshold estradiol level below which fracture risk increases in men [17]. Testosterone may also contribute to fracture risk, particularly in the setting of high SHBG levels. In men, sex steroid deficiency alone is sufficient to increase bone resorption markers, even in the setting of suppressed follicle-stimulating hormone (FSH) levels [34]. However, the precise role of increases in FSH with aging in mediating age-related bone loss remains unclear [17].

Growth hormone (GH) and IGF-1 have an anabolic effect on skeletal growth [15]. Their receptors in growth plate chondrocytes stimulate longitudinal bone growth with endochondral bone formation. Cell receptors for GH and IGF-1 are also found on both osteoblasts and osteoclasts [35]. With aging, GH and IGF-1 levels are reduced [36]; the alterations of GH production with age have been termed "somatopause." Daily GH secretion may be impaired in the elderly, reaching only 1/20 of its levels encountered in young adults [37]. Most of systemic and local IGF-1 is bound to specific binding proteins (IGFBPs). The fact that they inhibit IGF-1 function means that they are likely involved in the pathogenesis of osteoporosis. It has been found that IGFBP-2 increases significantly with aging in both men and women and is negatively correlated with BMD and positively with bone turnover biochemical markers [38]. The concomitant decrease in IGF-1 is associated more than any other factor with the changes observed in cancellous bone in men during the first two decades of adult life. Later in life these changes are mainly attributed to sex hormones [36].

13.3.1.3 Male Idiopathic Osteoporosis: Osteoblast Dysfunction

Osteoblast function was evaluated in vitro in cells isolated from bone specimens of men with osteoporosis [39]. A study by Pernow et al. [40] found that osteoblast-like cells isolated from men with idiopathic osteoporosis showed impaired bone formation and slightly decreased bone resorption, which might be due to the low expression levels of receptor activator of nuclear factor kappa-B ligand (RANKL) and runt-related transcription factor 2 (RUNX 2) as demonstrated in a study by Patsch et al. [41]. Pernow et al. [40] described osteoblast dysfunction with decreased osteocalcin and increased production of factors stimulating osteoclast activation.

In men with idiopathic osteoporosis, low levels of serum estradiol and high levels of SHBG have been reported [42, 43]. Moreover, a lower abundance of estrogen receptor alpha has been found in osteoblasts and osteocytes from male idiopathic osteoporosis patients [44].

Whereas the mechanisms of estrogen action on bone may be complex, the finding that osteoblasts express estrogen receptors suggests that this class of hormones exerts direct effects on bone cells; in vitro estrogen treatment coordinately increases DNA content and alkaline phosphatase activity. Estrogen increases both the levels of messenger RNA for alkaline phosphatase and type I collagen. Thus, estrogen promotes the formation of bone while reducing cellular responsiveness to hormones that may trigger bone resorption [45]. Furthermore, positive correlations between parameters of bone formation and estradiol levels have been demonstrated in men with idiopathic osteoporosis [46]. Low osteoid thickness and wall thickness are indicators of a low formative capacity of the osteoblast in the bone morphogenic unit, i.e., short osteoblast life span or low osteoblast number, leading to low bone mass. The bone structure, with thin wall and thin osteoid, was associated with low estradiol levels.

In addition to low estradiol levels, also low circulating IGF-1 levels could result in decreased bone formation in men with idiopathic osteoporosis [47]. Our current working model of the pathophysiology of idiopathic osteoporosis in men is shown in Fig. 13.3.

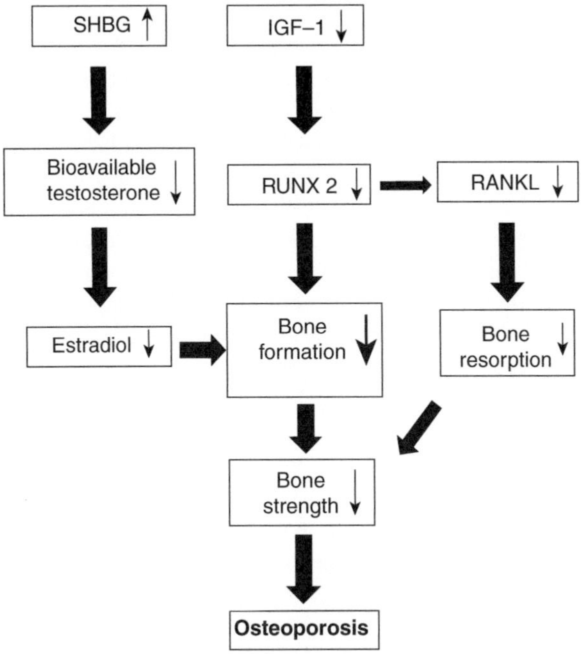

Fig. 13.3 Our hypothetical model of the pathophysiology of osteoporosis in men. *SHBG* sex hormone-binding globulin, *IGF-1* insulin-like growth factor 1, *RUNX 2* runt-related transcription factor 2, *RANKL* receptor activator of nuclear factor kappa-B ligand

13.3.2 Secondary Osteoporosis

The pathogenesis of secondary osteoporosis is heterogeneous encompassing induction by lifestyle conditions and habits, medications, or the consequences of underlying diseases [48]. Lifestyle conditions and habits such as smoking, excessive alcohol consumption, diet, and physical activity are associated with osteoporosis and considered to be risk factors which can be modified [49].

The most frequent secondary causes of osteoporosis in men are glucocorticoid use, hypogonadism, and excessive alcohol intake [50]. One of these causes is present in the majority of younger men with osteoporosis [20] and may be superimposed on primary osteoporosis [14]. In this line, the treatment with exogenous glucocorticoids is the most common cause of secondary osteoporosis in adult males [51, 52]. Synthetic glucocorticoids are widely used for treatment of patients with diverse conditions, including inflammatory bowel disease, rheumatoid arthritis, or chronic obstructive pulmonary disease that may also be precipitants of osteoporosis [53]. Glucocorticoid-induced osteoporosis occurs in two phases: a rapid decrease in BMD that appears to be due to an increase in bone resorption, followed by a slower, progressive phase of BMD decline likely a result of impaired bone formation [53, 54]. The mechanisms might be indirect, e.g., an upregulation of osteoclastogenesis via stimulation of RANKL and suppression of osteoblast OPG expressions [49, 55]. Moreover, a major effect of glucocorticoids is a profound impairment of bone formation through suppression of osteoblastogenesis and induction of osteoblast and osteocyte apoptosis [56]. The resulting increased risk of fracture is seen within 3 months after initiation of oral glucocorticoid therapy and is reflected by changes in the concentrations of various bone markers such as osteocalcin [54, 57].

Osteoporosis is regularly mentioned as a secondary consequence of alcoholism, and chronic alcohol abuse is established as an independent risk factor for osteoporosis [58]. Alcohol exhibits various direct effects on the activity of bone cells. Under the influence of alcohol, the growth of mesenchymal stem cells in the bone marrow and the transformation into osteoblasts are inhibited [59]. Furthermore, alcohol inhibits osteoblast growth in cell cultures and impaired DNA synthesis and cell proliferation of osteoblasts [60]. The modality of the decrease in bone mass and strength following alcohol consumption is mainly due to a bone remodeling imbalance, with a predominant decrease in bone formation [61]. Another factor that seems to be involved in mediating the impaired osteoblastic function appears to be sclerostin, which correlates with decreased markers of bone synthesis and increased markers of bone breakdown [62]. In contrast, estradiol has a protective influence on alcohol-induced bone loss through the inhibition of the upregulation of RANKL in osteoblasts [63]. On the other hand, alcohol may indirectly influence bone remodeling, including osteocyte apoptosis, oxidative stress, and Wnt signaling pathway modulation [58]. In this line, oxidase activity is increased through the alcohol-induced oxidative stress resulting in an increase of RANKL signaling, which enhances osteoclastogenesis [64].

13.4 Diagnosis

In the diagnostic workup of men with osteoporosis, it is important to determine possible secondary causes of the disease. For further details, the reader is referred to Chap. 7 "Osteoporosis: Diagnosis."

13.5 Treatment

The National Osteoporosis Foundation recommends that BMD testing should be performed in all men aged 70 years and older, as well as some aged 50–69 years depending on the risk factor profile [65, 66]. Moreover, the guidelines recommend osteoporosis treatment not only after hip or vertebral fractures or with *T*-scores ≤−2.5 but also in men aged >50 with osteopenia if FRAX-based 10-year hip or major osteoporotic fracture probability is >20% [67].

13.5.1 Calcium and Vitamin D

Vitamin D insufficiency and consequent secondary hyperparathyroidism are common in older men. It leads to bone loss, muscle weakness, decreased balance, and falls. All major osteoporosis trials have included calcium and vitamin D, which reduce fractures by 10–15% [68]. However, the adequate intake levels of calcium and vitamin D is still a controversial issue. For further details, see part III of this book: *Part III: Prevention and Treatment.*

13.5.2 Antiresorptive Drugs

Randomized controlled trials in male osteoporosis have been completed for all commonly used osteoporosis drugs, including alendronate and risedronate (daily and weekly), intravenous zoledronate and ibandronate, and most recently, denosumab and strontium ranelate [68, 69]. In practice, drug choice will depend on availability, cost, reimbursement criteria, disease severity, side effects, comorbidities, and (relative) contraindications.

13.5.2.1 Alendronate

Alendronate is a potent bisphosphonate that inhibits osteoclast-mediated bone resorption [70]. The 2-year double-blind trial study by Orwoll et al. [71] demonstrated that a daily dose of 10 mg of alendronate increased lumbar spine and hip BMD, reduced the rate of vertebral fractures, and prevented decreases in height in men with osteoporosis.

13.5.2.2 Zoledronic Acid

Zoledronic acid is a bisphosphonate administered intravenously. A once-yearly infusion of zoledronic acid at a dose of 5 mg was associated with a significant decrease in the risk of new vertebral fractures among men with osteoporosis [72].

13.5.2.3 Denosumab

Denosumab is a fully human monoclonal antibody that specifically binds to the receptor activator of nuclear factor-κB ligand, a key mediator of osteoclast formation, function, and survival [73]. Denosumab was studied in men with low bone mass; 2 years of denosumab therapy was associated with increased BMD at all skeletal sites, with maintained reductions in bone resorption, and was well tolerated [74].

Androgen-deprivation therapy is well-established for treating prostate cancer but is associated with bone loss and an increased risk of fracture [75–77]. Bone mineral density loss is rapid during the first year of androgen-deprivation therapy; up to 4.6% of total hip, femoral neck, and lumbar spine BMD loss has been reported in prostate cancer patients without bone metastases (nonmetastatic prostate cancer) [75]. Smith et al. [76] found that twice-yearly administration of denosumab increased BMD at all skeletal sites and significantly reduced the incidence of vertebral fractures.

13.5.3 Bone Anabolic Drugs

13.5.3.1 Intermittent Parathyroid Hormone (PTH) Therapy

Intermittent PTH with the 1–34 fragment teriparatide treatment has been approved as an anabolic agent for osteoporosis in men. The therapy is usually given for 2 years maximum (at which time bone resorption catches up and exceeds formation) followed by antiresorptive treatment to maintain benefits. Orwoll et al. [78] described that once-daily administration of teriparatide resulted in increased BMD at the spine and proximal femur, and increased bone mineral content in osteoporotic men, after a median treatment duration of 11 months. Furthermore, the effects of teriparatide on markers of bone turnover and BMD were similar to those seen in a trial in postmenopausal women, who experienced dramatic reductions in the risk of vertebral and non-vertebral fractures [79].

13.5.4 Undertreatment

Although in recent years significant progress in our knowledge on the treatment of osteoporosis has been made, only a small fraction of the patients receive adequate medication. Underdiagnosis and undertreatment of osteoporosis have been reported for both genders but appear to be particularly common in elderly subjects and men [80, 81]. With regard to the high incidence of postfracture disability and high mortality rate undertreatment of osteoporosis in men not only causes unnecessary suffering but also high healthcare costs.

Conclusion

Osteoporosis in men should be considered as a serious public health concern and as a potentially life-threatening disease. In contrast to osteoporosis in women, osteoporosis in men frequently is a secondary condition (e.g., due to glucocorticoid treatment, hypogonadism, or alcohol abuse). Osteoblast dysfunction appears to play the dominant role in the pathophysiology of primary osteoporosis in men.

The treatment of osteoporosis in men has been studied far less than in women; nevertheless, a reduction of the incidence of vertebral fractures in men has been demonstrated in three independent studies with three different compounds. However, further research, e.g., with regard to the reduction of non-vertebral fractures, is necessary.

Conflict of Interest Elena Nebot declares that there is no conflict of interest. Peter Pietschmann has received research support and/or honoraria from Amgen GmbH, Eli Lilly GesmbH, Fresenius Kabi, and MEDA Pharma GmbH.

Acknowledgments Elena Nebot was supported by a postdoctoral fellow awarded by the University of Granada (Spain). The work of Peter Pietschmann is supported by the Austrian Science Fund (Project # P28827-B30). The authors are grateful to Ursula Föger-Samwald, Katharina Wahl-Figlash, and Birgit Schwarz for their assistance.

References

1. NIH Consensus Development Panel on Osteoporosis Prevention, Diagnosis, and Therapy. Osteoporosis prevention, diagnosis, and therapy. JAMA. 2001;285(6):785–95.
2. Khosla S. Update in male osteoporosis. J Clin Endocrinol Metab. 2010;95(1):3–10.
3. Patsch JM, Deutschmann J, Pietschmann P. Gender aspects of osteoporosis and bone strength. Wien Med Wochenschr. 2011;161(5–6):117–23.
4. Melton LJ 3rd, et al. Effects of body size and skeletal site on the estimated prevalence of osteoporosis in women and men. Osteoporos Int. 2000;11(11):977–83.
5. Schuit SC, et al. Fracture incidence and association with bone mineral density in elderly men and women: the Rotterdam Study. Bone. 2004;34(1):195–202.
6. Wright NC, et al. The recent prevalence of osteoporosis and low bone mass in the United States based on bone mineral density at the femoral neck or lumbar spine. J Bone Miner Res. 2014;29(11):2520–6.
7. US Department of Health and Human Services. Bone health and osteoporosis: a report of the surgeon general. 2004. Rockville, MD.
8. Burge R, et al. Incidence and economic burden of osteoporosis-related fractures in the United States, 2005-2025. J Bone Miner Res. 2007;22(3):465–75.
9. Hernlund E, et al. Osteoporosis in the European Union: medical management, epidemiology and economic burden. Arch Osteoporos. 2013;8(1):1–115.
10. Center JR, et al. Mortality after all major types of osteoporotic fracture in men and women: an observational study. Lancet. 1999;353(9156):878–82.
11. Kannegaard PN, et al. Excess mortality in men compared with women following a hip fracture. National analysis of comedications, comorbidity and survival. Age Ageing. 2010;39(2):203–9.
12. D'Amelio P, Isaia GC. Male osteoporosis in the elderly. Int J Endocrinol. 2015;2015:907689.
13. Bass E, et al. Risk-adjusted mortality rates of elderly veterans with hip fractures. Ann Epidemiol. 2007;17(7):514–9.
14. Khosla S, Amin S, Orwoll E. Osteoporosis in men. Endocr Rev. 2008;29(4):441–64.
15. Stathopoulos IS, et al. A review on osteoporosis in men. Hormones (Athens). 2014;13(4):441–57.
16. Kirmani S, et al. Bone structure at the distal radius during adolescent growth. J Bone Miner Res. 2009;24(6):1033–42.
17. Khosla S. Pathogenesis of osteoporosis. Transl Endocrinol Metab. 2010;1(1):55–86.
18. Lips P. Vitamin D deficiency and secondary hyperparathyroidism in the elderly: consequences for bone loss and fractures and therapeutic implications. Endocr Rev. 2001;22(4):477–501.
19. Fink HA, et al. Association of testosterone and estradiol deficiency with osteoporosis and rapid bone loss in older men. J Clin Endocrinol Metab. 2006;91(10):3908–15.
20. Orwoll E, et al. Testosterone and estradiol among older men. J Clin Endocrinol Metab. 2006;91(4):1336–44.
21. Gagnon C, Li V, Ebeling PR. Osteoporosis in men: its pathophysiology and the role of teriparatide in its treatment. Clin Interv Aging. 2008;3(4):635–45.
22. Riggs BL, et al. A population-based assessment of rates of bone loss at multiple skeletal sites: evidence for substantial trabecular bone loss in young adult women and men. J Bone Miner Res. 2008;23(2):205–14.
23. Walsh JS, Eastell R. Osteoporosis in men. Nat Rev Endocrinol. 2013;9(11):637–45.
24. Seeman E. Structural basis of growth-related gain and age-related loss of bone strength. Rheumatology (Oxford). 2008;47(Suppl 4):iv2–8.
25. Burghardt AJ, et al. Age- and gender-related differences in the geometric properties and biomechanical significance of intracortical porosity in the distal radius and tibia. J Bone Miner Res. 2010;25(5):983–93.
26. Callewaert F, Boonen S, Vanderschueren D. Sex steroids and the male skeleton: a tale of two hormones. Trends Endocrinol Metab. 2010;21(2):89–95.
27. Khosla S, et al. Relationship of volumetric BMD and structural parameters at different skeletal sites to sex steroid levels in men. J Bone Miner Res. 2005;20(5):730–40.

28. Mellstrom D, et al. Older men with low serum estradiol and high serum SHBG have an increased risk of fractures. J Bone Miner Res. 2008;23(10):1552–60.
29. Falahati-Nini A, et al. Relative contributions of testosterone and estrogen in regulating bone resorption and formation in normal elderly men. J Clin Invest. 2000;106(12):1553–60.
30. Leder BZ, et al. Differential effects of androgens and estrogens on bone turnover in normal men. J Clin Endocrinol Metab. 2003;88(1):204–10.
31. LeBlanc ES, et al. The effects of serum testosterone, estradiol, and sex hormone binding globulin levels on fracture risk in older men. J Clin Endocrinol Metab. 2009;94(9):3337–46.
32. Khosla S. Testosterone: more is not always better. J Clin Endocrinol Metab. 2009;94(12):4665–7.
33. Khosla S. Estrogen and bone: insights from estrogen-resistant, aromatase-deficient, and normal men. Bone. 2008;43(3):414–7.
34. Sanyal A, et al. Regulation of bone turnover by sex steroids in men. J Bone Miner Res. 2008;23(5):705–14.
35. Giustina A, Mazziotti G, Canalis E. Growth hormone, insulin-like growth factors, and the skeleton. Endocr Rev. 2008;29(5):535–59.
36. Khosla S, et al. Hormonal and biochemical determinants of trabecular microstructure at the ultradistal radius in women and men. J Clin Endocrinol Metab. 2006;91(3):885–91.
37. Veldhuis JD, Bowers CY. Human GH pulsatility: an ensemble property regulated by age and gender. J Endocrinol Investig. 2003;26(9):799–813.
38. Amin S, et al. High serum IGFBP-2 is predictive of increased bone turnover in aging men and women. J Bone Miner Res. 2007;22(6):799–807.
39. Marie PJ, et al. Decreased DNA synthesis by cultured osteoblastic cells in eugonadal osteoporotic men with defective bone formation. J Clin Invest. 1991;88(4):1167–72.
40. Pernow Y, et al. Osteoblast dysfunction in male idiopathic osteoporosis. Calcif Tissue Int. 2006;78(2):90–7.
41. Patsch JM, et al. Trabecular bone microstructure and local gene expression in iliac crest biopsies of men with idiopathic osteoporosis. J Bone Miner Res. 2011;26(7):1584–92.
42. Pietschmann P, et al. Bone turnover markers and sex hormones in men with idiopathic osteoporosis. Eur J Clin Investig. 2001;31(5):444–51.
43. Gillberg P, Johansson AG, Ljunghall S. Decreased estradiol levels and free androgen index and elevated sex hormone-binding globulin levels in male idiopathic osteoporosis. Calcif Tissue Int. 1999;64(3):209–13.
44. Braidman I, et al. Preliminary evidence for impaired estrogen receptor-alpha protein expression in osteoblasts and osteocytes from men with idiopathic osteoporosis. Bone. 2000;26(5):423–7.
45. Majeska RJ, Ryaby JT, Einhorn TA. Direct modulation of osteoblastic activity with estrogen. J Bone Joint Surg Am. 1994;76(5):713–21.
46. Pernow Y, et al. Bone histomorphometry in male idiopathic osteoporosis. Calcif Tissue Int. 2009;84(6):430–8.
47. Kurland ES, et al. Insulin-like growth factor-I in men with idiopathic osteoporosis. J Clin Endocrinol Metab. 1997;82(9):2799–805.
48. Ebeling PR. Osteoporosis in men. Curr Opin Rheumatol. 2013;25(4):542–52.
49. Korpi-Steiner N, Milhorn D, Hammett-Stabler C. Osteoporosis in men. Clin Biochem. 2014;47(10–11):950–9.
50. Ebeling PR. Clinical practice. Osteoporosis in men. N Engl J Med. 2008;358(14):1474–82.
51. Adler RA. Osteoporosis in men: recent progress. Endocrine. 2013;44(1):40–6.
52. Kanis JA, et al. Towards a diagnostic and therapeutic consensus in male osteoporosis. Osteoporos Int. 2011;22(11):2789–98.
53. Canalis E, et al. Glucocorticoid-induced osteoporosis: pathophysiology and therapy. Osteoporos Int. 2007;18(10):1319–28.
54. Minisola S, et al. Biochemical markers in glucocorticoid-induced osteoporosis. J Endocrinol Investig. 2008;31(7 Suppl):28–32.
55. Hofbauer LC, et al. Stimulation of osteoprotegerin ligand and inhibition of osteoprotegerin production by glucocorticoids in human osteoblastic lineage cells: potential paracrine mechanisms of glucocorticoid-induced osteoporosis. Endocrinology. 1999;140(10):4382–9.
56. Pierotti S, et al. Pre-receptorial regulation of steroid hormones in bone cells: insights on glucocorticoid-induced osteoporosis. J Steroid Biochem Mol Biol. 2008;108(3–5):292–9.

57. Van Staa TP, et al. Use of oral corticosteroids and risk of fractures. J Bone Miner Res. 2000;15(6):993–1000.
58. Mikosch P. Alcohol and bone. Wien Med Wochenschr. 2014;164(1):15–24.
59. Suh KT, et al. Decreased osteogenic differentiation of mesenchymal stem cells in alcohol-induced osteonecrosis. Clin Orthop Relat Res. 2005;431:220–5.
60. Klein RF, Fausti KA, Carlos AS. Ethanol inhibits human osteoblastic cell proliferation. Alcohol Clin Exp Res. 1996;20(3):572–8.
61. Maurel DB, et al. Alcohol and bone: review of dose effects and mechanisms. Osteoporos Int. 2012;23(1):1–16.
62. Gonzalez-Reimers E, et al. Serum sclerostin in alcoholics: a pilot study. Alcohol Alcohol. 2013;48(3):278–82.
63. Chen JR, et al. Estradiol protects against ethanol-induced bone loss by inhibiting up-regulation of receptor activator of nuclear factor-kappaB ligand in osteoblasts. J Pharmacol Exp Ther. 2006;319(3):1182–90.
64. Chen JR, et al. Protective effects of estradiol on ethanol-induced bone loss involve inhibition of reactive oxygen species generation in osteoblasts and downstream activation of the extracellular signal-regulated kinase/signal transducer and activator of transcription 3/receptor activator of nuclear factor-kappaB ligand signaling cascade. J Pharmacol Exp Ther. 2008;324(1):50–9.
65. Cosman F, et al. Clinician's guide to prevention and treatment of osteoporosis. Osteoporos Int. 2014;25(10):2359–81.
66. Nayak S, Greenspan SL. Cost-effectiveness of osteoporosis screening strategies for men. J Bone Miner Res. 2016;31(6):1189–99.
67. Dawson-Hughes B, et al. The potential impact of the National Osteoporosis Foundation guidance on treatment eligibility in the USA: an update in NHANES 2005–2008. Osteoporos Int. 2012;23(3):811–20.
68. Laurent M, et al. Osteoporosis in older men: recent advances in pathophysiology and treatment. Best Pract Res Clin Endocrinol Metab. 2013;27(4):527–39.
69. Gielen E, et al. Osteoporosis in men. Best Pract Res Clin Endocrinol Metab. 2011;25(2):321–35.
70. Fisher JE, et al. Alendronate mechanism of action: geranylgeraniol, an intermediate in the mevalonate pathway, prevents inhibition of osteoclast formation, bone resorption, and kinase activation in vitro. Proc Natl Acad Sci U S A. 1999;96(1):133–8.
71. Orwoll E, et al. Alendronate for the treatment of osteoporosis in men. N Engl J Med. 2000;343(9):604–10.
72. Boonen S, et al. Fracture risk and zoledronic acid therapy in men with osteoporosis. N Engl J Med. 2012;367(18):1714–23.
73. Ellis GK, et al. Randomized trial of denosumab in patients receiving adjuvant aromatase inhibitors for nonmetastatic breast cancer. J Clin Oncol. 2008;26(30):4875–82.
74. Langdahl BL, et al. A 24-month study evaluating the efficacy and safety of denosumab for the treatment of men with low bone mineral density: results from the ADAMO trial. J Clin Endocrinol Metab. 2015;100(4):1335–42.
75. Higano CS. Androgen-deprivation-therapy-induced fractures in men with nonmetastatic prostate cancer: what do we really know? Nat Clin Pract Urol. 2008;5(1):24–34.
76. Smith MR, et al. Denosumab in men receiving androgen-deprivation therapy for prostate cancer. N Engl J Med. 2009;361(8):745–55.
77. Michaelson MD, Marujo RM, Smith MR. Contribution of androgen deprivation therapy to elevated osteoclast activity in men with metastatic prostate cancer. Clin Cancer Res. 2004;10(8):2705–8.
78. Orwoll ES, et al. The effect of teriparatide [human parathyroid hormone (1–34)] therapy on bone density in men with osteoporosis. J Bone Miner Res. 2003;18(1):9–17.
79. Neer RM, et al. Effect of parathyroid hormone (1-34) on fractures and bone mineral density in postmenopausal women with osteoporosis. N Engl J Med. 2001;344(19):1434–41.
80. Kamel HK, et al. Failure to diagnose and treat osteoporosis in elderly patients hospitalized with hip fracture. Am J Med. 2000;109(4):326–8.
81. Kiebzak GM, et al. Undertreatment of osteoporosis in men with hip fracture. Arch Intern Med. 2002;162(19):2217–22.

Rheumatic Diseases and Osteoporosis 14

Ombretta Di Munno, Nazzarena Malavolta, and Giovanni Minisola

14.1 Introduction

Inflammatory joint diseases, such as seronegative spondyloarthropathies (SnSp), rheumatoid arthritis (RA), systemic lupus erythematosus (SLE), systemic sclerosis, and vasculitides, are characterized by bone complications including osteoporosis (OP) and fragility fractures (FF).

The course of OP is closely connected with the activity of the underlying disease and other risk factors, including low body mass index (BMI) (<18 kg/m^2), early menopause (<45 years), low-energy fractures, renal failure, diabetes, smoking and alcohol use, high bone turnover, vitamin D deficiency, low intake or impaired absorption of calcium, and low calcium concentration. However, active inflammation, glucocorticoids (GC) therapy, long disease duration, immobilization, and reduced physical activity are considered the main risk factors altering both the quality and the amount of bone mineral density (BMD) associated to these diseases [1]. It is well-known that inflammatory cytokines, such as the tumor necrosis factor (TNF)-α, interleukin (IL)-1, IL-6, IL-7, and IL-17, are involved in the regulation of the bone homeostasis, with increasing osteoclast activity through receptor activator of the nuclear factor kappa-B ligand (RANKL) and receptor activator of the nuclear factor kappa-B (RANK) pathway, with the prevalence of bone resorption on bone formation in rheumatic diseases [2]. Therefore, treatment with synthetic and

O. Di Munno
University of Pisa, Pisa, Italy
e-mail: ombretta.dimunno@med.unipi.it

N. Malavolta
"Sant'Orsola-Malpighi" Hospital, Bologna, Italy
e-mail: nazzarena.malavolta@aosp.bo.it

G. Minisola (✉)
"San Camillo" Hospital, Rome, Italy
e-mail: GMinisola@scamilloforlanini.rm.it

A. Lenzi, S. Migliaccio (eds.), *Multidisciplinary Approach to Osteoporosis*,
https://doi.org/10.1007/978-3-319-75110-8_14

biological disease-modifying antirheumatic drugs (DMARDs) is of major importance, not only to control disease activity but also to limit generalized bone loss. GC are frequently used in the treatment of rheumatic diseases because they suppress the systemic inflammation with a subsequent beneficial effect on bone mass, even though one of the principal complications of GC long-term use consists of an important alteration of bone metabolism. FF risk is positively related to their daily dose and increases during the first 6 months of therapy, and the relative risk of fractures is higher for forearm, hip, and vertebral sites and depends on the duration of GC therapy itself [3].

This paper focuses on three inflammatory joint diseases, SnSp, RA and SLE, because OP and FF represent the main extra-articular complications of these diseases.

14.2 Osteoporosis in Seronegative Spondyloarthropathies

SnSp are a heterogeneous group of disorders with clinical features that include axial and peripheral arthritis, psoriasis, inflammatory bowel disease, and uveitis. The group, which affects approximately 0.5–1.5% of the Western population, comprises chronic inflammatory diseases such as ankylosing spondylitis (AS), psoriatic arthritis (PsA), reactive arthritis, inflammatory bowel disease-related spondyloarthropathies, and undifferentiated spondyloarthritis. In the context of SnSp, AS and PsA are the most frequently observed conditions; both are immunoinflammatory disorders characterized by bone involvement and associated with different prevalence of low bone mineral density (BMD), OP, and an increased risk of OP-related FF.

Chronic and persistent inflammation is an important risk factor for bone loss in AS and PsA due to its deleterious effect on bone remodelling. As a consequence, bone balance is negatively affected; indeed, imbalance between osteoblast bone formation and osteoclast bone resorption with net prevalence of osteoclastogenesis occurs [1]. Furthermore, additional and relevant risk factors for OP and FF to take into account are GC treatment, low levels of vitamin D, sarcopenia, intestinal malabsorption, hypo(immo)bilization, and reduced physical activity due to compromised mobility, joint pain, and functional impairment.

Emerging and increasing evidence highlights the harmful role on the bone played by inflammatory cytokines, such as tumor necrosis factor (TNF)-α, interleukin (IL)-1, IL-6, IL-17, and IL-23. In fact, chronic inflammation is characterized by overexpression of inflammatory cytokines involved in the upregulation of the receptor activator of the nuclear factor kappa-B ligand (RANKL); RANKL is responsible for inducing osteoclastogenesis by binding to receptor activator of the nuclear factor kappa-B (RANK) on the surface of cells of the osteoclast lineage [2, 4].

It is not fully defined the role of dickkopf-1 (Dkk-1), the potent inhibitor of the Wnt/β-catenin pathway, whose levels in AS are below those of the healthy control population. It was speculated that the decrease in Dkk-1 results in increased Osteoprotegerin (OPG) and up-regulation of the Wnt pathway leading to activation of β-catenin, which transcriptionally enhances OPG gene expression [5]. Even less known is the role of Dkk-1 in PsA.

Since TNF-α, IL-17, and IL-23 are cytokines involved in the pathogenic mechanism of the typical lesions of AS and PsA, including the skeletal ones, it follows that neutralizing their effects with more innovative drugs can provide favourable results on maintaining bone homeostasis. Available data suggest that the anti-inflammatory treatment with TNF-α inhibitors, while having a positive effect on BMD at the spine and the hip, is less effective in reducing the risk of fracture [6].

Traditional anti-osteoporotic drugs for OP and FF prevention according to local recommendations and in combination with calcium and vitamin D are indicated.

14.3 Osteoporosis in Ankylosing Spondylitis

AS, the prototype disease in the spectrum of SnSp, is a progressive inflammatory rheumatic disorder that primarily affects the axial skeleton, including the sacroiliac joints. AS usually presents during the third decade of life and rarely after the age of 45 years. Its prevalence is generally reported between 0.1 and 1.4%. There is some gender disparity with a 2–3:1 male-to-female ratio rather than the previously thought 5–6:1.

Many studies have shown decreased BMD levels by dual-energy X-ray absorptiometry (DEXA), with an OP prevalence range from 19 to 62% [6]. The frequencies differ widely as a consequence of different duration, activity and extent of disease and of the degree of the impaired back mobility.

One of the main features of bony damage in early AS is the excessive loss of the trabecular bone in the centre of the vertebral body causing osteopenia or OP [7]. In long-standing disease the presence of structural bone lesions, such as syndesmophytes (new bone formation "bridging" two or more adjacent vertebrae), may be responsible for increased BMD. Therefore, in early AS, DEXA measurements should include both the spine and the hip, while in long-standing disease, only the hip BMD level should be considered; however, active or past hip osteoarthritis can represent a confounding factor.

Generally low BMD levels are associated with high disease activity expressed by relevant inflammation indices and abnormal values of Bath Ankylosing Spondylitis Functional Index (BASFI), Bath Ankylosing Spondylitis Disease Activity Index (BASDAI) and Bath Ankylosing Spondylitis Metrology (BASMI) [8]. In early SA, risk factors for low BMD seem to be related to male gender and decreased functional capacity [9].

A systematic review showed a high prevalence of osteopenia versus OP for the lumbar spine (39% and 16%, respectively) and for the femoral neck (38% and 13% respectively), particularly in patients with a short disease duration. This high prevalence was not expected in a relatively young and predominantly male population [10].

A study in a cohort of 204 patients (57% men, mean age 50 ± 13 years) found a prevalence of OP of 21% in participants aged ≥50 [11]. Low BMD was associated with age, disease duration, and inflammatory parameters.

In a study of 103 patients, osteopenia at the hip and spine was found in 56% and 41%, respectively, of patients with disease duration <5 years, with an additional 11 and 15% having OP. In patients with a longer disease duration (>10 years), 29% were osteoporotic at the hip and only 4% at the lumbar spine [12].

Given the low BMD, the alteration of the biomechanical properties of the spine, and the structural bony damage, patients with AS have a fourfold FF risk, during their lifetime, compared with the general population, even from minor injury.

Vertebral FF are a common finding in AS, but their prevalence is highly variable up to more than 40% [13]. The discrepancies in prevalence rate reflect inadequate design or lack of power of the studies, inconsistency in the definition of vertebral FF, differences in recruitment, sex distribution, age, and vertebral FF assessment methods. Vertebral FF may depend on the low BMD and/or the increased spine vulnerability secondary to the bone lesions, with reduced shock absorption, induced by the disease; however, they appear to be related more to the duration and structural severity of the disease rather than to BMD. Vertebral FF should be promptly and carefully considered in any patient with neck or back pain that is changed in intensity or character as they are often associated with neurological signs and symptoms.

A case-control study of 53,108 patients with fractures concluded that the risk of fractures was higher in AS than in rheumatoid arthritis (RA), with the largest increase for vertebral fractures (odds ratios 7.1 and 2.7, respectively) [14].

Recent data suggest both low BMD and high prevalence of vertebral FF even in patients with early-onset disease [15].

Patients with AS are also at increased risk of nonvertebral FF; in a large study, this risk was found to be statistically significant, even after adjustment for potential confounding factors (smoking, alcohol consumption, body mass index, and use of oral steroids) [16]. According to the results of the same study, the regular use of nonsteroidal anti-inflammatory drugs (NSAIDs) seems to eliminate the excess vertebral and nonvertebral FF risk with an unknown mechanism.

Increased levels of RANKL and low levels of OPG have been detected in the sera of patients with AS. Furthermore, cross-sectional studies have highlighted an association between low vitamin D concentrations and both susceptibility and disease activity, suggesting a potential role of vitamin D related to its skeletal and immunological effects [17]. Paradoxically, although subjects with AS generally exhibit localized regions of enhanced bone formation at sites of spinal involvement, some of them may have low BMD at the spine [18]. It is possible to speculate that this happens when and if the local inflammatory process is still active and persistent.

TNF-α inhibitors appear to increase lumbar spine and hip BMD [5]; so far there is no clear evidence of an anti-fracture effect. It is likely that also the novel biotechnological drugs targeting IL-17 and IL-23/17 axis can exert the same effects. More research is needed to assess the effects of these agents on bone quality and fracture risk.

14.4 Osteoporosis in Psoriatic Arthritis

PsA is an inflammatory chronic rheumatic disease affecting both peripheral and axial joints in addition to skin. PsA usually occurs in the age of 40–50 years old; male-to-female ratio is from 0.7:1 to 2.1:1.

Prevalence of low BMD is not well defined; studies addressing the topic have shown conflicting results as far as the prevalence of OP in patients with PsA is concerned. Though most of the studies have found no significant increase in OP concluding that the magnitude of the problem seems to be mild, others suggest a higher prevalence than previously thought [19, 20].

OP, when present, recognizes pathophysiological mechanisms similar to those of AS and appears to be related to the duration, extent, and activity of the disease.

A study of 155 patients found no differences in BMD values between patients and reference population [21]. Prevalence of OP was 16%; it was higher in postmenopausal women (28%) than in men (9%) or premenopausal women (4%). Prevalence of clinical fractures was 13%, mainly found in postmenopausal women; however, spine X-ray was not performed so that morphometric vertebral FF were not considered.

A study including 91 patients found no significant differences in mean lumbar spine and femoral neck BMD between PsA patients and controls; however, the prevalence of FF was significantly higher in patients (14.3%) than in controls (4.4%) [22].

A previous study carried out in 45 postmenopausal women with PsA concluded that patients did not have lower BMD even if they had a higher prevalence of FF [23]. In contrast, a study in 100 postmenopausal women with PsA showed that the prevalence of vertebral and nonvertebral FF on radiographic readings did not differ between cases and controls [24].

The higher prevalence of fractures compared with controls found in some studies indicates that alterations of bone quality are a characteristic of the disease, regardless of BMD values.

According to a recent systematic review, high likelihood of bias and inconsistent results of the available studies suggest a need for well-designed longitudinal studies on bone health in PsA [25].

Limited available data on vitamin D status in PsA suggest that patients have low levels of vitamin D with an inverse correlation between the serum level and the activity of the disease [26].

There are limited data on the effect of traditional therapies for OP in PsA patients. However, treatment with the currently available TNF-α inhibitors can potentially positively interfere on skeletal damage related to the disease; it is likely that a similar favourable effect can be exerted by the novel inhibitors of IL-17, IL-23/17 axis, and phosphodiesterase 4.

14.5 Osteoporosis in Rheumatoid Arthritis

RA is an autoimmune, systemic disease that is characterized by distal and symmetrical synovitis with joint destructions. It affects 0.5–2% of the general population, with a female preponderance and an increased prevalence with age. This disease is associated with subchondral bone erosion, cartilage degradation, and systemic bone loss. Periarticular bone loss, adjacent to the inflamed and swelling joints, is a key feature of RA and the result of local inflammation [27]. Generalized bone loss, leading to OP, is the main extra-articular manifestation of RA and may lead to the occurrence of FF, exacerbating pain and disability and impairing the quality of life of these patients [28]. In the USA, data from the National Data Bank for Rheumatic Diseases indicated that FF are the third cause of mortality in RA patients, after respiratory problems and myocardial infarctions, and the second cause of invalidity, after depression [29].

Even if the patients with RA are at high risk of OP and FF, having several well-known risk factors, such as menopausal status, low BMI, reduced physical activity and disability, vitamin D deficiency, and GC therapy, the inflammatory disease activity may be the most important factor associated with bone loss in RA [30, 31]. Another risk factor for developing OP is represented by the rheumatoid factor (RF) status: the frequency of OP and reduced bone mass is higher in RF-positive than RF-negative patients [32].

The prevalence of OP in RA patients is reported to be approximately twice that in the general population [32]. The frequency of OP in patients with RA ranges from 12.3 to 38.9% at the lumbar spine and from 6.3 to 36.3% at the hip [33–34]. According to a recent report, the frequency of OP in Korean postmenopausal women with RA was of 46.8% [31]. Above all, there is at least a twofold increase in the risk of vertebral FF in RA patients, and a higher risk, up to sixfold, has been reported in patients with a long-standing disease [34–36]. Recently, RA has been taken into account as an independent risk factor in the assessment of fracture risk [37, 38].

An important part of the accountability for the increased fracture risk is the reduced bone strength, which can be explained by disturbances in bone remodelling. It is known that upregulation of pro-inflammatory cytokines, such as TNF-α, IL-1, Il-6, and IL-17, is responsible for the overexpression of RANKL that promotes osteoclasts differentiation and leads to an increased bone resorption. More recently, it became known that formation of the bone is also hampered in RA patients [39]. This is orchestrated by osteocytes, which send their molecular signals based upon loading and unloading forces, resulting in changes in RANKL/OPG and the Wnt pathway. Inhibitors of the Wnt signalling pathway, such as Dkk-1 and sclerostin, result to be upregulated in active RA [40], leading to apoptosis of osteoblasts and hence to a decreased bone formation. Additionally, OPG is inhibited by increased receptor activation for RANKL expression, which leads to a prolonged lifespan of osteoclastic cells.

GC are frequently used in the treatment of RA. It is well demonstrated that GC have an action both in retarding the progression of erosive joint damage in early RA and a control of disease activity [41–43]. The use of GC is restrained by the occurrence of their side effects, and one of the principal complications of long-term GC use consists of an important alteration of bone metabolism. GC mainly suppress bone formation because they determine a decrease in osteoblastogenesis, interfering with osteoblastic differentiation and maturation and inducing loss of function and apoptosis of osteocytes [44, 45]. Risk of fracture in patients who received long-term GC therapy is about 33–50%, positively relating to daily and cumulative dose [46, 3].

Several studies have shown a lower BMD in RA as compared to controls [47–49], the largest effect being measured at the hip. The observed BMD reduction is approximately of 2–17% at the hip and from no reduction to 10% at the spine; in a population of 394 female RA patients, no significant reduction in spine BMD was found, in contrast with a significant reduction of 3.7–8.5% at the hip and 4.2–5.0% at the femoral neck (according to the age group) [32]. In a study focused on perimenopausal women, a BMD reduction of 5.5% was observed at the lumbar spine [50]. In the largest study conducted on 94 male patients with RA, no reduction was observed at the spine BMD, and a significant decrease at the hip (6.9%) was observed in the oldest patients only [51]; one longitudinal result suggests that BMD loss is lower in males than in pre- and postmenopausal women [52]. A recent study showed that in premenopausal women with RA both spine and hip BMD values were significantly lower than in age-matched controls and that such a difference was maintained at the hip after adjustment of BMD for GC therapy and disease activity indices [53]. This suggests that the disease itself is responsible of the significant bone loss, in particular at predominantly cortical skeletal sites. An association between low-dose GC use (≥6 months) and OP has not been observed [54]. This may be explained by a control of the disease activity and an improvement of function of the co-treatment with low-dose GC and GC-induced OP (GIO) preventive therapy [55, 56].

A common observation in all studies is the large interindividual variations, explaining why there is an apparent discrepancy between a relatively modest mean reduction in BMD and a high prevalence of OP. Among the confounding factors affecting the interpretation of BMD results in RA patients is the long duration of the disease, including the course of the disease itself, and an association has been observed between the severity of RA and the risk of OP [57].

Patients with RA are at increased risk of FF at the hip, vertebrae, and pelvis [35, 58, 59]. Humerus and tibia/fibula fracture risk is also increased in some but not all the [35, 58] studies. The risk of wrist fracture seems not to be increased in RA as compared to controls [35, 58].

In the General Practice Research Database, 30,262 patients with RA (ages ≥40 years) were compared to controls, with a mean duration of follow-up of 4.3 years; the increased risk of clinical fracture was of 1.5 (1.4–1.6) [35]. Indicators of a substantially elevated risk of hip fracture were the long duration of the disease, low BMI, and the use of oral GC. Two important observations for the potential mechanisms of bone fragility have been made in this study: the risk of fracture is the same in men and women; the fracture risk remains elevated after excluding patients who had taken GC at any time during the follow-up.

RA is characterized by a higher severity of spine involvement with a higher risk of having two or more fractures compared to controls [34, 60]. The incidence of vertebral FF is 6.7 per 100 patient-years according to a study with a mean follow-up of 2–3 years [61]. Patients with incident vertebral FF are those with older age, lower BMD, higher disability, and previous nonvertebral fractures. Being diagnosed as having RA, the risk is related to vertebral deformities independent of BMD and GC use [34]. Presence of vertebral FF is inversely related to the use of DMARDs and GC, enhancing the hypothesis that an appropriate control of the disease may be a protective factor against bone fragility [60]. Low bone quality might be the cause of the frequent prevalence of vertebral FF in patients with RA [62]. Vertebral FF may not emerge to clinical attention in RA because of analgesics use for painful joints. Thus, vertebral fracture assessment technology on DEXA devices should be used in these patients at the time of BMD measurement.

The incidence rate of nonvertebral FF in IORRA cohort study is 3.5/100 patient-years and does not change in 10 years, despite a striking improvement in RA disease control [63]. This study could indicate that OP treatment and nonvertebral fracture prevention remain important, regardless of RA disease activity.

DMARDs, as methotrexate (MTX), and biotherapies, as anti-TNF therapies, have proved to be successful in retarding joint destruction in RA while being able to control inflammation. The goal of the treatments is the remission of the disease and the prevention of the structural damage; prevention of bone complications is therefore expected.

Infliximab was able to decrease bone resorption; at its introduction as therapy in a population of patients with RA for 11 ± 7 years and failure of other DMARDs, an increase in the ratio between markers of bone formation and bone resorption was observed [64]. There was no BMD change over 1 year. In a small group of 20 patients, with early and active disease, BMD loss was significantly reduced in patients receiving MTX and infliximab, as compared to those treated by MTX alone, at the femoral neck and the hip: −0.35 vs. −3.43% and −0.23 vs. −2.62% [65]¸ there was no change at the spine level. Other studies showed that infliximab and etanercept were able to arrest BMD loss at the spine [66, 67]. The BeSt study compared prospectively the efficacy of four treatment strategies in RA: (a) sequential monotherapy of several DMARDs, (b) step-up combination therapy, (c) initial combination therapy with tapered high-dose prednisone, and (d) initial combination therapy with infliximab. In the group with better suppression of inflammation, the BMD loss was less than in other groups [68]. In a study of 50 patients with active RA who started adalimumab in addition to stable MTX e prednisone (less than 10 mg/day) at baseline, BMD was associated with disease activity and duration; after 12 months, adalimumab arrested further decrease in BMD, with an inverse association between decrease in serum C reactive protein (CRP) levels and increase in BMD, but a greater increase at femur BMD was observed in patients who received concomitant low doses of prednisone [69]. While most studies were of short duration, up to 1 year, the BMD sparing effect seemed to maintain thereafter in a cohort of 184 established RA patients: only a small decrease of hip BMD and a stable spine BMD was shown after a mean follow-up of 4 years of anti-TNF treatment [70]. In a large sample size study, the use of biologic DMARDs (infliximab, adalimumab, etanercept, golimumab, certolizumab, rituximab, abatacept, tocilizumab, anakinra) did not lead to a reduction in the risk of nonvertebral osteoporotic fractures [71]. In a group of 8419 RA women, it was found that the use of anti-TNF in combination with MTX was not associated with a reduction in the risk of FF [72]. Another recent study also did not report any advantages of TNF inhibitors over traditional nonbiologic therapies for the prevention of bone loss and fracture in RA patients [73].

At this stage, there is increasing evidence on the beneficial effect of anti-TNF agents to prevent bone loss, even if the clinical impact, in terms of fracture risk reduction, has yet to be confirmed. Therefore, the administration of bisphosphonates

(BP), as well as other agents, such as teriparatide and denosumab (a monoclonal antibody against RANKL), might be important for OP treatment and consequent fracture reduction in RA patients.

14.6 Osteoporosis in Systemic Lupus Erythematosus

SLE is an autoimmune disease characterized by chronic inflammation and the production of a wide array of autoantibodies. SLE can virtually involve any organ/system; in its clinical picture, active disease, chronic damage, and comorbidities overlap [74].

SLE typically affects young women in their childbearing age, with a peak of incidence between 15 and 40 years of age and a male to female ratio of 1:9. Disease onset is less common in childhood and in elderly population with female to male ratios of 2–6:1 and 3–8:1, respectively [74]. Because the survival of patients with SLE has improved dramatically over recent decades, attention is now focused on disease complications leading to increased morbidity and mortality.

Of note, the musculoskeletal system is frequently involved, and OP is one of the most common comorbidities, found in 1.4–68% of this population [75–77]. This wide variation in prevalence may be related to the study design, sample size, GC use, disease activity and duration, patient demographics, and under-recognition as more than 75% of patients are thought to have suboptimal screening [78]. A systematic review and meta-analysis, which evaluated the mean difference of the BMD level between SLE patients and controls, has been recently published [79]. Literature showed that SLE patients had significantly lower BMD levels than controls ($p < 0.001$).

In SLE, FF also occur in younger patients as compared with those with primary OP, and 4–30% of patients may develop FF despite normal BMD [76, 77, 80–82]. The most common sites of FF are the hip, vertebra, ankle, rib, foot, and arm [76, 80]. OP and associated FF may result in severe pain, disability, impaired quality of life, and increased mortality [83, 84].

The pathogenesis of OP and the occurrence of FF in SLE are likely to be multifactorial, involving both non-disease-related and disease-related factors.

It has been established that the old age, postmenopausal status, low body mass index, reduced physical activity, and constitutional symptoms are the possible risk factors for OP [75–77, 85, 86].

Pro-inflammatory cytokines including IL-6, IL-1, and TNF-α are overexpressed by activated immune cells in SLE patients and have a direct action on the bone, increasing on one side osteoclastic bone resorption and on the other reducing osteoblastic bone formation [2, 7, 77, 85, 87]. It is well known that upregulated RANKL/RANK/OPG signalling and downregulated Wnt/β-catenin pathway are responsible for bone loss associated with inflammatory rheumatic diseases [2, 7, 85, 87]; in addition, polymorphisms in the RANKL and OPG genes appear to play an important role in bone remodelling process and in FF occurrence in SLE [88].

OP and atherosclerosis are common clinical problems and share bidirectional correlation [89, 90]. Cardiovascular disease is a well-recognized complication of

SLE, and there has been a growing interest in the biology and mechanisms underlying premature and accelerated atherosclerosis in this disease [91, 92]. To date, the role of inflammatory immunological pathways has been recognized for both the increased risk of cardiovascular disease and low BMD [86, 92, 93]. Oxidized low-density lipoprotein (LDL) and LDL cholesterol (LDL-c) play an important role in the generation and progression of atherosclerosis; additionally, it has been shown that high serum LDL-c level may also be a risk factor for low BMD and for nonvertebral FF [80, 86]. Oxidized lipids are able to activate T cells, which in turn can induce increased production of TNF-α and RANKL; moreover, oxidized lipids may negatively influence osteogenesis by reducing osteoblast differentiation and maturation. As a consequence, LDL and LDL-c may be considered the link between OP and atherosclerosis, and in fact in active SLE patients, high serum levels of LDL and LDL-c were inversely correlated with BMD [80, 86, 93].

Although some clinical and cross-sectional studies failed to demonstrate a relationship between disease activity and bone loss in SLE [80, 94, 95], a recent 5-year prospective study in Chinese women with SLE demonstrated an association between high disease flare rate and increased bone loss in spine and hip [96]. In addition, low complement C4 levels were a predictor of low lumbar spine BMD in the Hopkins Lupus Cohort, and low complement C4 was an independent contributor to the association between low BMD and carotid atherosclerosis [93, 97].

The relationship between organ damage and reduced BMD is still debated. While several studies report such a relation [96, 98], the results of other studies [75] failed to identify organ damage as a risk factor for OP and FF [76, 94, 95]. Lupus nephritis occurs in up to 60% of SLE patients during the disease course and can result in renal failure. In chronic renal failure, the development of both secondary hyperparathyroidism and low 1,25[OH]2D levels will adversely affect bone mass. However, an association between impaired renal function and low BMD was reported in only one study, in older female SLE patients [99].

Hypovitaminosis D is highly prevalent in SLE as a result of avoidance of sunshine, photoprotection, renal insufficiency, and the use of GC, anticonvulsants, calcineurin inhibitors, and, probably, antimalarials which alter the metabolism of vitamin D or downregulate the functions of the vitamin D receptor [82, 87, 100]. Studies that included healthy controls reported lower vitamin D levels in SLE patients in 12/14 (86%) [101]. Vitamin D insufficiency (25OH-D serum levels <30 ng/mL) was also recently documented in 60% of non-supplemented female SLE patients in the Mediterranean region [102]. A cross-sectional evaluation of bone metabolism parameters in 186 SLE patients showed vitamin D insufficiency in 79% with a mean level of 21.8 ± 15.7 ng/mL; of note, 25OH-D levels <20 ng/mL were found in 52.2% of patients [82].

With respect to bone mass, hypovitaminosis D, which predisposes to secondary hyperparathyroidism, represents an additional risk factor for OP. A significant association between low 25OH-D levels and low vertebral BMD was found in [103]. A positive correlation was also observed between 25OH-D levels and lumbar spine and total hip BMD in Chinese young male SLE patients [104]. Furthermore, a 6-year prospective study in 126 Dutch SLE patients confirmed that low 25OH-D levels at baseline were significantly associated with bone loss in the lumbar spine and hip [105].

The active form of vitamin D [1.25(OH)2D] is a steroid hormone that, in addition to its actions on calcium and bone metabolism, exhibits a wide spectrum of immunomodulatory and anti-inflammatory effects, as extensively documented by experimental studies [100, 101, 106–108]. Although these effects have been also reported in clinical studies and reviews specifically evaluating SLE patients, the relationship between vitamin D status and the onset, activity, and complications of the disease is currently theoretical, and further well-designed trials are needed [100, 101, 106, 108–110].

Most patients develop SLE in their premenopausal years, and some of them do so in the years preceding the achievement of peak bone mass. Both the disease and its treatment (e.g., cyclophosphamide) can also induce amenorrhoea and premature menopause, which cause bone loss. Furthermore, it has been suggested that other endocrine dysfunctions may affect negatively bone mass in SLE. The hormonal status of SLE patients has been described as a relatively high oestrogenic and low androgenic state; low plasma androgens in active and inactive SLE and an association between low dehydroepiandrosterone sulphate levels and low BMD have been reported [80, 85, 87].

The antimalarial drugs chloroquine (CQ) and hydroxychloroquine (HCQ) are frequently used in SLE patients as immunosuppressants. The mechanism of action has been linked to an effect on DNA, antigen processing, cytokines, lysosomal membranes, and T-cell proliferation [85]. Additionally, CQ and HCQ were thought to interfere with the synthesis of 1,25(OH)2D, by inhibiting hydroxylase α1 [85, 87].

With regard to the skeletal effects, studies in SLE patients demonstrated conflicting results [77, 80, 85]. Two cross-sectional studies in SLE female patients reported a significant correlation between HCQ and higher BMD in the spine and hip [111, 112]; additionally, treatment duration was significantly associated with higher BMD in the spine [112]. Conversely, a cross-sectional and a 6-year prospective study in Dutch SLE patients showed a negative correlation between BMD and HCQ use [105, 113]. In a 5-year prospective study, no influence of HCQ treatment on BMD was found [96]. Thus, it is still unclear whether the antimalarial drugs ultimately affect bone metabolism, and further studies on this possible adverse effect are needed [77, 80, 85, 87].

In SLE patients, GC, commonly used at high doses for the treatment of disease flares, significantly improved survival and the quality of life [85]. However, there is no doubt that GC and other immunosuppressants could represent an additional risk factor for bone loss and FF [3, 44, 45, 77, 85, 114]. Longer duration of GC therapy and cumulative and high-dose GC use appear to be associated with bone loss and FF in SLE patients [3, 44, 45, 77, 80, 82, 96, 114, 115]. Moreover, cumulative dose [116] and duration of GC therapy independently predicted higher FF risk in SLE patients compared with controls, using the FRAX tool, the most widely used algorithm for assessing the 10-year individual FF risk [37, 117, 118].

For cyclosporine A (CyA), a possible deleterious effect on the skeleton has also been suggested based on the high frequency of FF occurring in transplant recipients treated with this drug. However, in rheumatic diseases including SLE, CyA is used at lower doses than in transplant recipients, and present data do not allow to confirm the relationship between CyA and bone loss in SLE patients [77, 82, 85].

Cyclophosphamide, commonly used to treat severe SLE comorbidities including renal and neurologic involvement, may contribute to treatment-related OP by inducing amenorrhoea and premature menopause secondary to ovarian failure [77].

Chronic treatment with antiepileptics and anticoagulants may also contribute to bone loss and FF occurrence by negatively affecting bone mass, as documented in some studies [77, 80, 82, 85].

Although estimates for the prevalence of OP and FF in SLE patients indicate that their burden may be dramatically elevated, bone health care in SLE is still suboptimal, and quality-improvement efforts should address OP screening, prevention, and treatment [78]. There is no consensus regarding the optimal method of identifying bone loss and risk of FF in SLE; the FRAX and the DeFRA (the Italian algorithm derived from FRAX) could represent useful tools to establish the need for pharmacological treatments [38].

At present, there are no specific guidelines regarding OP prevention and treatment in SLE patients.

Calcium and vitamin D are recommended in all patients treated with GC [44, 45, 114, 119, 120]; special attention must be paid to obtain the target 25OH-D serum level above 30 ng/mL, as recommended by multiple scientific societies [121, 122].

BP are considered the first choice to prevent bone loss and reduce FF risk in GIO [44, 45, 114, 119, 120].

However, when considering premenopausal women, there is no generally recommended treatment, and BP should only be prescribed in patients with high risk of FF, as these drugs may be long term stored in the bone and are associated with foetal abnormalities in animal models [77, 85, 87, 119].

Teriparatide, which counteracts the most relevant pathophysiological mechanisms of GIO [45, 114, 119, 120], has been shown to be superior to BP in both FF rate and BMD in patients with GIO [114, 119, 120] and SLE [123].

Denosumab could represent an attractive effective agent in the treatment of GIO [114, 120, 123]; additionally, since denosumab is not incorporated in the bone, this drug may be also advantageous in premenopausal patients [77, 114, 119, 120, 124]. A recent study has shown that denosumab is superior to BP in SLE [125].

Conclusion

Several, if not all, inflammatory rheumatic diseases may be complicated by increased bone loss and elevated FF risk. We focus on RA, SLE, AS, and PsA because OP and associated FF are largely documented in these diseases.

The pathogenesis of OP and the occurrence of FF are likely to be multifactorial, involving both non-disease-related and disease-related factors. In addition to disease state, several factors including genetic, metabolic, and hormonal factors may have a deleterious effect on the bone. Increasing evidence highlights the role of complex interactions involving chronic inflammation, RANKL/RANK/OPG signalling, and Wnt/β-catenin pathway. Even if clinical studies have demonstrated that adequate immunosuppressive therapy prevents both local and generalized bone loss, there is no doubt that the chronic use of GC and other immunosuppressants could represent an additional risk factor for bone health.

There are no specific guidelines regarding OP prevention and treatment in rheumatic diseases.

A healthy lifestyle and calcium and vitamin D supplementations are diffusely recommended in almost all patients; BP are considered the first choice in patients at risk of FF with caution in their use both in premenopausal and younger patients. Denosumab and teriparatide might be an attractive additional option.

Whether TNF-α inhibitors and other biologic agents are ultimately effective in reducing FF risk remains so far inconclusive.

References

1. Maruotti N, Corrado A, Cantatore FP. Osteoporosis and rheumatic diseases. Reumatismo. 2014;66:125–35.
2. Schett G, Saag KG, Bijlsma JWJ. From bone to biology to clinical outcome: state of the art and future perspectives. Ann Rheum Dis. 2010;69:1415–9.
3. Van Staa TP, Leufkens HG, Abenhaim L, Zhang B, Cooper C. Use of oral corticosteroids and risk fractures. J Bone Miner Res. 2000;15:993–1000.
4. Briot K, Roux C. Inflammation, bone loss and fracture risk in spondyloarthritis. RMD Open. 2015;1(1):e000052. https://doi.org/10.1136/rmdopen-2015-000052.
5. Diarra D, Stolina M, Polzer K, et al. Dickkopf-1 is a master regulator of joint remodeling. Nat Med. 2007;13:156–63.
6. Haroon NN, Sriganthan J, Al Ghanim N. Effect of TNF-alpha inhibitor treatment on bone mineral density in patients with ankylosing spondylitis: a systematic review and meta-analysis. Semin Arthritis Rheum. 2014;44:155–61.
7. Amarasekara DS, Yu J, Rho J. Bone loss triggered by the cytokine network in inflammatory autoimmune diseases. J Immunol Res. 2015;2015:832127. https://doi.org/10.1155/2015/832127.
8. Ghozlani I, Ghazi M, Nouijai A, et al. Prevalence and risk factors of osteoporosis and vertebral fractures in patients with ankylosing spondylitis. Bone. 2012;44:772–6.
9. van der Weijden MA, van Denderen JC, Lems WF, et al. Low bone mineral density is related to male gender and decreased functional capacity in early spondylarthropathies. Clin Rheumatol. 2011;30:497–503.
10. van der Weijden MA, Claushuis TA, Nazari T, et al. High prevalence of low bone mineral density in patients within 10 years of onset of ankylosing spondylitis: a systematic review. Clin Rheumatol. 2012;31:1529–35.
11. Klingberg E, Geijer M, Göthlin J, et al. Vertebral fractures in ankylosing spondylitis are associated with lower bone mineral density in both central and peripheral skeleton. J Rheumatol. 2012;39:1987–95.
12. Karberg K, Zochling J, Sieper J, et al. Bone loss is detected more frequently in patients with ankylosing spondylitis with syndesmophytes. J Rheumatol. 2005;32:1290–8.
13. Leone A, Marino M, Dell'Atti C, et al. Spinal fractures in patients with ankylosing spondylitis. Rheumatol Int. 2016;5(1):51–5. [Epub ahead of print].
14. Weiss RJ, Wick MC, Ackermann PW, et al. Increased fracture risk in patients with rheumatic disorders and other inflammatory diseases – a case-control study with 53,108 patients with fracture. J Rheumatol. 2010;37:2247–50.

15. van der Weijden MA, van der Horst-Bruinsma IE, van Denderen JC, et al. High frequency of vertebral fractures in early spondylarthropathies. Osteoporos Int. 2012;23:1683–90.
16. Muñoz-Ortego J, Vestergaard P, Rubio JB, et al. Ankylosing spondylitis is associated with an increased risk of vertebral and nonvertebral clinical fractures: a population-based cohort study. J Bone Miner Res. 2014;29:1770–6.
17. Zhao S, Duffield SJ, Moots RJ, et al. Systematic review of association between vitamin D levels and susceptibility and disease activity of ankylosing spondylitis. Rheumatology. 2014;53:1595–603.
18. Goldring SR. Osteoimmunology and bone homeostasis: relevance to spondyloarthritis. Curr Rheumatol Rep. 2013;15:342–7.
19. Ogdie A, Schwartzman S, Eder L, et al. Comprehensive treatment of psoriatic arthritis: managing comorbidities and extraarticular manifestations. J Rheumatol. 2014;41:2315–22.
20. Borman P, Babaoğlu S, Gur G, et al. Bone mineral density and bone turnover in patients with psoriatic arthritis. Clin Rheumatol. 2008;27:443–7.
21. Busquets N, Vaquero CG, Moreno JR, et al. Bone mineral density status and frequency of osteoporosis and clinical fractures in 155 patients with psoriatic arthritis followed in a university hospital. Rheumatol Clin. 2014;10:89–93.
22. Riesco M, Manzano F, Font P, et al. Osteoporosis in psoriatic arthritis: an assessment of densitometry and fragility fractures. Clin Rheumatol. 2013;32:1799–804.
23. Pedreira PG, Pinheiro MM, Szejnfeld VL. Bone mineral density and body composition in postmenopausal women with psoriasis and psoriatic arthritis. Arthritis Res Ther. 2011;13:R16. https://doi.org/10.1186/ar3240.
24. Del Puente A, Esposito A, Costa L, et al. Fragility fractures in patients with psoriatic arthritis. J Rheumatol Suppl. 2015;93:36–9.
25. Chandran S, Aldei A, Johnson SR, et al. Prevalence and risk factors of low bone mineral density in psoriatic arthritis: a systematic review. Semin Arthritis Rheum. 2016;46(2):174–82. https://doi.org/10.1016/j.semarthrit.2016.05.005. [Epub ahead of print].
26. Kincse G, Bhattoa PH, Herédi E, et al. Vitamin D_3 levels and bone mineral density in patients with psoriasis and/or psoriatic arthritis. J Dermatol. 2015;42:679–84.
27. McInnes IB, Schett G. The pathogenesis of rheumatoid arthritis. N Engl J Med. 2015;365:2205–19.
28. Deodhar AA, Woolf AD. Bone mass measurement and bone metabolism in rheumatoid arthritis: a review. Br J Rheumatol. 1996;35:309–22.
29. Michaud K, Wolfe F. Comorbidities in rheumatoid arthritis. Best Pract Res Clin Rheumatol. 2007;21:885–906.
30. Kleyer A, Schett G. Arthritis and bone loss: a hen and egg story. Curr Opin Rheumatol. 2014;26:80–4.
31. Lee JH, Sung YK, Choi CB, et al. The frequency of and risk factors for osteoporosis in Korean patients with rheumatoid arthritis. BMC Musculoskelet Disord. 2016;17:98. https://doi.org/10.1186/s12891-016-0952-8.
32. Haugeberg G, Uhlig T, Falch JA, et al. Bone mineral density and frequency of osteoporosis in female patients with rheumatoid arthritis: results from 394 patients in the Oslo County rheumatoid arthritis register. Arthritis Rheum. 2000;43:522–30.
33. Sinigaglia L, Nervetti A, Mela Q, et al. A multicenter cross sectional study on bone mineral density in rheumatoid arthritis. Italian Study Group on Bone Mass in Rheumatoid Arthritis. J Rheumatol. 2000;27:2582–9.
34. Ørstavik RE, Haugeberg G, Uhlig T, et al. Vertebral deformities in rheumatoid arthritis: a comparison with population based controls. Arch Intern Med. 2004;164:420–5.
35. van Staa T, Geusens P, Bijlsma JW, et al. Clinical assessment of the long-term risk of fracture in patients with rheumatoid arthritis. Arthritis Rheum. 2006;54:3104–12.
36. Pell NF, Moore DJ, Barrington NA, et al. Risk of vertebral fracture and relationship to bone mineral density in steroid treated rheumatoid arthritis. Ann Rheum Dis. 1995;54:801–6.
37. Kanis JA, Johnell O, Oden A, et al. FRAX and the assessment of fracture probability in men and women from the UK. Osteoporos Int. 2008;19:385–97.

38. Adami S, Bianchi G, Brandi ML, et al. Validation and further development of the WHO 10-year fracture risk assessment tool in Italia postmenopausal women: project rationale and description. Clin Exp Rheumatol. 2010;28:561–70.
39. Vis M, Guler-Yuksel M, Lems WF. Can bone loss in rheumatoid arthritis be prevented? Osteoporos Int. 2013;24:2541–53.
40. Miao CG, Yang YY, He X, et al. Wnt signaling pathway in rheumatoid arthritis, with special emphasis on the different roles in synovial inflammation and bone remodeling. Cell Signal. 2013;25:2069–78.
41. Kirwan JR. The effect of glucocorticoids on joint destruction in rheumatoid arthritis. The Arthritis and Rheumatism Council Low-Dose Glucocorticoid Study Group. N Engl J Med. 1995;333:142–6.
42. Wassenberg S, Rau R, Steinfeld P, et al. Very low-dose prednisolone in early rheumatoid arthritis retards radiographic progression over two years: a multicenter, double-blind, placebo-controlled trial. Arthritis Rheum. 2005;52:3371–80.
43. Svensson B, Boonen A, Albertsson K, et al. Low-dose prednisolone in addition to the initial disease-modifying antirheumatic drug in patients with early active rheumatoid arthritis reduces joint destruction and increases the remission rate: a two-year randomized trial. Arthritis Rheum. 2005;52:3360–70.
44. Canalis E, Mazziotti G, Giustina A, et al. Glucocorticoid-induced osteoporosis: pathophysiology and therapy. Osteoporos Int. 2013;18:1319–28.
45. Compston J. Management of glucocorticoid-induced osteoporosis. Nat Rev Rheumatol. 2010;6:82–8.
46. Pereira RMR, de Carvalho JF, Canalis E. Glucocorticoid-induced osteoporosis in rheumatic diseases. Clinics. 2010;65:1197–205.
47. Martin JC, Munro R, Campbell MK. Effects of disease and corticosteroids on appendicular bone mass in postmenopausal women with rheumatoid arthritis: comparison with axial measurements. Br J Rheumatol. 1997;36:43–9.
48. Hall GM, Spector TD, Griffin AJ, et al. The effect of rheumatoid arthritis and steroid therapy on bone density in postmenopausal women. Arthritis Rheum. 1993;36:1510–6.
49. Sambrook PN, Eisman JA, Champion GD, Yeates MG, et al. Determinants of axial bone loss in rheumatoid arthritis. Arthritis Rheum. 1987;30:721–8.
50. Kroger H, Honkanen R, Saarikoski S, et al. Decreased axial bone mineral density in perimenopausal women with rheumatoid arthritis—a population based study. Ann Rheum Dis. 1994;53:18–23.
51. Haugeberg G, Uhlig T, Falch JA, et al. Reduced bone mineral density in male rheumatoid arthritis patients. Arthritis Rheum. 2000;43:2776–84.
52. Gough AK, Lilley J, Eyre S, et al. Generalised bone loss in patients with early rheumatoid arthritis. Lancet. 1994;344:23–7.
53. Fassio A, Idolazzi L, Jaber MA, et al. The negative bone effects of the disease and of chronic corticosteroid treatment in premenopausal women affected by rheumatoid arthritis. Reumatismo. 2016;68:65–71.
54. Peng J, Gong Y, Zhang Y, et al. Bone mineral density in patients with rheumatoid arthritis and 4-year follow-up results. J Clin Rheumatol. 2016;22:71–4.
55. van Everdingen AA, Jacobs JW, Siewertsz Van Reesema DR, et al. Low-dose prednisone therapy for patients with early active rheumatoid arthritis: clinical efficacy, disease-modifying properties, and side effects: a randomized, double-blind, placebo-controlled clinical trial. Ann Intern Med. 2002;136:1–12.
56. Bakker MF, Jacobs JW, Welsing PM, et al. Low-dose prednisone inclusion in a methotrexate-based, tight control strategy for early rheumatoid arthritis: a randomized trial. Ann Intern Med. 2012;156:329–39.
57. Lodder MC, de Jong Z, Kostense PJ, et al. Bone mineral density in patients with rheumatoid arthritis: relation between disease severity and low bone mineral density. Ann Rheum Dis. 2004;63:1576–80.

58. Orstavik RE, Haugeberg G, Uhlig T, et al. Self reported non-vertebral fractures in rheumatoid arthritis and population based controls: incidence and relationship with bone mineral density and clinical variables. Ann Rheum Dis. 2004;63:177–82.
59. Huusko TM, Korpela M, Karppi P, et al. Threefold increased risk of hip fractures with rheumatoid arthritis in Central Finland. Ann Rheum Dis. 2001;60:521–2.
60. Ghazi M, Kolta S, Briot K, et al. Prevalence of vertebral fractures in patients with rheumatoid arthritis: revisiting the role of glucocorticoids. Osteoporos Int. 2012;23:581–7.
61. Orstavik RE, Haugeberg G, Mowinckel P, et al. Vertebral deformities in rheumatoid arthritis. Arch Intern Med. 2004;164:420–5.
62. Okano T, Inui K, Tada M, et al. High frequency of vertebral fracture and low bone quality in patients with rheumatoid arthritis—results from TOMORROW study. Mod Rheumatol. 2016;2:1–7. [Epub ahead of print].
63. Ochi K, Inoue E, Furuya T, Ikari K, et al. Ten-year incidences of self-reported non-vertebral fractures in Japanese patients with rheumatoid arthritis: discrepancy between disease activity control and the incidence of non-vertebral fracture. Osteoporos Int. 2015;26:961–8.
64. Chopin F, Garnéro P, le Henanff A, et al. Long-term effects of infliximab on bone and cartilage turnover markers in patients with rheumatoid arthritis. Ann Rheum Dis. 2008;67:353–7.
65. Haugeberg G, Conaghan PG, Quinn M, et al. Bone loss in patients with active early rheumatoid arthritis: infliximab and methotrexate compared with methotrexate treatment alone. Explorative analysis from a 12-month randomised, double-blind, placebo-controlled study. Ann Rheum Dis. 2009;68:1898–901.
66. Vis M, Havaardsholm EA, Haugeberg G, et al. Evaluation of bone mineral density, bone metabolism, osteoprotegerin and receptor activator of the NFkB ligand serum levels during treatment with infliximab in patients with rheumatoid arthritis. Ann Rheum Dis. 2006;65:1495–9.
67. Seriolo B, Paolino S, Sulli A, et al. Bone metabolism changes during anti-TNF-alpha therapy in patients with active rheumatoid arthritis. Ann N Y Acad Sci. 2006;1069:420–7.
68. Güler-Yüksel M, Bijsterbosch J, Goekoop-Ruiterman YPM, et al. Bone mineral density in patients with recently diagnosed, active rheumatoid arthritis. Ann Rheum Dis. 2007;66:1508–12.
69. Wijbrandts CA, Klaasen R, Dijkgraaf MGW, et al. Bone mineral density in rheumatoid arthritis patients 1 year after adalimumab therapy: arrest of bone loss. Ann Rheum Dis. 2009;68:373–6.
70. Krieckaert CL, Nurmohamed MT, Wolbink G, et al. Changes in bone mineral density during long-term treatment with adalimumab in patients with rheumatoid arthritis: a cohort study. Rheumatology (Oxford). 2013;52:547–53.
71. Roussy JP, Bessette L, Bernatsky S, et al. Biologic disease-modifying anti-rheumatic drugs and the risk of nonvertebral osteoporotic fractures in patients with rheumatoid arthritis aged 50 years and over. Osteoporos Int. 2013;24:2483–92.
72. Coulson KA, Reed G, Gilliam BE, et al. Factors influencing fracture risk, T score, and management of osteoporosis in patients with rheumatoid arthritis in the Consortium of Rheumatology Researchers of North America (CORRONA) registry. J Clin Rheumatol. 2009;15:155–60.
73. Kim SY, Schneeweiss S, Liu J, et al. Effects of disease-modifying antirheumatic drugs on nonvertebral fracture risk in rheumatoid arthritis: a population-based cohort study. J Bone Miner Res. 2012;27:789–96.
74. Lisnevskaia L, Murphy G, Isenberg D. Systemic lupus erythematosus. Lancet. 2014;384:1878–88.
75. Bultink IEM, Harvey NC, Lalmohamed A, et al. Elevated risk of clinical fractures and associated risk factors in patients with systemic lupus erythematosus versus matched controls: a population-based study in the United Kingdom. Osteoporos Int. 2014;25:1275–83.
76. Cramarossa C, Urowitz MB, Su J, et al. Prevalence and associated factors of low bone mass in adults with systemic lupus erythematosus. Lupus. 2016;26(4):365–72. pii: 0961203316664597. [Epub ahead of print].

77. Edens C, Robinson AB. Systemic lupus erythematosus, bone health, and osteoporosis. Curr Opin Endocrinol Diabetes Obes. 2015;22:422–31.
78. Schmajuk G, Yelin E, Chakravarty E, et al. Osteoporosis screening, prevention and treatment in systemic lupus erythematosus: application of systemic lupus erythematosus quality indicators. Arthritis Care Res (Hoboken). 2010;62:993–1001.
79. Wang X, Yan S, Liu C, et al. Fracture risk and bone mineral density levels in patients with systemic lupus erythematosus: a systemic review and meta-analysis. Osteoporos Int. 2016;27:1413–23.
80. Bultink IEM, Lems WF. Systemic lupus erythematosus and fractures. RMD Open. 2016;1(Suppl 1):e000069. [Epub ahead of print].
81. Li EK, Tam LS, Griffith JF, et al. High prevalence of asymptomatic vertebral fractures in Chinese women with systemic lupus erythematosus. J Rheumatol. 2009;36:1646–52.
82. Carli L, Tani C, Spera V, et al. Risk factors for osteoporosis and fragility fractures in patients with systemic lupus erythematosus. Lupus Sci Med. 2016;3(1):e000098. [Epub ahead of print].
83. García-Carrasco M, Mendoza-Pint C, Riebeling C, et al. Influence of prevalent vertebral fractures on the quality of life patients with systemic lupus erythematosus. Isr Med Assoc J. 2011;13:333–7.
84. Meacock R, Dale N, Harrison MJ. The humanistic and economic burden of systemic lupus erythematosus: a systematic review. PharmacoEconomics. 2013;31:49–61.
85. Di Munno O, Mazzantini M, Delle Sedie A, et al. Risk factors for osteoporosis in female patients with systemic lupus erythematosus. Lupus. 2004;13:724–30.
86. Sun YN, Feng XY, He L, et al. Prevalence and possible risk factors of low bone mineral density in untreated female patients with systemic lupus erythematosus. Biomed Res Int. 2015;2015:510514. [Epub ahead of print].
87. Bultink IEM, Vis M, van der Horst-Bruinsma IE, et al. Inflammatory rheumatic disorders and bone. Curr Rheumatol Rep. 2012;14:224–30.
88. Bonfá AC, Seguro LPC, Caparbo V, et al. RANKL and OPG gene polymorphisms: associations with vertebral fractures and bone mineral density in premenopausal systemic lupus erythematosus. Osteoporos Int. 2015;26:1563–71.
89. Fisher A, Srikusalanukul W, Davis M, et al. Cardiovascular diseases in older patients with osteoporotic hip fracture: prevalence, disturbances in mineral and bone metabolism, and bidirectional links. Clin Interv Aging. 2013;8:239–56.
90. Farhat GN, Newman AB, Sutton-Tyrrell K. The association of bone mineral density measures with incident cardiovascular disease in older adults. Osteoporos Int. 2007;18:999–1008.
91. Schoenfeld SR, Kasturi S, Costenbader KH. The epidemiology of atherosclerotic cardiovascular disease among patients with SLE: a systematic review. Semin Arthritis Rheum. 2013;43:77–95.
92. Magder LS, Petri M. Incidence of and risk factors for adverse cardiovascular events among patients with systemic lupus erythematosus. Am J Epidemiol. 2012;176:708–19.
93. Ajeganova S, Gustafsson T, Jogestrand T, et al. Bone mineral density and carotid atherosclerosis in systemic lupus erythematosus: a controlled cross-sectional study. Arthritis Res Ther. 2015;17:84–96.
94. Bultink IEM, Lems WF, Kostense PJ, et al. Prevalence of and risk factors for low bone mineral density and vertebral fractures in patients with systemic lupus erythematosus. Arthritis Rheum. 2005;54:2044–50.
95. Bhattoa HP, Kiss E, Bettembuk P, et al. Bone mineral density, biochemical markers of bone turnover, and hormonal status in men with systemic lupus erythematosus. Rheumatol Int. 2001;21:97–102.
96. Zhu TY, Griffith JF, Au SK. Bone mineral density change in systemic lupus erythematosus: a 5-year followup study. J Rheumatol. 2014;41:1990–7.
97. Petri M. Musculoskeletal complications of systemic lupus erythematosus in the Hopkins lupus cohort: an update. Arthritis Care Res. 1995;8:137–45.

98. Mendoza-Pinto C, García-Carrasco M, Sandoval-Cruz H, et al. Risk factors of vertebral fractures in women with systemic lupus erythematosus. Clin Rheumatol. 2009;28:579–85.
99. Almehed K, Forsblad d'Elia H, Kvist G, et al. Prevalence and risk factors of osteoporosis in female SLE patients-extended report. Rheumatology (Oxford). 2007;46:1185–90.
100. Mok CC. Vitamin D and systemic lupus erythematosus: an update. Expert Rev Clin Immunol. 2013;9:453–63.
101. Reynolds JA, Bruce IN. Vitamin D treatment for connective tissue diseases: hope beyond the hype? Rheumatology (Oxford). 2016;56(2):178–86. pii: kew212. [Epub ahead of print].
102. Salman-Monte TC, Torrente-Segarra V, Almirall M, et al. Prevalence and predictors of vitamin D insufficiency in supplemented and non-supplemented women with systemic lupus erythematosus in the Mediterranean region. Rheumatol Int. 2016;36:975–85.
103. Yeap SS, Othman AZ, Zain AA, et al. Vitamin D levels: its relationship to bone mineral density response and disease activity in premenopausal Malaysian systemic lupus erythematosus patients on corticosteroids. Int J Rheum Dis. 2012;15:17–24.
104. Guo Q, Fan P, Luo J, et al. Assessment of bone mineral density and bone metabolism in young male adults recently diagnosed with systemic lupus erythematosus in China. Lupus. 2016;26(3):289–93. pii: 0961203316664596. [Epub ahead of print].
105. Jacobs J, Korswagen LA, Schilder AM, et al. Six-years follow-up study of bone mineral density in patients with systemic lupus erythematosus. Osteoporos Int. 2013;24:1827–33.
106. Cutolo M. Further emergent evidence for the vitamin D endocrine system involvement in autoimmune rheumatic disease risk and prognosis. Ann Rheum Dis. 2013;72:473–5.
107. Prietl B, Treiber G, Pieber TR, et al. Vitamin D and immune function. Forum Nutr. 2013;5:2502–21.
108. Watad A, Neumann SG, Soriano A, et al. Vitamin D and systemic lupus erythematosus: myth or reality? Isr Med Assoc J. 2016;18:177–82.
109. Ritterhouse LL, Crow SR, Niewold TB, et al. Vitamin D deficiency is associated with an increased autoimmune response in healthy individuals and in patients with systemic lupus erythematosus. Ann Rheum Dis. 2011;70:1569–74.
110. Durcan L, Petri M. Immunomodulators in SLE: clinical evidence and immunologic actions. J Autoimmun. 2016;74(16):30088–9. https://doi.org/10.1016/j.jaut.2016.06.010. [Epub ahead of print].
111. Mok CC, Mak A, Ma KM. Bone mineral density in postmenopausal Chinese patients with systemic lupus erythematosus. Lupus. 2015;14:106–12.
112. Lakshminarayanan S, Walsh S, Mohanraj M, et al. Factors associated with low bone mineral density in female patients with systemic lupus erythematosus. J Rheumatol. 2001;28:102–8.
113. Mok CC, Ying SK, To CH, et al. Bone mineral density and body composition in men with systemic lupus erythematosus: a case control study. Bone. 2008;43:327–31.
114. Mazzantini M, Di Munno O. Glucocorticoid-induced osteoporosis: 2013 update. Reumatismo. 2014;66:144–52.
115. Zhu TY, Griffith JF, Qin L, et al. Cortical thinning and progressive cortical porosity in female patients with systemic lupus erythematosus on long-term glucocorticoids: a 2-year case-control study. Osteoporos Int. 2015;26:1759–71.
116. Mak A, Lim JQ, Liu Y, et al. Significantly higher estimated 10-year probability of fracture in lupus patients with bone mineral density comparable to that of healthy individuals. Rheumatol Int. 2013;33:299–307.
117. Lee JJ, Aghdassi E, Cheung AM, et al. Ten-year absolute fracture risk and hip bone strength in Canadian women with systemic lupus erythematosus. J Rheumatol. 2012;39:1378–84.
118. FRAX® tool. http://www.shef.ac.uk/FRAX. Assessed 9 Sept 2011
119. Grossman JM, Gordon R, Ranganath VK, et al. American College of Rheumatology 2010 recommendations for the prevention and treatment of glucocorticoid-induced osteoporosis. Arthritis Care Res (Hoboken). 2010;62:1515–26.
120. Rizzoli R, Adachi JD, Cooper C, et al. Management of glucocorticoid-induced osteoporosis. Calcif Tissue Int. 2012;91:225–43.

121. Francis RM, Aspray TJ, Boering CE, et al. National Osteoporosis Society practical clinical guideline on vitamin D and bone health. Maturitas. 2015;80:119–21.
122. Holick MF, Binkley NC, Bischoff-Ferrari HA, et al. Evaluation, treatment, and prevention of vitamin D deficiency: an Endocrine Society clinical practice guideline. J Clin Endocrinol Metab. 2011;96:1911–30.
123. Saag KG, Zanchetta JR, Devogelaer JP, et al. Effects of teriparatide versus alendronate for treating glucocorticoid-induced osteoporosis: thirty-six-month results of a randomized, double-blind, controlled trial. Arthritis Rheum. 2009;60:3346–55.
124. Baron R, Ferrari S, Graham R, et al. Denosumab and bisphosphonates: different mechanisms of actions and effects. Bone. 2011;48:677–92.
125. Mok CC, Ho LY, Ma KM. Switching of oral bisphosphonates to denosumab in chronic glucocorticoid users: a 12-month randomized controlled trial. Bone. 2015;75:222–8.

Part II

Prevention and Treatment

15 Nutrition and Skeletal Health

Chiara Marocco, Rachele Fornari, Andrea Lenzi, and Emanuela A. Greco

15.1 Introduction

During the last decades, in industrialized countries was observed a significant increase in average life expectancy with a gradual aging of the population. The prolonged life expectancy, lifestyle and improper eating behaviors have contributed to increase the incidence of illnesses, often resulting of well-being, such as obesity, dysmetabolism, cardiovascular disease, osteoporosis, which contribute heavily to both quality of life of those affected and significant increase in social costs.

Osteoporosis is one of these chronic diseases and it is defined as a metabolic disorder of the skeletal tissue characterized by a decrease in bone strength, leading to an increased risk of developing traumatic and/or spontaneous fractures [1], due to a reduction in both bone quantity and quality [2–5], that include alterations in micro- and macro-architecture, turnover and changes of ultra-structural material. The decrease in skeletal tissue strength makes the subject more susceptible to vertebral, non-vertebral fractures and, especially in the most advanced decades, femoral fractures associated with high morbidity and mortality.

The integrity of the skeletal tissue is maintained by a sophisticated highly dynamic process called remodeling, characterized by balanced osteoclast activity, monocyte-macrophage origin cells, bone resorption and osteoblast cells, mesenchymal origin cells, responsible for bone neoformation.

Bone tissue is a highly specialized connective tissue that owes its peculiarity to being mineralized, since the intercellular substance (composed of collagen fibers

C. Marocco (✉)
Department of Movement, Human and Health Sciences, University of Foro Italico of Rome, Rome, Italy

R. Fornari · A. Lenzi · E. A. Greco
Department of Experimental Medicine, Section of Medical Pathophysiology, Endocrinology and Nutrition, University Sapienza of Rome, Rome, Italy

A. Lenzi, S. Migliaccio (eds.), *Multidisciplinary Approach to Osteoporosis*, https://doi.org/10.1007/978-3-319-75110-8_15

and amorphous substance) is mostly impregnated with mineral crystals (predominantly calcium phosphate) arranged around the collagen fibers, which constitute an organic scaffold for the formation of the crystals themselves. Calcium phosphate crystals are very resistant, but anelastic and rather friable, while collagen fibers are flexible and can be easily elongated or folded. This particular combination of proteins and crystals gives the bone exceptional mechanical properties: hardness and at the same time, flexibility, lightness and traction and twist resistance.

Several factors can act on bone cells by modulating their activity, optimizing skeletal tissue health, but also affecting the different phases of bone remodeling in periods of life or in pathological conditions. The rate of bone loss in adults reflects the interactions of genetic, hormonal, environmental and lifestyle factors, such as diet, alcohol, smoking and physical activity, which also influence the extent of bone acquisition and play a key role in maintaining physiological skeletal homeostasis.

In particular, the nutritional aspect is crucial not only during adulthood, but also in the early stages of life as a proper diet can guarantee an adequate supply of macro and micronutrients [6–9]. A very important factor that needs to be considered, but often omitted, is the optimization of bone mass peak reached within the third decade of life. After the first three decades of life our skeleton arrives at a balance in adulthood. In other words, the greater the bone mass obtained during the growth stages, the lower the risk of developing osteoporosis in the most advanced phases of life [10–13]. For this reason osteoporosis must be considered as many other chronic pathologies a disease to be cured, but even more a pathology for which primary prevention can play an important role.

Our skeleton forms before birth, it sustains us in life, and can withstand a long time after death. Throughout life the size of our skeleton and the amount of bone will change in meaningful way. During the first 10–12 years of life, bone mass increases steadily, both in boys and girls. During puberty, the accumulation rate of bone mass accelerates, with a faster increase in men, and at least half of the bone mineral density is acquired, making it a critical time to optimize conditions that contribute to proper skeletal growth, thus achieving the peak of bone mass (PBM) in the mid-20 s. Infact, the bone mass acquired at the beginning of adulthood acts as a bone bank for the rest of life (Fig. 15.1 Modified by https://www.iofbonehealth.org/news/bone-healthy-lifestyle-teenageyears-pays) [14]. The main goals for good bone health in the various phases of life are the following:

Kids and teens: to reach the potential genetic bone mass peak;
Adults: avoid premature bone loss and keep a healthy skeleton;
Elderly: prevention and treatment of osteoporosis.

Proper nutrition for the construction and the maintaining the skeleton is essential for the achieving these goals. A balanced diet provides the body with all the essential macro- and micro nutrients for the well-being of the body and the specific skeletal tissue. The most important nutrients are calcium, vitamin D and proteins.

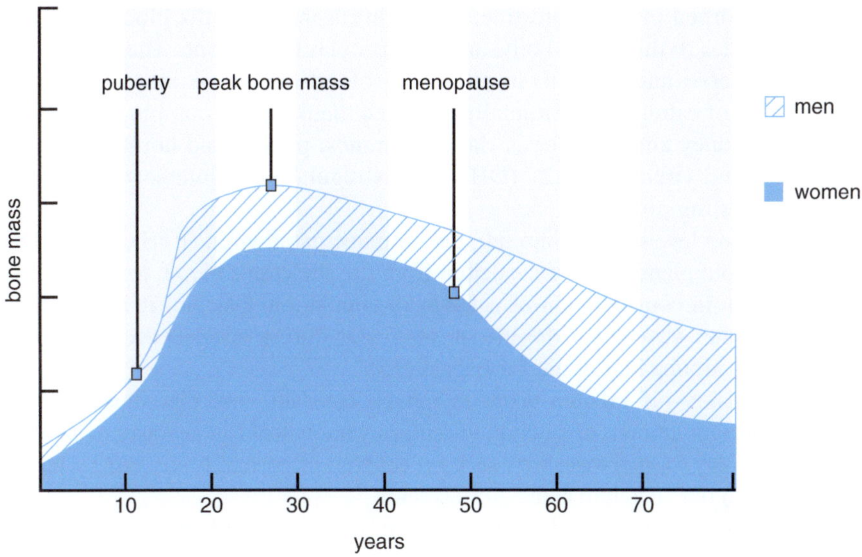

Fig. 15.1 Peak bone mass through out life

15.2 Calcium

Calcium ion is among the fundamental micronutrients for maintaining a physiological skeletal homeostasis. Calcium is absolutely the most important mineral presents in our body, and it is about 1.5–2% of the total weight of an adult. So, depending on their weight, men contain on average about 950–1300 g of calcium, women about 770–920 g. 99% of the total calcium of our body is contained in the skeleton and in the teeth. The remaining 1% is in solution in the blood, which distributes it to various tissues according to their needs. Calcium is present in bone in the form of a complex mineral, called hydroxyapatite, that gives resistance to the skeleton.

The concentration of calcium in all districts must be kept by the body under close control, and the central mechanism for doing so is the control of calcium concentration in the blood (calcium). Under normal conditions, calcium is maintained by the body within precise limits. This is necessary to ensure vital functions such as muscle contraction, blood clotting, nerve impulse conduction, and others. The calcic pool of the organism is divided into a ionized, metabolically active portion and a protein bound, predominantly albumin or salts. The ionized and anion-linked calcium together constitute the ultrafiltration fraction of plasma calcium, which represents the fraction filtered by the glomeruli. Protein-bound fraction may also vary considerably in relation to pH values and plasma concentration of bicarbonates and proteins. Calcium is introduced with food, is absorbed into the intestine, passed into solution in the blood, and with blood it comes to the whole body, and in particular to the bone. The bone is our calcium reserve and calcium levels in the blood are maintained in balance. Calculation of calcium is continually achieved thanks to the combined action on the bone, kidney and intestine of three hormones: parathyroid hormone (PTH), calcitonin and vitamin D 1.25 (OH) 2. This regulation is intersected with the bone remodeling process.

If the blood levels of calcium fall, the hormone parathyroid (PTH), secreted by the parathyroid glands, releases calcium from the skeleton's blood, to compensate the reduction in concentration of calcium in circulation. Calcium is important to health of bones throughout the life, in particular during adolescence, when it is accumulated around half of our bone mass [15].

In conclusion—if calcium needs to remain constant—our diet should always contain the right amount of calcium to replace what is lost (on average, in an adult 300 mg per day). Otherwise, we can keep calcium at normal levels just by taking calcium from our "calcium bank", the skeleton.

As long as plasma calcium deficiency persists (for example due to insufficient food intake or bad bowel absorption), calcium withdrawal from the bone continues. This causes a progressive loss of bone tissue, which, if significant, will be very difficult to correct. Often you can no longer return to the original levels. If the calcium loss process lasts long, its inevitable consequence is the appearance of osteoporosis. Conversely, when these needs are met, available calcium can be deposited in the bone, replenishing the reserve and maintaining the robustness of the skeleton.

The food calcium requirements vary widely with age (Table 15.1) [15]. It is very high in growing subjects especially in relation to body weight; increases in particular during pregnancy and during lactation. Calcium requirements may increase frequently in the elderly for the occurrence of malabsorption.

Children and adolescents, whose skeleton is growing, must take up each day with much more calcium than what they lose with urine. And the same goes for pregnant women, especially during the third trimester, where the child's skeleton is built.

Adults, who no longer have to grow, should only cover urinary calcium loss. But the intestine absorbs only part of the calcium contained in the foods (Table 15.2) [16, 17].

Table 15.1 Recommended daily calcium intakes

Infancy to adolescence	*Calcium (mg/day)*
0–8 years	700–1000
9–18 years	1300
Women	*Calcium (mg/day)*
19–50 years	1000
During pregnancy/lactation	1200–1500
Post-menopause (50+ years)	1200
Men	*Calcium (mg/day)*
19–65 years	1000
65+ years	1200

Table 15.2 Calcium content of common foods

Food	Serving size	Calcium (mg)
Milk, whole	200 ml	236
Milk, semi-skimmed	200 ml	240
Milk, skimmed	200 ml	244
Soy drink (non-enriched)	200 ml	26
Soy drink, calcium enriched	200 ml	240
Rice drink	200 ml	22
Almond drink	200 ml	90
Yoghurt (with whole milk)	125 ml	154
Yoghurt (with semi-skimmed milk)	125 ml	148
Hard cheese (cheddar, parmesa, gruyere, emmental)	30 g	240
Fresh cheese (mascarpone, ricotta, cottage cheese)	200 g	138
Eggs	60 g	27
Sardines in oil (canned)	60 g	240
Oysters	100 g	186
Shrimps	150 g	45
Chick peas	80 g raw/200 g cooked	100
White beans	80 g raw/200 g cooked	132
Almonds	30 g	75
Walnuts	30 g	28
Sesame seeds	15 g	22
Bok choy	50 g (raw)	20
Broccoli	120 g (raw)	112
Cress	120 g (raw)	188
Orange	150 g	60
Figs, dried	60 g	96

15.3 Vitamin D

Vitamin D is closely linked to calcium requirements and daily intake. In fact, scientific studies have shown that the administration of vitamin D in the presence of low calcium intake is not equally effective [18]. Vitamin D plays two key roles in development and in maintaining bone health: it helps absorb calcium from food in the gut and ensures the correct renewal and the mineralization of the bones. Vitamin D was discovered in 1922 and it was called so by mistake. Indeed it is not a real vitamin but it should be more properly defined as the precursor of the hormone. Vitamin D is synthesized directly in our skin by the action of ultraviolet light B sunlight (UVB) on a substance called 7-dehydro-cholesterol, but can also be obtained from foods like the blue fish (Table 15.3) [17]. In some countries it is normally added to milk and baby foods. Vitamin D is the only vitamin we are able to produce on its own, but if necessary it can be given as a "supplement".

Vitamin D is strongly lipophilic, so both the food source and the amount of skin synthesis remain very low. The circulating vitamin D is immediately deposited mainly in the fatty tissue, where the storage capacity is very high. This is the reason for which vitamin D can be administrated as a bolus that can cover the needs even for many months. Vitamin D that passes through the liver is immediately hydroxylated at 25 and becomes 25OH-vitamin D. This process does not require "energy",

Table 15.3 Approximate vitamin D levels in food

Food	Serving size	Mcg per serving	IU per serving	RNI[a]
Cod liver oil	1 tablespoon	23.1	924	231
Salmon, grilled	100 g	7.1	284	71
Mackerel, grilled	100 g	8.8	352	88
Tuna, canned in brine	100 g	3.6	144	36
Sardines, canned in brine	100 g	4.6	184	46
Margarine, fortified	20 g	1.6	62	16
Egg	60 g	0.9	36	9
Liver	100 g	0.9	36	9

[a]The RNI (recommended nutrient intake) is defined by the FAO/WHO as "the daily intake which meets the nutrient requirements of almost all (97.5%) apparently healthy individuals in an age- and sex-specific population group". Daily intake corresponds to the average over a period of time

but it provides it and therefore does not compromise in case of hepatic failure. The 25OH-Vitamin D is actually the most important circulating metabolite, deposited in the liver and muscles in sufficient quantities to guarantee the need for no more than 10 days. The 25OH-Vitamin D can then be activated at 1.25 (OH) 2 Vitamin D or degraded at 24.25 (OH) 2 Vitamin D. This alternative hydroxylation process is rigidly controlled by PTH, calcium and phosphoremia. Vitamin D deficiency in children can lead to late growth and bone deformity, known as "rachitism". The same processes in adults lead to "osteomalacia", which is a 'softening' of bones due to poor mineralization. Vitamin D is needed both to ensure good absorption of calcium in the intestine and for proper mineralization of the bone.

The hypovitaminosis D causes bone mineralization alterations depending on the severity of the deficiency and its duration, as well as calcium intake. It is known that vitamin D deficiency especially if prolonged in time can produce proximal myopathy and sarcopenia, with increased risk of falls [19]. It is likely that vitamin D exerts physiological actions in other organs and apparatus other than calcium metabolism as demonstrated by the presence of calcitriol receptors in different organs, particularly at the prostate, colon, breast and in different cell types, where the expression of the 1-hydroxylase renal activity was documented, necessary to raise levels of 1.25 (OH) 2 vitamin D. Vitamin D actions are due to calcitriol, its active metabolite. At the muscle tissue level, 1.25 (OH) 2 Vitamin D is able to activate calcium transport mechanisms at the level of the sarcoplasmic reticulum, which are fundamental to muscle contraction [20]. The 25-OH-vitamin D (25OHD) serum concentrations adequately express the levels of vitamin deposits. Vitamin D deficiency is extremely common in Italy [21, 22], especially for the type of Mediterranean diet, less rich in animal fat or following the introduction of vegetarian or vegan diets, which is not adequately corrected for vitamin D intake. It is estimated that supplementation of foods with vitamin D is not greater than 200 U/l/day [23]. In the Nordic countries, the situation is better because traditionally dairy products are supplemented with vitamin D since childhood.

To ensure year-round vitamin D levels of 40 ng/ml, daily doses of vitamin D of at least 1000 U are recommended. Over the last few years, a steady increase in recommended daily vitamin D levels has been reported, starting with from 200 to 400 U in growth at up to 600 U in subjects over the age of 18 [24–26]. Clinical studies have shown that only doses around 800 U are associated with a significant reduction in the risk of femoral fractures in the elderly population [27]. Vitamin D supplementation can change and it must be personalized to the risk of hypovitaminosis D and calcium dietary intake [28]. Regarding the safety issue, a homeostatic physiological mechanism acts to control the circulating levels of vitamin D up to the administration of 10,000 U daily and to avoid overdose [23] at the same time.

15.4 Protein

If an important role in the approach of a proper diet is given by a fair amount of macro- and micro nutrients it is crucial to remember the role of a correct equilibrium of all nutrients as indicated by the nutrition pattern of the Mediterranean diet. Within the macronutrients, it seems that a correct and appropriate amount of proteins plays an important role both in achieving a good bone mass peak and for maintaining adequate bone mass in adult life and during aging.

Food proteins are a source of important aminoacids necessary to maintain the bone structure. They also have an effect favorable on the bone, stimulating the release of the insulin-like growth factor I (IGF-I), which plays a major role in bone formation, increasing the activity of osteoblasts and so the production of bone matrix [29]. In 2009 the first systematic review and a meta-analysis were published on the relationship between proteins food and health of healthy bitches in healthy adults [30]. The researchers found a positive association between protein intake, BMD and BMC, and one reduction of bone resorption markers. Variations in protein intake during childhood and adolescence may have an impact on skeletal growth and affect the genetic potential of achieving PBM. In the elderly, the lower protein intake is associated with loss of bone mineral density (BMD) at the level of the hip and spine.

15.5 Vitamin K

Vitamin K is necessary to create osteocalcin, the second most important protein in the bone after collagen. Epidemiological studies have showed that high-diets Vitamin K is associated with less risk of fractures in the elderly [31]. Good food sources of vitamin K include green leafy vegetables—like lettuce, spinach and cabbage -, liver, some fermented foods–such as fermented cheese and natto (fermented soy)–and dried fruit (plums).

Randomized controlled studies on the intake of vitamin K1 or K2 supplements do not have showed BMD increase at the major skeletal sites [32]. Consequently, they are necessary further studies to determine the role of Vitamin K supplements for prevention and treatment of osteoporosis.

15.6 Vitamin B and Homocysteine

Homocysteine is an amino acid that can interfere with the synthesis of collagen, the main protein bone. When the blood levels of vitamin B6, vitamin B12 and folic acid are low, homocysteine levels may increase. Consequently vitamin B deficiency could compromise bone health. This concept is supported by observational studies that have found an association between high levels of homocysteine, low levels of BMD [33] and an increased risk fracture of the hip in the elderly [34].

However, a 2014 review concluded that inconsistencies within current data require definitive studies to evaluate the role of vitamin Group B in the prevention of osteoporosis. [35].

15.7 Vitamin A

The role of vitamin A in bone health is controversial [36]. The high intake of vitamin preformed, which can be obtained from food sources of animal origin such as liver, other offal and fish oils, was associated with osteoporosis and hip fracture. However, carotenoids, which are vitamin A precursors, were associated with the improvement of health of the bones. Carotenoids can be obtained from green leafy vegetables, carrots, pumpkins, red and yellow peppers, mango, papaya and apricots. The simultaneous intake of oil supplements fish and a multivitamin supplement could lead to excessive intake of vitamin A.

15.8 Magnesium

About half the total body magnesium is stored in the skeleton [37]. Magnesium plays an important role in bone formation, stimulating the proliferation of osteoblasts. Magnesium deficiency is rare in well nutrited populations. However, since its absorption decreases with age, seniors may be at risk of a slight shortage. Good sources of magnesium are green vegetables, legumes, nuts, seeds, cereals refined, fish and dried fruit (apricots, plums, raisins).

15.9 Zinc

Zinc plays a role in the renewal of bone tissue and mineralization. The shortage of zinc is usually associated with malnutrition, deficiency calories and proteins, and has been reported as widespread in elderly people living in the community [38].

Although vegetarian diets do not behave necessarily a lower intake of zinc, for vegetarians can be bioavailability of zinc lower, so hiring may be required maggiori. Zinc sources are red meat lean, poultry, whole grains, legumes and dried fruits (peaches, plums, apricots).

15.10 Modifiable Risks

Talking about nutritional aspects there are foods that can adversely affect bone health, such as alcool and caffeine.

More than two alcohol-per-day units may increase the risk of having a fragility fracture, while more than four units per day can double the risk of fracture [39]. For those who drink alcohol, moderation is the healthiest choice for bone health. Up to two glasses of 120 ml wine per day do not affect negatively affecting the health of the bones.

Caffeine increases urinary and fecal calcium losses and so, in combination with a low diet calcium content, has the potential to negatively affect bone health. A Swedish study suggests that a caffeine intake of 330 mg per day (i.e. four 600 ml cups) could be associated with a 20% increase in risk of osteoporotic fractures compared to caffeine intake less than 200 mg per day [40]. However, increasing by 40 mg the calcium intake for each cup of coffee with caffeine drink, counterbalance the potential loss of calcium [41].

15.11 Pregnancy

Over the last two decades, the idea that the environmental influences of intrauterine life and the onset of postnatal life may have implications for health in adulthood. The environment of the first years of life has consequences to long term in musculoskeletal development [42, 43] in fact, little growth during childhood is associated with a reduced bone mineral content in the bone mass peak and adult life [44], as well as a an increased risk of fracture. During the third quarter, much of the bone development in the fetus, a process that requires a total 30 g of calcium [45]. During pregnancy the calcium intestinal absorption of the mother increases and a too low take-up may be one risk factor for a low bone mass in the newborns, especially in areas where the content of calcium in the diet is chronically low [46].

During the gestation development of the bone of the offspring appears related to maternal diet: the healthiest diets are associated with a greater bone mass of the prole, [47] and the micronutrient more closely associated with the bone development of the offspring in the period gestational is vitamin D. Vitamin D deficiency is common during the pregnancy. A controlled, randomly controlled trial scale, "UK Maternal Vitamin D Osteoporosis Study (MAVIDOS) ", is testing whether mothers' offspring that have supplemented vitamin D in pregnancy has a greater bone mass at moment of birth with respect to the mothers' offspring who did not take it [48]. The American Academy of Pediatrics (AAP) [49], the Endocrine Society [50] and the National Osteoporosis Foundation [51], have proposed some strategies to reach the daily dose recommended (RDA—Recommended Dietary Allowance) of vitamin D, including: consumption of fortified foods, the extension of the range of milk products fortified and in some cases, the use of a vitamin D supplement or a multivitamin that understands it. Strategies to improve calcium intake include an increase in dairy consumption or fortified products.

15.12 Children

A clinical report published in 2014 by American Academy of Pediatrics highlighted some modifiable factors that influence accumulation bone mass in children and adolescents [49]: nutrition, exercise and lifestyle, body weight, body composition and hormonal status. Most important nutrients to optimize your health of bones in children and adolescents are calcium, vitamin D and proteins. Among the food choices that can adversely affect the health of bone there is the so-called 'displacement of milk'—for where carbonated drinks are consumed in place of milk—and high-sodium diets. The consumption of carbonated beverages is increasing in all the world and a meta-analysis showed that it is associated with a lower intake of milk, calcium and other nutrients [52]. The main source of nutrition for children in the first year of life is breast milk or formula. Insufficient calcium intake is a problem spread all over the world [53], found in particular among women of fertil age and pregnant women [54]. Milk and dairy products provide up to 80% of the dose daily calcium for children from second year of life. The daily reference dose (RDA) of vitamin D recommended by IOM for children is shown in [55].

Food proteins are a source of amino acids necessary to build the bone matrix. The milk provides high-quality protein, mostly casein, but also whey proteins, which they contain promoters of growth [56]. The children healthy people who received extra doses of milk in the diet, and therefore more protein, they have Significant increases of the IGF-l compared to the control subjects [57]. The change in the assumption of proteins, within the normal range of children and teenagers well-fed, can influence skeletal growth and so have an impact on the ability of each child to reach its PBM genetic potential. For optimal bones health it takes a weight healthy body in childhood and adolescence. A body mass index (BMI) at the extremities of the spectrum can pose a threat to it skeletal development.

It has been shown that nervous anorexia has a strong negative impact on bone mineral density in the teens and boys [58], as well as indexes of skeletal force [59, 60]. Overweight and obese children have a low bone mass and bone surface compared to weight [61] and have more likely to meet repeatedly wrist fractures. [62]

15.13 Mediterranean Diet and Bone

A balanced diet plays a key role in maintaining the well-being of the individual, preventing chronic metabolic diseases and optimizing the individual's genetic heritage. A balanced diet involves the presence of all macro- and micronutrients distributed in a balanced manner in the various daily meals. No food alone provides all the essential nutrients to maintain the body's well-being, including that of bone tissue, so it's fundamental that a proper diet is as much varied as possible to optimize skeletal homeostasis. The ideal dietary diet model is the Mediterranean Diet (MeDi). The first studies on the Mediterranean diet and the importance of a proper diet to correct cardiovascular risk factors such as cholesterol are those implemented by Ancel Keys in the 1950s in Italy, in the Salento region [63]. These studies showed that a diet rich in vegetable products, poor in animal foods (preferably fish and white meat), poor in fat, except for extra virgin olive oil, was associated with a reduced risk, in the population studied, of chronic metabolic pathologies and longer life expectancy [64]. After these initial studies, many researches published over the last decades, have focused their interest in evaluating and characterizing the mechanisms behind MeDi 's positive effect on the well-being of the organism [65]. First of all, it has been shown that MeDi is also based on an optimal distribution of nutrients [66]: 45–60% of daily calories should from carbohydrates, preferably complex, by limiting simple sugars (OMS 2016), less than 30% of calories must come from fat, mostly unsaturated, and about 12–18% of proteins mainly of vegetal origin.

There are many clinical studies that have shown a positive effect of MeDi on reducing the risk of developing chronic metabolic pathologies [67–71], presumably through an inhibition of mechanisms related to a chronic subclinical inflammation. In recent years, several studies have shown that MeDi components can modulate skeletal homeostasis. A recent study in an animal model evaluated the possible role of specific MeDi components, such as olive oil as a source of polyphenols, that played an important role in skeletal well-being [72].

But if the results obtained in animal models are even more interesting, studies that associate adherence to MeDi with maintaining skeletal well-being, bone mineral density and reduced risk of fragility fracture are even more interesting [73–75]. Recent results, published by an Italian group, demonstrate a positive correlation between bone health and adherence to MeDi, suggesting that a high adherence to MeDi favors bone health [76]. In a recently published study, Benetou and colleagues assessed association of MeDi membership with hip fracture incidence in a cohort in eight European countries. A total of nearly 200,000 participants were evaluated in a prospective study on cancer and nutrition. Data extrapolated from the study showed that increased adhesion to MeDi was associated with a 7% decrease in hip fracture. Newly published studies have is confirmed a positive role of MeDi in preventing skeletal and fractures of fragility [77, 78].

Finally a particularly interesting recent study by Mousavi et al. that has shown that mice fed with a MeDi during pregnancy and different concentrations of olive oil have led to an increase in osteoblastic cell proliferation in the skeleton of births during neonatal life [79], suggesting an important role in the diet even during the embryonic stage of life that could thus have important repercussions in adult life.

Further studies will be needed to confirm the protective role of MeDi on the skeleton and to characterize the mechanisms by which this effect will be implemented but the observations in the literature still confirm that a specific dietary approach, such as MeDi, can represent an editable environmental factor for the prevention of osteoporosis.

15.14 Vegetarian Diet and Bone

The adoption of a vegetarian diet has become increasingly popular in recent years. Some data suggest that about 3–5% of the US population is vegetarian. Vegetarianism is associated with many health benefits such as reducing the incidence of obesity, diabetes, hypertension, cardiovascular disease and some types of cancer [80]. However, the rather restrictive typology of this diet promptly raised some concerns about a possible shortage of some nutrients and an increased risk of osteoporosis [81].

Vegetarians are those who exclude meat, fish and all their derivatives from their diet [82]. Generally, the vegetarian diet is classified based on the foods included or excluded. For example, we talk about lacto-ovo-vegetarian diet when we include dairy and egg, lacto-vegetarian diet that includes only dairy products and vegan diet which excludes all animal derivatives. However, even on the basis of this subdivision there are numerous heterogeneities also linked to the variation of individual choice. In addition, despite the fact that most vegetarians lead a healthy and active lifestyle, various studies indicate that vegetarianism may have a negative impact on bone health due to reduced vitamin B12, calcium and vitamin D intake [83–85].

15.14.1 Calcium, Protein, and Vitamin D in the Vegetarian Diet

Public opinion generally believes that vegetarians, especially vegans, do not need the same calcium intake of non vegetarians for their dietary regime with low protein content. Since there is no scientific evidence to support this hypothesis, it is recommended that vegetarians respect the same dietary guidelines and the same references as dietary intake of non vegetarians.

Although dairy products are widely recognized as an important source of dietary calcium, various plant-derived foods contain a good source of absorbable calcium. Among them are bock choy, cabbage, broccoli, tofu and fortified foods such as vegetable lettuce, orange juice and energy bars [86]. The bioavailable calcium derived from vegetable foods is affected by the presence of oxalic acid and phytic acid contained in some foods, like legumes. High-oxalic foods include spinach, rhubarb, beetroot; calcium absorption from these foods can be very low, equal to 5% compared to low oxalic acid plants such as broccoli and bock choy where.

It is well known that increased protein intake with the diet causes increased urinary calcium excretion [87]. As a result, vegetarians, whose diet is low in protein, should have reduced urinary calcium loss and thus require less calcium; However, recent studies suggest that the relationship between protein intake and calcium requirement is much more complex and that however, a protein rich diet offers greater benefits in terms of bone health [88, 89]. Proteins have countless positive effects on the bone. A higher protein intake improves calcium absorption, especially in low-calorie diets. Proteins also help maintain bone structure by suppressing parathyroid hormone (PTH) and improving muscle strength [90]. Vegetarians can take high amounts of protein through soy, corn, wheat and rice containing sulphate amounts per gram, similar to meat, milk and eggs, and may therefore exhibit high levels of excreted calcium in the urine [91]. However, there are various foods that neutralize acids such as fruit and vegetables, and therefore a fairly balanced supply of protein, fruit, vegetables, and calcium-rich foods can still be protected against the bone. Fruits and vegetables are good sources of various nutrients such as magnesium, calcium, potassium, vitamin K and vitamin C; the presence of antioxidants in such foods could protect the bone by reducing the absorption related to oxidative stress [92].

Generally, non-vegetarian protein intake varies from 1% to 18% of energy input, where protein intakes in lacto-ovo-vegetarians and vegans are about 12–14% and 10–12% respectively. The sources of protein also vary according to the type of diet; for example, in a study, animal proteins varied from 6.3% in non-vegetarians to 2.4% in lacto-ovo-vegetarians up to 0.6% in vegans [93].

Vitamin D plays a key role in bone homeostasis by stimulating calcium reabsorption and promoting proper bone mineralization. Dairy products are often fortified with vitamin D and therefore constitute a good source of food for lacto-ovo-vegetarians and lacto-vegetarians. Even vegetable milk can be fortified with vitamin D constituting a source of such vitamin for vegans. However these types of foods are recently introduced and not available everywhere. For example, in Finland, dietary intake of vitamin D in vegans and lacto-ovo-vegetarians was insufficient to maintain both the 25OH vitamin D and PTH levels in the normal range in the winter months with possible long-term negative effects on BMD [94]. The identification of a good vitamin D diet is therefore clearly a priority in vegetarian and vegan subjects to keep bone homeostasis. Although fortified foods and UV rays are vegetable sources of vitamin D, however, the amount they provide is limited and insufficient to meet the currently recommended RDA of 600 UI/d for subjects between 19 and 70 years of age and 800 UI/d for subjects over 70 years, indicating the need for vitamin D supplementation in vegetarian subjects.

In addition, vegans are generally at risk of vitamin B12 deficiency due to reduced dietary intake, as the main source of this vitamin is animal food. Vegetarians have low levels of vitamin B12 and increased levels of homocysteine than non vegetarians. A European study compared lacto-ovo-vegetarians and vegans to omnivorous subjects and showed a deficiency of vitamin B12 in 11% of omnivores, 77% of lacto-ovo-vegetarians and 92% of vegans [95]. Similarly, high serum methylmalonic acid levels, functional indicators of Vitamin B12 deficiency, were present in 5% of omnivorous, 68% of the vegetarian side and 67% of vegans. It is therefore clear that ensuring an adequate supply of vitamin B12 is essential for vegetarians. Non-animal sources of this vitamin are fortified cereals, yeast and fortified soy products. Since vitamin deficiency is very common in vegetarians, it is advisable to periodically control the serum levels of methylmalonic acid or adequate supplementation.

In conclusion, it is always advisable for vegetarians to follow some dietary recommendations such as an adequate calcium and vitamin D intake by fortified foods or specific supplements, an adequate protein intake, an abundant intake of fruits and vegetables, and an adequate supply of vitamin B12.

References

1. NIH Consensus Development Panel on Osteoporosis. JAMA. 2001;285:785–95.
2. Migliaccio S, Falcone S, Spera G. Bone modeling and remodeling: new roles for an old game. Aging Clin Exp Res. 2004;16(Suppl 3):20–2.
3. Seeman E. Bone quality. Osteoporos Int. 2003;14(S5):3–7.
4. Boivin G, Meunier PJ. The mineralization of bone tissue: a forgotten dimension in osteoporosis research. Osteoporos Int. 2003;14(3):S19–24.
5. Dempster DW. The contribution of trabecular architecture to cancellous bone quality. J Bone Miner Res. 2000;15:20–4.
6. Kitchin B, Morgan S. Nutritional considerations in osteoporosis. Curr Opin Rheumatol. 2003;15:476–80.
7. Javaid MK, Cooper C. Prenatal and childhood influences on osteoporosis. Best Pract Res Clin Endocrinol Metab. 2002;16:349–67.
8. Migliaccio S, Migliaccio PA. Attuali orientamenti della dietoterapia in gravidanza per la salute della donna e del bambino. Atti Congresso Nazoinale SIGO. 2001.
9. Wosje KS, Khoury PR, Claytor RP, Copeland KA, Hornung RW, Daniels SR, Kalkwarf HJ. Dietary patterns associated with fat and bone mass in young children. Am J Clin Nutr. 2010;92(2):294–303.
10. Bonjour JP, Ammann P, Chevalley T, Rizzoli R. Protein intake and bone growth. Can J Appl Physiol. 2001;26:S153–66.
11. Earl S, Cole ZA, Holroyd C, Cooper C, Harvey NC. Session 2: other diseases: dietary management of osteoporosis throughout the life course. Proc Nutr Soc. 2010;69:25–33.
12. Cooper C, Harvey N, Cole Z, Hanson M, Dennison E. Developmental origins of osteoporosis: the role of maternal nutrition. Adv Exp Med Biol. 2009;646:31–9.
13. Kalkwarf HJ, Khoury JC, Lanphear BP. Milk intake during childhood and adolescence, adult bone density, and osteoporotic fractures in US women. Am J Clin Nutr. 2003;77:257–65.
14. Cooper C, Melton LJ 3rd. Epidemiology of osteoporosis. Trends Endocrinol Metab. 1992;3:224–9.
15. Institute of Medicine. Dietary reference intakes for calcium and vitamin D. Washington, DC: National Academies Press; 2011.
16. Table Ciqual de composition des aliments, ANSES (French agency for food, environmental and occupational health and safety), France. 2012. Accessed September 2017.
17. Food Standards Agency. McCance and Widdowson's the composition of foods. 6th Summary ed. Cambridge: Royal Society of Chemistry; 2002.
18. Adami S, Viapiana O, Gatti D, Idolazzi L, Rossini M. Relationship between serum parathyroid hormone, vitamin D sufficiency, age, and calcium intake. Bone. 2008;42:267–70.
19. Schott GD, Willis MR. Muscle weakness in osteomalacia. Lancet. 1976;1:626–7.
20. Boland R. Role of vitamin D in skeletal muscle function. Endocr Rev. 1986;7:434–48.
21. Rossini M, Mattarei A, Braga V, Viapiana O, Zambarda C, Benini C, Pancheri S, Spanevello MC, Lovato R, Sella S, Giannini S, Olivi P, Lavini F, Giulini GM, Fracassi E, Gatti D, Adami S. Risk factors for hip fracture in elderly persons. Reumatismo. 2010;62:273–82.
22. Isaia G, Giorgino R, Rini GB, Bevilacqua M, Maugeri D, Adami S. Prevalence of hypovitaminosis D in elderly women in Italy: clinical consequences and risk factors. Osteoporos Int. 2003;14:577–82.
23. Vieth R. Vitamin D supplementation, 25-hydroxyvitamin D concentrations, and safety. Am J Clin Nutr. 1999;69:842–56.
24. Malabanan A, Veronikis IE, Holick MF. Redefining vitamin D insufficiency. Lancet. 1998;351:805–6.
25. Holick MF. Vitamin D Deficiency. N Engl J Med. 2007;357:266–81.
26. Holick MF, Binkley NC, Bischoff-Ferrari HA, Gordon CM, Hanley DA, Heaney RP, Murad MH, Weaver CM. Evaluation, treatment, and prevention of vitamin D deficiency: an Endocrine Society clinical practice guideline. J Clin Endocrin Metab. 2011;7:1911–30.

27. Bischoff-Ferrari HA, Willett WC, Wong JB, Giovannucci EG, Dietrich T, Dawson-Hughes B. Fracture prevention with vitamin D supplementation. A meta-analysis of randomized controlled trials. JAMA. 2005;293:2257–64.
28. Adami S, Romagnoli E, Carnevale V, Scillitani A, Giusti A, Rossini M, Gatti D, Nuti R, Minisola S. Linee guida su prevenzione e trattamento dell'ipovitaminosi D con colecalciferolo. Reumatismo. 2011;63:129–147.2.
29. Heaney RP. Dairy and bone health. J Am Coll Nutr. 2009;28(Suppl 1):82S–90S.
30. Darling AL, Millward DJ, Torgerson DJ, Hewitt CE, Lanham-New SA. Dietary protein and bone health: a systematic review and meta-analysis. Am J Clin Nutr. 2009;90:1674–92.
31. Booth SL, Colditz GA. Vitamin K intake and hip fractures in women: a prospective study. Am J Clin Nutr. 1999;69:74–9.
32. Hamidi MS, Gajic-Veljanoski O, Cheung AM. Vitamin K and bone health. J Clin Densitom. 2013;16:409–13.
33. Morris MS, Jacques PF, Selhub J. Relation between homocysteine and B-vitamin status indicators and bone mineral density in older Americans. Bone. 2005;37:234–42.
34. McLean RR, Jacques PF, Selhub J, Tucker KL, Samelson EJ, Broe KE, Hannan MT, Cupples LA, Kiel DP. Homocysteine as a predictive factor for hip fracture in older persons. N Engl J Med. 2004;350:2042–9.
35. Clarke M, Ward M, Strain JJ, Hoey L, Dickey W, McNulty H. B-vitamins and bone in health and disease: the current evidence. Proc Nutr Soc. 2014;73:330–9.
36. Tanumihardjo SA. Vitamin a and bone health: the balancing act. J Clin Densitom. 2013;16:414–9.
37. de Baaij JH, Hoenderop JG, Bindels RJ. Magnesium in man: implications for health and disease. Physiol Rev. 2015;95:1–46.
38. Kvamme JM, Gronli O, Jacobsen BK, Florholmen J. Risk of malnutrition and zinc deficiency in community-living elderly men and women: the Tromso study. Public Health Nutr. 2014;18(11):1–7.
39. Kanis JA, Johansson H, Johnell O, Oden A, De Laet C, Eisman JA, Pols H, Tenenhouse A. Alcohol intake as a risk factor for fracture. Osteoporos Int. 2005;16:737–42.
40. Hallstrom H, Wolk A, Glynn A, Michaelsson K. Coffee, tea and caffeine consumption in relation to osteoporotic fracture risk in a cohort of Swedish women. Osteoporos Int. 2006;17:1055–64.
41. Barrett-Connor E, Chang JC, Edelstein SL. Coffee-associated osteoporosis offset by daily milk consumption. The rancho Bernardo study. JAMA. 1994;271:280–3.
42. Holroyd C, Harvey N, Dennison E, Cooper C. Epigenetic influences in the developmental origins of osteoporosis. Osteoporos Int. 2012;23:401–10.
43. Harvey N, Dennison E, Cooper C. Osteoporosis: a lifecourse approach. J Bone Miner Res. 2014;29:1917–25.
44. Baird J, Kurshid MA, Kim M, Harvey N, Dennison E, Cooper C. Does birthweight predict bone mass in adulthood? A systematic review and meta-analysis. Osteoporos Int. 2011;22:1323–34.
45. Namgung R, Tsang RC. Bone in the pregnant mother and newborn at birth. Clin Chim Acta. 2003;333:1–11.
46. Ganpule A, Yajnik CS, Fall CH, et al. Bone mass in Indian children--relationships to maternal nutritional status and diet during pregnancy: the Pune maternal nutrition study. J Clin Endocrinol Metab. 2006;91:2994–3001.
47. Cole ZA, Gale CR, Javaid MK, Robinson SM, Law C, Boucher BJ, Crozier SR, Godfrey KM, Dennison EM, Cooper C. Maternal dietary patterns during pregnancy and childhood bone mass: a longitudinal study. J Bone Miner Res. 2009;24:663–8.
48. Harvey NC, Javaid K, Bishop N, Kennedy S, Papageorghiou AT, Fraser R, Gandhi SV, Schoenmakers I, Prentice A, Cooper C. MAVIDOS maternal vitamin D osteoporosis study: study protocol for a randomized controlled trial. The MAVIDOS study group. Trials. 2012;13:13.
49. Golden NH, Abrams SA, Committee on N. Optimizing bone health in children and adolescents. Pediatrics. 2014;134:e1229–43.

50. Holick MF, Binkley NC, Bischoff-Ferrari HA, Gordon CM, Hanley DA, Heaney RP, Murad MH, Weaver CM, Endocrine S. Evaluation, treatment, and prevention of vitamin D deficiency: an Endocrine Society clinical practice guideline. J Clin Endocrinol Metab. 2011;96:1911–30.
51. National Osteoporosis Foundation. Calcium and vitamin D: what you need to know. 2015. http://nof.org/articles/10 Accessed 24 Feb 2015.
52. Vartanian LR, Schwartz MB, Brownell KD. Effects of soft drink consumption on nutrition and health: a systematic review and metaanalysis. Am J Public Health. 2007;97:667–75.
53. Peterlik M, Boonen S, Cross HS, Lamberg-Allardt C. Vitamin D and calcium insufficiencyrelated chronic diseases: an emerging world-wide public health problem. Int J Environ Res Public Health. 2009;6:2585–607.
54. Dietary Guidelines Advisory Committee. Scientific Report of the 2015 Dietary Guidelines Advisory Committee: Advisory Report to the Secretary of Health and Human Services and the Secretary of Agriculture. In: U.S. Department of Agriculture, Department of Health and Human Services – USA, editors. Washington DC; 2015.
55. Institute of Medicine. Dietary reference intakes tables and application. 2015. http://www.iom.edu/Activities/Nutrition/SummaryDRIs/DRI-Tables.aspx. Accessed 24 Feb 2015.
56. Rizzoli R. Nutrition: its role in bone health. Best Pract Res Clin Endocrinol Metab. 2008;22:813–29.
57. Cadogan J, Eastell R, Jones N, Barker ME. Milk intake and bone mineral acquisition in adolescent girls: randomised, controlled intervention trial. BMJ. 1997;315:1255–60.
58. Misra M, Katzman DK, Cord J, Manning SJ, Mendes N, Herzog DB, Miller KK, Klibanski A. Bone metabolism in adolescent boys with anorexia nervosa. J Clin Endocrinol Metab. 2008;93:3029–36.
59. DiVasta AD, Feldman HA, Beck TJ, LeBoff MS, Gordon CM. Does hormone replacementnormalize bone geometry in anorexia nervosa? J Bone Miner Res. 2014;29:151–7.
60. Misra M, Katzman DK, Clarke H, Snelgrove D, Brigham K, Miller KK, Klibanski A. Hip structural analysis in adolescent boys with anorexia nervosa and controls. J Clin Endocrinol Metab. 2013;98:2952–8.
61. Goulding A, Taylor RW, Jones IE, McAuley KA, Manning PJ, Williams SM. Overweight and obese children have low bone mass and area for their weight. Int J Obes Relat Metab Disord. 2000;24:627–32.
62. Goulding A, Grant AM, Williams SM. Bone and body composition of children and adolescents with repeated forearm fractures. J Bone Miner Res. 2005;20:2090–6.
63. Keys A, Fidanza F, Scardi V, Bergami G, Keys MH, Di Lorenzo F. Studies on serum cholesterol and other characteristics of clinically healthy men in Naples. AMA Arch Intern Med. 1954;93(3):328–36.
64. Keys A, Menotti A, Karvonen MJ, Aravanis C, Blackburn H, Buzina R, Djordjevic BS, Dontas AS, Fidanza F, Keys MH, et al. The diet and 15-year death rate in the seven countries study. Am J Epidemiol. 1986;124(6):903–15.
65. Mancini M, Parillo M, Rivellese A, Riccardi G. Nutrition and cardiovascular risk: the Mediterranean experience. Acta Cardiol. 1989;44(6):466–7.
66. Alberti-Fidanza A. Mediterranean meal patterns. Bibl Nutr Dieta. 1990;45:59–71.
67. FerroLuzzi A, Ghiselli A. Protective aspects of the Mediterranean diet. Adv Exp Med Biol. 1993;348:137–44.
68. Santoro A, Pini E, Scurti M, Palmas G, Berendsen A, Brzozowska A, Pietruszka B, Szczecinska A, Cano N, Meunier N, de Groot CP, Feskens E, Fairweather-Tait S, Salvioli S, Capri M, Brigidi P, Franceschi C, NU-AGE Consortium. Combating inflammaging through a Mediterranean whole diet approach: the NU-AGE project's conceptual framework and design. Mech Ageing Dev. 2014;136-137:3–13.
69. Mattioli AV, Palmiero P, Manfrini O, Puddu PE, Nodari S, Dei Cas A, Mercuro G, Scrutinio D, Palermo P, Sciomer S, Di Francesco S, Novo G, Novo S, Pedretti RFE, Zito A, Parati G, Pedrinelli R, Farinetti A, Maiello M, Moscucci F, Tenaglia RL, Sucato V, Triggiani M, Cugusi L, Scicchitano P, Saba PS, Ciccone MM. Mediterranean diet impact on cardiovascular diseases: a narrative review. J Cardiovasc Med (Hagerstown). 2017;18(12):925–35.

70. Dinu M, Pagliai G, Casini A, Sofi F. Mediterranean diet and multiple health outcomes: an umbrella review of meta-analyses of observational studies and randomised trials. Eur J Clin Nutr. 2017. https://doi.org/10.1038/ejcn.2017.58.
71. Veronese N, Stubbs B, Noale M, Solmi M, Rizzoli R, Vaona A, Demurtas J, Crepaldi G, Maggi S. Adherence to a Mediterranean diet is associated with lower incidence of frailty: a longitudinal cohort study. Clin Nutr. 2017. pii: S0261-5614(17)30311-4.
72. Tagliaferri C, Davicco MJ, Lebecque P, Georgé S, Amiot MJ, Mercier S, Dhaussy A, Huertas A, Walrand S, Wittrant Y, Coxam V. Olive oil and vitamin D synergistically prevent bone loss in mice. PLoS One. 2014;9(12):e115817. https://doi.org/10.1371/journal.pone.0115817.
73. Kontogianni MD, Melistas L, Yannakoulia M, Malagaris I, Panagiotakos DB, Yiannakouris N. Association between dietary patterns and indices of bone mass in a sample of Mediterranean women. Nutrition. 2009;25:165–71.
74. Benetou V, Orfanos P, Pettersson-Kymmer U, Bergström U, Svensson O, Johansson I, Berrino F, Tumino R, Borch KB, Lund E, Peeters PH, Grote V, Li K, Altzibar JM, Key T, Boeing H, von Ruesten A, Norat T, Wark PA, Riboli E. Trichopoulou Mediterranean diet and incidence of hip fractures in a European cohort. Osteoporos Int. 2013;24(5):1587–98.
75. Romero Pérez A, Rivas Velasco A. Adherence to Mediterranean diet and bone health. Nutr Hosp. 2014;29(5):989–96.
76. Savanelli MC, Barrea L, Macchia PE, Savastano S, Falco A, Renzullo A, Scarano E, Nettore IC, Colao A, Di Somma C. Preliminary results demonstrating the impact of Mediterranean diet on bone health. J Transl Med. 2017;15(1):81.
77. Kunutsor SK, Laukkanen JA, Whitehouse MR, Blom AW. Adherence to a Mediterranean-style diet and incident fractures: pooled analysis of observational evidence. Eur J Nutr. 2017. https://doi.org/10.1007/s00394-017-1432-0.
78. Byberg L, Bellavia A, Larsson SC, Orsini N, Wolk A, Michaëlsson K. Mediterranean diet and hip fracture in Swedish men and women. J Bone Miner Res. 2016;31(12):2098–105.
79. Mousavi SN, Koohdani F, Eslaminejad MB, Izadi P, Eshraghian M, Sayahpour FA, Neek LS, Shidfar F. Extra virgin olive oil in maternal diet increases osteogenic genes expression, but high amounts have deleterious effects on bones in mice offspring at adolescence. Iran J Basic Med Sci. 2016;19(12):1299–307. https://doi.org/10.22038/ijbms.2016.7915.
80. Dewell A, Weidner G, Sumner MD, Chi CS, Ornish D. A very-low-fat vegan diet increases intake of protective dietary factors and decreases intake of pathogenic dietary factors. J Am Diet Assoc. 2008;108:347–56.
81. New SA. Do vegetarians have a normal bone mass? Osteoporosis Int. 2004;15:679–88.
82. Craig WJ, Mangels AR, American Dietetic Association. Position of the American dietetic association: vegetarian diets. J Am Diet Assoc. 2009;109:1266–82.
83. Spencer EA, Appleby PN, Davies GK, Key TJ. Diet and body-mass index in 38000 EPIC-Oxford meat-eaters, fish-eaters, vegetarians, and vegans. Int J Obes Relat Metab Disord. 2003;27:728–34.
84. Crowe FL, Steur M, Allen NE, Appleby PN, Travis RC, Key TJ. Plasma concentrations of 25-hydroxyvitamin D in meat eaters, fish eaters, vegetarians and vegans: results from the EPIC-Oxford study. Public Health Nutr. 2011;14:340–6.
85. Pawlak R, Parrott SJ, Raj S, Cullum-Dugan D, Lucus D. How prevalent is vitamin B(12) deficiency among vegetarians? Nutr Rev. 2013;71:110–7.
86. Food and Nutrition Board, Institute of Medicine. Dietary reference intakes for calcium and vitamin D. Washington, DC: National Academies Press; 2011.
87. Kerstetter JE, Allen LH. Dietary protein increases urinary calcium. J Nutr. 1990;120:134–6.
88. Thorpe MP, Evans EM. Dietary protein and bone health: harmonizing conflicting theories. Nutr Rev. 2011;69:215–30.
89. Kerstetter JE, Kenny AM, Insogna KL. Dietary protein and skeletal health: a review of recent human research. Curr Opin Lipidol. 2011;22:16–20.
90. Genaro PS, Martini LA. Effect of protein intake on bone and muscle mass in the elderly. Nutr Rev. 2010;68:616–23.
91. Massey LK. Dietary animal and plant protein and human bone health: a whole foods approach. J Nutr. 2003;133:862S–5S.

92. Hamidi M, Boucher BA, Cheung AM, Beyene J, Shah PS. Fruit and vegetable intake and bone health in women aged 45 years and over: a systematic review. Osteoporos Int. 2011;22:1681–93.
93. Rizzo NS, Jaceldo-Siegl K, Sabate J, Fraser GL. Nutrient profiles of vegetarian and nonvegetarian dietary patterns. J Acad Nutr Diet. 2013;113:1610–9.
94. Outila TA, Kärkkäinen MU, Seppänen RH, Lamberg-Allardt CJ. Dietary intake of vitamin D in premenopausal, healthy vegans was insufficient to maintain concentrations of serum 25-hydroxyvitamin D and intact parathyroid hormone within normal ranges during the winter in Finland. J Am Diet Assoc. 2000;100:434–41.
95. Herrmann W, Schorr H, Obeid R, Geisel J. Vitamin B-12 status, particularly holotranscobalamin II and methylmalonic acid concentrations, and hyperhomocysteinemia in vegetarians. Am J Clin Nutr. 2003;78:131–6.

Different Physical Activity Protocols in the Subjects Affected by Osteoporosis

16

Gian Pietro Emerenziani, Emanuela A. Greco, Laura Guidetti, and Carlo Baldari

16.1 Introduction

The bone is a dynamic tissue that responds to the external and internal environments to which it is exposed across the life course. The skeleton serves many important purposes in the body. For instance, it provides a framework for the body and consequently allows us to stand upright and move about in our environment. The skeleton should be strong enough not only to support our weight but also to exercise daily. Moreover, it protects vital organs such as the brain and heart from trauma.

Age, gender, genetics, and lifestyle may influence bone mass, structure, and strength. During growth, exercise is associated with an increase in bone shape, strength, and density; during adulthood, exercise may help to maintain bone strength, while at older age, exercise may attenuate the physiological (natural) decline in bone mass [1].

Osteoporosis is a bone metabolism alteration characterized by a decrease in bone strength, due to decreased bone density and quality, which lead to a significant increase in the risk of fracture risk [2]. These injuries are a significant source of morbidity and mortality. International Osteoporosis Foundation (IOF) highlight the importance of physical activity or exercise for the prevention on bone loss and

G. P. Emerenziani (✉)
Department of Experimental and Clinical Medicine,
University of Catanzaro "Magna Græcia", Catanzaro, Italy
e-mail: emerenziani@unicz.it

E. A. Greco
Department of Experimental Medicine, Section of Medical Pathophysiology, Endocrinology and Nutrition, Sapienza University of Rome, Rome, Italy

L. Guidetti
Department of Movement, Human and Health Sciences, University of Foro Italico of Rome, Rome, Italy

C. Baldari
University eCampus, Novedrate, Italy

A. Lenzi, S. Migliaccio (eds.), *Multidisciplinary Approach to Osteoporosis*,
https://doi.org/10.1007/978-3-319-75110-8_16

the maintenance of bone health [3]. However, when subjects with high risk of fracture start to exercise, many issues should be addressed. For instance, specific questions might be the following: Will the exercise increase the risk of falls? Which intensity should be chosen in order to reach the positive effects on skeletal metabolism? How exercise should be modified in order to be adaptable for subjects with osteoporosis?

To address these questions, it is very important to know how physical activity could influence bone health.

It is well known that chronic reduction in mechanical loading, such as it occurs following prolonged bed rest, results in a generalized bone mass loss, particularly in skeletal sites that bear weight under normal conditions [4]. Evidences supporting the role of weight bearing on the skeleton came from observations of bone loss in astronauts [5]. Therefore, non-weight-bearing exercises such as swimming or cycling may not be the best to improve bone health. However, they might have a role in muscle strength maintenance and in sarcopenia prevention in aging population. A large number of cross-sectional studies have shown that bone density depends on customary activity levels [6, 7]. However, the World Health Organization [8] affirms that these studies could be misleading since it is not clear whether physical attributes determine activity levels or the other way around. While bone density is related to exercise levels, it is much less clear that customary exercise levels affect fracture risk. In fact, research evidences show different results. In particular, the European Vertebral Osteoporosis Study (EVOS) [9] suggested that high levels of physical activity were associated with increased risk of fracture in men, but not in women. In contrast, the Tromsø study [10] suggested that high levels of physical activity were protective against axial fractures in middle-aged men but not in women. We may justify these opposite results by the interaction of the effects of exercise on bone density, on the one hand, and on exposure to skeletal trauma on the other. Because of the difficulties associated with observational studies mentioned above, randomized controlled studies have been used to determine the effects of exercise on the bone. Evidences suggest that exercise has positive effects on bone density at all ages. Several results showed that exercise confers the greatest long-term benefit when initiated in the prepubertal years [11]. Kannus et al. [12] showed that the bones of the playing extremity clearly benefit from active tennis and squash training, which increases their mineral mass. The benefit of playing is about two times greater if females start playing at or before menarche rather than after it. However, the minimal duration of activity necessary to produce positive results on bone mineral density should be studied further. On the other hand, Slemenda et al. [13] found no relationship between physical activity and bone mineral density in peripubertal girls indicating that during puberty, other factors such as sex steroids become more influential on bone acquisition. Nordström et al. [14] showed that variations in bone mineral density response to different activities reflect the different loading patterns of each sport and the phenomenon of site specificity. Regarding adults, weight-bearing exercise at relatively high intensities has consistently greater bone mineral density than subjects that exercise at low intensity or did not exercise [15].

Also for adults the higher bone mineral density of athletes is observed predominantly at the skeletal sites loaded during their respective activities. However, some activities may not apply a sufficient stimulus to the skeleton to induce an adaptive response such as swimming. We may suggest that physical activity could lead to positive effects on bone health throughout life. The magnitude of this effect depends on the nature and intensity of the physical activity and the number of years spent in training and in contrasting the sedentary behavior. However, while exercise should be encouraged, it is not by itself an adequate and safe therapy for those at higher risk of fractures.

16.2 Physical Activity Principles

To understand the relation between physical activities and skeletal health, it is very important to be familiar with the physical activity principles such as specificity, overload, and progression. Drinkwater [16] suggests to incorporate five principles into exercise study design for osteoporosis: specificity, overload, reversibility, initial values, and diminishing returns.

Specificity: this principle states that the type of exercise should be chosen to best meet the desired goal of the exercise program. In an exercise program for osteoporosis condition, the exercise protocol should be carefully designed to load the target bone, i.e., be specific to the site measured.

Overload: this principle states that the target system of interest must be sufficiently challenged for it to adapt to exercise training. For instance, exercise must overload the bone in order to properly stimulate bone remodelling.

Reversibility: sometimes it is renamed "use it or lose it" principle. This principle states that if a subject stops exercising, he/she will lose the gained benefits from exercise training. Osteoporosis conditions refer to the reversal in bone response once a stimulus is removed.

Initial values: it refers to the fact that responses from the bone are greatest when bone mass at baseline is lower than average.

Diminishing returns: it means that once a given training level is achieved, further responses will probably be slower and of smaller magnitude.

Another important parameter is the *progression of the load*. It means that an exercise program must continue to be challenging once the effect is obtained in order to keep improving. In other words if you want to see even greater improvements after your initial gains, your program has to progress by increasing the overload.

Since the bone is influenced by several factors, its mass, structure, and strength vary considerably between individuals. For this reasons, it is very important that the physical activity training design for osteoporosis must be individualized according to the subject's characteristics. To do this, the physical activity protocols should be realized taking into consideration the frequency, the intensity, the duration, and the type of exercise.

Frequency: it refers to the number of workouts a subject performs over a specific time period. It is usually expressed as a day per week of exercise. It can be easily manipulated to produce bone overload.

Intensity: intensity refers to how much effort a subject put forth during exercise and how hard is the exercise. The bone is most influenced by this parameter. In fact, a study developed by Robinson et al. [17] showed that bone mass at both the hip and spine is 30–40% higher in gymnasts than in runners. This result could be justified by the higher intensity of exercise in gymnasts than in runners. Gymnasts can experience forces at the ground reaction of more than 12 times body weight, whereas only three to five times in runners. If we analyze walking exercise, we could affirm that it is a low-intensity activity, creating ground reaction forces of approximately one time body weight [18], and it has a little or no effects on bone mass.

Duration: it refers to how much exercise is performed during one session. Together with the other parameters, it can be varied in order to produce different bone overload. Usually duration of session depends on the number of repetitions, the sets, and the recovery time between each sets.

Type: it refers to the kind of exercise that the subjects do. First, as previously mentioned, exercise must be site specific. Second, exercise incurring impact, such us jumping or squash, has been shown to best stimulate bone mass accretion [19]. Therefore bone mineral density is strongly associated with the type of activity performed [20].

16.3 Physical Activity Program

Exercise prescription needed to benefit the bone will differ across the life span according to age and health of participant. In children and adults, activities with high magnitude and high loading rate promote bone gain. These exercises include impact activities such as jumping and resistance activities such as weight training. Whereas high-magnitude impact activities are recommended for younger and adults, they are not recommended for elderly with low bone mineral density. Elderly should not be involved in jumping activities, but the training program should promote resistance exercise, balance, and flexibility in order to reduce the risk of falling. Any individuals should start the physical activity program with caution and with an appropriate progression. Exercise that produces severe joint pain or muscle soreness that lasts more than 2 days should be avoided and changed with a new exercise that can be better tolerated. Moreover, exercise should also be aimed at reinforcing muscle that is important for posture. In order to reach the positive effects of exercise on bone mineral density, it is very important that subjects perform the exercise continuously throughout their life. To accomplish this aim, the most appropriate exercise prescription should also take into consideration the enjoyment, cost, and accessibility.

It may be not correct to make strong recommendations for exercise prescription in subjects with osteoporosis. Individuals with osteoporosis should be engaged in a multicomponent exercise program that includes resistance training in combination with balance and with low potential risk of fall. Moreover, a combination of aerobic exercise with resistance or balance training should be chosen.

16.3.1 Resistance Training

Progressive resistance training program is strongly recommended for individuals with osteoporosis, at least twice a week. The intensity and the type of exercise should be tailored to subjects' capacity, especially in the presence of pain. It is suggested to perform two sets of at least one exercise for each major muscle group, at the target intensity of 8–12 repetitions maximum. Obviously, sedentary subjects with low level of fitness should begin training at lower intensity. In order to provide the resistance load, it is possible to use bands or cables, free weights, body weight, and machines. The latter should be used with caution in subjects with high risk of fractures. Regarding the velocity of the movement, slow, controlled movements are recommended.

Figure 16.1 shows a progressive resistance exercise program for thighs and buttocks.

16.3.2 Balance Training

It should be suggested to perform daily balance training to accumulate 2 h of balance training weekly. Balance exercise may be incorporated into daily activities or performed all at once. According to the overload principle, balance exercise should

Squat	**Chair stand**	**Leg press**
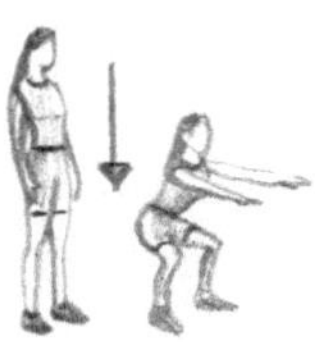	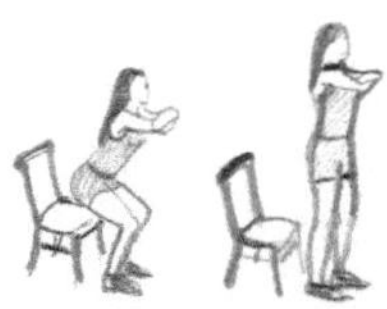	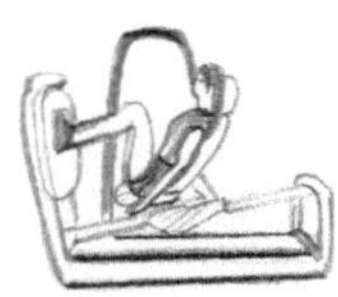
Starting position: Stand with your back straight and your feet a little wider than shoulder width apart.	**Starting position:** Sit at the edge of a stable, straight-backed chair with your back straight and your feet a little wider than shoulder width apart and directly under your knees. Corss your arm across your chest.	**Starting position:** Start the exercise in a seated position and adjust the seat on order that your torso and upper legs and your upper and lower legs are at right angles. Cross your arms across the chest.
Movement: Slowly lower your buttocks toward the floor, as if you were going to sit down in a chair, until your legs are bent between 45 and 90°. Slowly return to the starting position	**Movement:** Slowly raise yourself out of the chair to a full stand. Slowly return to the starting position	**Movement:** Slowly extend your legs until there is just a slight bend in your knees. Return to the starting position

Fig. 16.1 Progressive resistance exercise program for thinghs and buttocks

Semi Tandem Stand	Tandem Stand	One Leg Stance
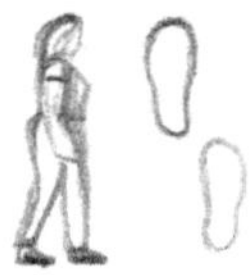	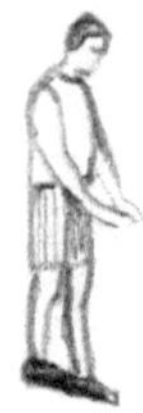	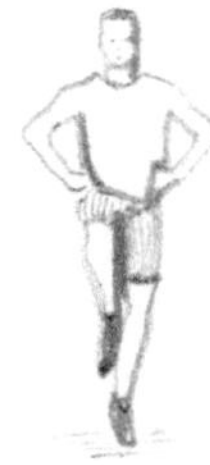
Starting position and movement stand with the side of the heel of one foot touching the big toe of the other foot for about 10 seconds. You may put either foot in front, whichever is more comfortable for you.You may use your arms, bend your knees, or move your body to maintain your balance, but try not to move your feet. Try to hold this position.To make this exercise more challenging, close your eyes.	**Starting position and movement** stand with the heel of one foot in front of and touching the toes of the other foot for about 10 seconds. You may put either foot in front, whichever is more comfortable for you.You may use your arms, bend your knees, or move your body to maintain your balance, but try not to move your feet. Try to hold this position. To make this exercise more challenging, close your eyes.	**Starting position and movement** Begin with your feetshoulder-width apart and one foot slightly off the floor. Rise one foot off the floor so that the knee is slightly in front and the foot a few centimeters off the ground. Hold the position for up to 30 seconds and then swith legs. Repeat up to three to five times on each leg. To make this exercise more challenging, close your eyes.

Fig. 16.2 Progressive balance exercise program

be chosen in order to provide a sufficient challenge to balance. For example, reducing the person's base of support or amount of sensory input.

Figure 16.2 shows a progressive balance exercise program

Conclusion

Physical activity may play an important role for bone health during all stages of life. In children it is very important to do exercise in order to acquire and develop bone mass, in adult age to maintain bone density and quality, and in older age to contrast the loss of bone mass. To reach the positive effects on bone health, it is very important that physical activity should be programmed on the subjects' clinical and physical characteristics. Thus, multicomponent exercise that includes aerobic training plus resistance training and balance training is strongly suggested. In addition, specific exercises on spinal extensor daily, and guidance on safe movement and how to empower desire to do, may lead to the best physical activity approach.

References

1. Nikander R, Sievänen H, Heinonen A, Daly RM, Uusi-Rasi K, Kannus P. Targeted exercise against osteoporosis: a systematic review and meta-analysis for optimising bone strength throughout life. BMC Med. 2010;8:47. Review.
2. Giangregorio LM, Papaioannou A, Macintyre NJ, Ashe MC, Heinonen A, Shipp K, Wark J, McGill S, Keller H, Jain R, Laprade J, Cheung AM. Too fit to fracture: exercise recommendations for individuals with osteoporosis or osteoporotic vertebral fracture. Osteoporos Int. 2014;25(3):821–35.
3. International Osteoporosis Foundation (IOF). Preventing Osteoporosis. https://www.iofbonehealth.org/preventing-osteoporosis.
4. Lupsa BC, Insogna K. Bone health and osteoporosis. Endocrinol Metab Clin N Am. 2015;44(3):517–30. Review.
5. Rabin R, Gordon SL, Lymn RW, Todd PW, Frey MA, Sulzman FM. Effects of spaceflight on the musculoskeletal system: NIH and NASA future directions. FASEB J. 1993;7(5):396–8. Review.
6. Välimäki MJ, Kärkkäinen M, Lamberg-Allardt C, Laitinen K, Alhava E, Heikkinen J, Impivaara O, Mäkelä P, Palmgren J, Seppänen R, et al. Exercise, smoking, and calcium intake during adolescence and early adulthood as determinants of peak bone mass. Cardiovascular Risk in Young Finns Study Group. BMJ. 1994;309(6949):230–5.
7. Lee I, Ha C, Kang H. Association of sarcopenia and physical activity with femur bone mineral density in elderly women. J Exerc Nutrition Biochem. 2016;20(1):23–8.
8. World Health Organization. Prevention and management of osteoporosis. World Health Organ Tech Rep Ser. 2003;921:1–164. back cover.
9. Silman AJ, O'Neill TW, Cooper C, Kanis J, Felsenberg D. Influence of physical activity on vertebral deformity in men and women: results from the European Vertebral Osteoporosis study. J Bone Miner Res. 1997;12(5):813–9.
10. Joakimsen RM, Fønnebø V, Magnus JH, Størmer J, Tollan A, Søgaard AJ. The Tromsø Study: physical activity and the incidence of fractures in a middle-aged population. J Bone Miner Res. 1998;13(7):1149–57.
11. Khan KM, Bennell KL, Hopper JL, Flicker L, Nowson CA, Sherwin AJ, Crichton KJ, Harcourt PR, Wark JD. Self-reported ballet classes undertaken at age 10-12 years and hip bone mineral density in later life. Osteoporos Int. 1998;8(2):165–73.
12. Kannus P, Haapasalo H, Sankelo M, Sievänen H, Pasanen M, Heinonen A, Oja P, Vuori I. Effect of starting age of physical activity on bone mass in the dominant arm of tennis and squash players. Ann Intern Med. 1995;123(1):27–31.
13. Slemenda CW, Reister TK, Hui SL, Miller JZ, Christian JC, Johnston CC Jr. Influences on skeletal mineralization in children and adolescents: evidence for varying effects of sexual maturation and physical activity. J Pediatr. 1994;125(2):201–7.
14. Nordström P, Nordström G, Thorsen K, Lorentzon R. Local bone mineral density, muscle strength, and exercise in adolescent boys: a comparative study of two groups with different muscle strength and exercise levels. Calcif Tissue Int. 1996;58(6):402–8.
15. Tønnesen R, Schwarz P, Hovind PH, Jensen LT. Physical exercise associated with improved BMD independently of sex and vitamin D levels in young adults. Eur J Appl Physiol. 2016;116(7):1297–304.
16. Drinkwater BL. 1994 C. H. McCloy Research Lecture: does physical activity play a role in preventing osteoporosis? Res Q Exerc Sport. 1994;65(3):197–206. Review.
17. Robinson TL, Snow-Harter C, Taaffe DR, Gillis D, Shaw J, Marcus R. Gymnasts exhibit higher bone mass than runners despite similar prevalence of amenorrhea and oligomenorrhea. J Bone Miner Res. 1995;10(1):26–35.
18. Röhrle H, Scholten R, Sigolotto C, Sollbach W, Kellner H. Joint forces in the human pelvis-leg skeleton during walking. J Biomech. 1984;17(6):409–24.

19. Bassey EJ, Rothwell MC, Littlewood JJ, Pye DW. Pre- and postmenopausal women have different bone mineral density responses to the same high-impact exercise. J Bone Miner Res. 1998;13(12):1805–13.
20. Heinonen A, Oja P, Kannus P, Sievänen H, Haapasalo H, Mänttäri A, Vuori I. Bone mineral density in female athletes representing sports with different loading characteristics of the skeleton. Bone. 1995;17(3):197–203.

Pharmacological Therapy: Past, Present, and Future

17

Silvia Migliaccio, Andrea Lenzi, and Emanuela A. Greco

17.1 Introduction

Osteoporosis is a bone metabolic disease characterized by a skeletal fragility, due to decreased of both bone density and quality, leading to an increased risk of developing spontaneous and traumatic fractures [1]. Osteoporosis has been defined a social disease due to its high impact on mortality and morbidity, to its significant alterations of the quality of life of patients, and to its high economic impact [2, 3].

The bone is a highly specialized connective tissue, whose primary functions are mechanical support, physical protection for organs and soft tissue, and storage for systemic mineral homeostasis [4, 5].

Several different causes and risk factors influence bone strength leading to skeletal fragility: (1) failure to reach an optimal peak bone mass in terms of mass and strength, (2) excessive bone resorption leading to decreased bone density and microarchitectural weakening, and (3) insufficient formation upon an augmented resorption during bone remodeling. Thus, osteoporosis is the consequence of an imbalance of the physiological process of bone turnover, with the loss of the equilibrium between the activity of specialized cells as osteoblasts and osteoclasts [6]. In fact, this sophisticated equilibrium is due to and maintained by a dynamic process, called remodeling, characterized by a balance, referred to as coupling, between the activity of osteoclasts, the bone resorbing cells, and osteoblasts, the bone forming cells [4, 7].

S. Migliaccio (✉)
Department of Movement, Human and Health Sciences, Unit of Endocrinology, University "Foro Italico" of Rome, Rome, Italy
e-mail: silvia.migliaccio@uniroma4.it

A. Lenzi · E. A. Greco
Department of Experimental Medicine, Section of Medical Pathophysiology, Endocrinology and Nutrition, University "Sapienza" of Rome, Rome, Italy

A. Lenzi, S. Migliaccio (eds.), *Multidisciplinary Approach to Osteoporosis*,
https://doi.org/10.1007/978-3-319-75110-8_17

Pharmacological therapies lead to correct remodeling imbalance, modulating the activity of bone target cells, to increase skeletal strength, and reduce the risk of fractures [8, 9]. Thus, anti-osteoporotic drugs can be classified as anti-resorptive agents, aimed at reducing or blocking bone density loss through mechanism(s) of action based on modulating osteoclastogenesis or osteoclast activity [9–14], and drugs that stimulate osteoblast activity, classified as anabolic agents, exerting their stimulus on osteoblasts, determining bone formation, and restoring skeletal micro-architecture with increase in both cortical thickness and connectivity [15].

On the basis of these considerations, optimal anti-fracture efficacy results when drug therapy is targeted to the underlying cellular abnormality, anabolic therapy for osteoporotic individuals with reduced bone formation, and anti-resorptive therapy for patients with increased bone resorption.

Moreover, it is important to underline that the adequacy of calcium intake and vitamin D status are priority measures before starting osteoporosis treatment with specific drugs, as well as encouraging physical activity and prevention of falls.

17.2 Hormone Replacement Therapy (HRT)

Bone loss starts 2–3 years prior to menopause; it is accelerated by estrogen deprivation during menopause and continues for up to 5–10 years later. It is known that estrogen deficiency is associated with an increase in the lifespan of osteoclasts and a concomitant decrease in osteoblast lifespan. It is also associated with increases in bone marrow levels in a number of osteoclastogenic cytokines, which expand the pool of osteoclast precursor cells, and increase expression of the key molecule regulating osteoclast development, activity, and lifespan, the receptor activator of nuclear factor B ligand (RANKL) [16].

Suppression of osteoclast activity by estrogen replacement therapy has been used for decades and was the mainstay of prevention and treatment of postmenopausal osteoporosis. Numerous indications have been demonstrated that estrogen was significantly more effective than placebo in preserving and increasing bone mineral density (BMD), and reducing incidence of vertebral and non-vertebral fractures, and that the discontinuation of estrogen resulted in bone loss at a rate similar to that seen in early menopause [17]. However, the primary indication for estrogen replacement therapy is the treatment of moderate and severe menopausal symptoms (i.e., vasomotor symptoms, vaginal atrophy), probably because of its association with an increased risk of adverse health outcomes in the long-term therapy, such as stroke and venous thromboembolic events [18].

17.3 Selective Estrogen Receptor Modulators (SERMS)

SERMs bind to the estrogen receptor (ER) with high affinity and mediate transcriptional events as agonist (bone and cardiovascular system) or antagonist (breast and endometrium), depending on target tissues. Raloxifene is approved for the prevention and treatment of postmenopausal osteoporosis (60 mg/day). However, the effects of raloxifene on BMD and bone turnover markers have generally been lower than bisphosphonate therapy [19]. The MORE (Multiple Outcomes of Raloxifene Evaluation) study demonstrated a 30% reduction of vertebral fracture risk, but not non-vertebral fractures during a follow-up of 3 years [12]. In the CORE study, an extension of the MORE study, it has been shown that raloxifene therapy had no effect on non-vertebral fracture risk after 8 years but reduced the risk of ER-positive invasive breast and endometrial cancer [20]. Finally, the RUTH (Raloxifene Use for The Heart) study, involving for 5 years postmenopausal women with high risk of cardiovascular disease, showed an increased risk of fatal stroke and venous thromboembolism [21]. These studies show that raloxifene is well tolerated, with transient occurrence of hot flushes and leg cramps in <10% of patients; thus it is not recommended to symptomatic postmenopausal women [12].

Other new SERMs, such as bazedoxifene, have been developed in recent years, having good efficacy, safety, and/or tolerability profiles.

17.4 Bisphosphonates

Bisphosphonates, which decrease bone turnover leading osteoclasts to apoptosis, are the most prescribed anti-resorptive agents in the world for the treatment of osteoporosis and are in use from last three decades. They are synthetic analogues of pyrophosphate, with high affinity for hydroxyapatite, which strongly bind to the mineralized tissue, especially in the active remodeling sites. They are removed from the bone by osteoclasts during resorption and are not metabolized for excretion; thus they can be rebound by the mineralized tissue again and can remain as long as 10 years in the skeleton. Variations in the structure of the amino side chains of these drugs affect their pharmacological activity in terms of bone affinity and potency. The most potent molecules have a nitrogen-containing chain, such as alendronate, risedronate, ibandronate, and zoledronate. Skeleton-binding affinity increases in this rank order: risedronate, ibandronate, alendronate, and zoledronate [22].

Alendronate can be given orally once a week (70 mg), ibandronate once a month (150 mg), and risedronate once a week or once a month (35 mg and 150 mg, respectively). Oral bisphosphonates have to be taken with plain water only, after an overnight fast, and followed by 30–60 min without eating or drinking. The patients need to stand upright for 1 h to prevent gastroesophageal reflux and damage to the mucosa [22]. Ibandronate can also be taken intravenously every 3 months (3 mg) and zoledronate once a year (5 mg). The main side effect of this administration is an auto-limited flu-like syndrome (acute phase reaction) due to release of cytokines (TNF-α, IFN-γ, and IL-6), causing mild fever and muscle pain that can be controlled with antipyretic drugs. This reaction usually ends in 1 or 2 days and gets milder with the subsequent infusions. Fifty percent of the absorbed dose binds to the bones, and the rest is excreted in the urine. Renal toxicity may occur with rapid intravenous administration; thus it is not recommended for patients with creatinine clearance lower than 30–35 mL/min [22].

Alendronate was the first bisphosphonate approved by the FDA for the prevention and treatment of osteoporosis. The once-weekly administration (70 mg) improved the use and tolerability with the same or better efficacy than the daily therapy (10 mg) [23]. In the FIT (Fracture Intervention Trial) study, there was a 47% reduction in new morphometric vertebral fractures and 51% in hip fractures in individuals with one prior vertebral fracture at least [24]. In those without fractures, alendronate reduced the risk of radiographic vertebral fractures in 4 years [25]. In the FOSIT (Fosamax International Trial) study, alendronate reduced 47% the risk of non-vertebral fractures [26]. In the FLEX (Fracture Intervention Trial Long-term Extension) study, the subjects treated with alendronate switched to placebo for 5 years, showing a decline in BMD, both at spine and total hip, but mean levels remained at or above pretreatment levels 10 years earlier. After 5 years, the cumulative risk of non-vertebral fractures was not significant. Among those who continued, there was a significantly lower risk of clinically recognized vertebral fractures, but no significant reduction in morphometric vertebral fractures [27].

Risedronate, which is taken once a week (35 mg) or monthly (150 mg), was evaluated in the US and the multinational VERT (Vertebral Efficacy With Risedronate Therapy) studies, showing a reduction of new vertebral (41% and 49%, respectively) and non-vertebral fractures (39% and 33%, respectively) during 3 years, at least in women with prior vertebral fracture [28]. In the Hip Intervention Program Study Group, risedronate showed a reduction of fracture risk of 40% in women with osteoporosis [29].

An oral daily dose (2.5 mg) and an intermittent dose (20 mg every other day for 12 doses every 3 months) of ibandronate were evaluated in the BONE (oral iBandronate Osteoporosis vertebral fracture trial in North America and Europe) study. After 3 years, daily and intermittent oral ibandronate significantly reduced the risk of new morphometric vertebral fractures by 62% and 50%, respectively, versus placebo. The overall population was at low risk of osteoporotic fractures. Consequently, the incidence of non-vertebral fractures was similar between the ibandronate and placebo groups. However, findings from a post hoc analysis showed that the daily regimen reduced the risk of non-vertebral fractures (69%) in a higher-risk subgroup (femoral neck BMD *T*-score < -3.0) [30]. The MOBILE (Monthly Oral IBandronate In LadiEs) study evaluated the monthly dose (50/50, 100, and 150 mg) compared with the daily regimen during 2 years. All monthly regimens were proven to be similar, and the 150 mg regimen is better than the daily regimen. All monthly regimens produced similar hip BMD gains, which were greater than those of the daily regimen [31]. The DIVA (Dosing IntraVenous Administration) study compared two regimens of intermittent intravenous injections of ibandronate (2 mg every 2 months and 3 mg every 3 months) with a regimen of 2.5 mg of oral ibandronate daily, which are at least as effective as the daily regimen of 2.5 mg by oral route [32].

The HORIZON (Health Outcomes and Reduced Incidence with Zoledronic Acid Once Yearly) study evaluated the efficacy of 5 mg zoledronate during 3 years. There was a reduction of the risk of morphometric vertebral fracture by 70% and hip fracture by 41%. Non-vertebral fractures, clinical fractures, and clinical vertebral fractures were reduced by 25%, 33%, and 77%, respectively [33]. A reduction of 35%

in new clinical fractures in patients with prior fractures was documented in another study, along with a reduction in mortality (28%) [34]. Recently, the extension FPT (HORIZON-Pivotal Fracture Trial) study showed the benefits of a 6-year treatment of zoledronate. In 3–6 years, femoral neck BMD remained constant in the zoledronate group, and dropped slightly in the discontinuing group, but remained above pretreatment levels. Other BMD sites showed similar differences. New morphometric vertebral fractures were lower in the zoledronate group, whereas other fractures were not different [35].

The most common adverse events reported with the use of oral bisphosphonates are related with gastroesophageal intolerance, reported in up to 10% of trial participants [36, 37]. An increased risk of atrial fibrillation was reported in the HORIZON trial [33], but other observational studies have failed in detecting an increased risk with any of the bisphosphonates [37].

Osteonecrosis of the jaw (ONJ) has been reported primarily in patients with cancer who have received large and cumulative doses of intravenous bisphosphonates. This condition is defined as exposure of necrotic bone in the oral cavity, not healing for 6–8 weeks, in the absence of radiotherapy and jaw metastases. In patients with osteoporosis treated with bisphosphonates, ONJ is rare, accounting for 0.8–5.0% of the reported cases, and no cases have been identified in clinical trials with alendronate, ibandronate, or risedronate. In the HORIZON-FPT, two cases of ONJ were reported among 7765 patients, one in the placebo and one in the zoledronate group [33]. The incidence of ONJ is estimated at 0.9/100,000 patient years of treatment among patients who receive oral bisphosphonate therapy, and the causal association is unproven [36, 37]. No validated diagnostic technique exists to determine which patients are at increased risk of developing ONJ, and discontinuing bisphosphonate therapy may not lower the risk but may have a negative effect on low-bone mass-treatment outcomes.

Cases of atypical low-trauma subtrochanteric and femoral shaft fractures have been reported in patients receiving long-term bisphosphonates. Prior to the fracture, patients reported prodromal symptoms of pain (typically groin or thigh). Radiographic findings are the thickening of the cortex in the lateral aspect of the proximal femur, which is the site of high tensional stresses. A complete atypical fracture is displayed in addition to a straight transverse fracture line and median cortical spiking [38]. Attention has been drawn to an association between this kind of fractures and the use of bisphosphonates, possibly related to long-term suppression of bone turnover [22]. However this hypothesis comes from retrospective case series with small numbers of patients involved. There is no randomized controlled trial evidence of an increase in the risk of atypical fractures. There is also a possible association of reduced bone turnover induced by bisphosphonates and the other risk factors, such as younger age at beginning or concomitant therapy with corticosteroids, proton pump inhibitors, or other anti-resorptive agents [22].

At the present time, the ideal duration of treatment with bisphosphonates is uncertain. There is considerable evidence showing that anti-resorptive agents are effective in reducing fracture risk and that they are well tolerated for over 3–5 years. It is a reasonable question when considering bisphosphonate therapy, however, because these drugs accumulate in the skeleton, leading to a reservoir that continues to be released for months or years after treatment is discontinued. Stopping alendronate after 10 years of treatment at a dose of 10 mg daily (which should be the same of 70 mg weekly), the amount of alendronate released from the bone over the next several months or years would be equivalent to taking one fourth of the usual dose (2.5 mg daily or 70 mg once a month). There is a concern that long-term treatment has the potential to oversuppress bone remodeling and inhibit repair of microdamage, cause excessive mineralization, and cause an increase in microcracks. The data from the FLEX trial [27] suggest that a subset of patients may safely take a break from alendronate after 5 years of therapy without experiencing a rapid decline in BMD. The data suggest that, although there is some residual benefit in terms of fracture reduction for some time after a 3- to 5-year course of bisphosphonate therapy, continuing treatment for 10 years is better for some patients (high risk of fracture). Decisions regarding discontinuation must be individualized and based upon the assessment of ongoing fracture risk [22].

17.5 Calcitonin

The PROOF (Prevent Recurrence Of Osteoporotic Fractures) study showed that a dose of 200 IU of salmon calcitonin nasal spray significantly reduced the risk of new vertebral fractures by 33% and 36% in women with prevalent fractures. Occasional rhinitis can occur. Headache, flushing, nausea, and diarrhea have been reported more commonly with subcutaneous dose than with intranasal calcitonin. There is no data on hip or non-vertebral fracture risk reduction [13]. Nowadays, calcitonin is used as second or third place of choice for the treatment of osteoporosis.

17.6 Denosumab

Denosumab is a human monoclonal antibody that inhibits RANKL and, consequently, osteoclastogenesis. It is administered as a 60 mg subcutaneous injection every 6 months. Its clearance occurs by means of the reticuloendothelial system and not by renal excretion. Therefore, denosumab can be taken by patients with renal impairment. The FREEDOM (Fracture Reduction Evaluation of Denosumab in Osteoporosis Every 6 Months) trial evaluated the efficacy of denosumab during 3 years; the treated group showed significant gains in lumbar spine and total hip BMD with a reduction of new radiographic vertebral fracture (68%), hip fracture (40%), and non-vertebral fracture (20%). Cellulitis was more frequent in patients taking denosumab compared with the placebo (0.3% vs. <0.1%), although the absolute risk was very low [39]. In the long-term group, BMD further increased in cumulative 6-year gains of 15.2% (lumbar spine) and 7.5% (total hip). In the long-term group, fracture incidence remained low and rare cases of ONJ have been reported [40]. Patients discontinuing denosumab experienced a fast decrease in BMD during the first 12 months, with the subsequent rate of BMD losses being similar to the placebo, demonstrating that denosumab does not confer a residual effect following cessation of therapy [41]. Long-term treatment with denosumab was associated with a sustained increase on BMD, as well as low bone markers, and maintained the vertebral and non-vertebral anti-fracture efficacy over 6 years [40].

17.7 Teriparatide

Intermittent administration of low-dose PTH enhances osteoblast activity and bone formation. Two PTH peptides have been approved for the treatment of osteoporosis: teriparatide (PTH 1-34) and PTH 1-84. Teriparatide is administered as a 20 mcg subcutaneous daily injection, and the data show a 65% and 54% reduction in fracture risk in vertebral and non-vertebral fractures [42]. The concomitant use of bisphosphonates may attenuate bone mass improvement seen with PTH alone, but the administration of an anti-resorptive agent has to be considered after the treatment in order to maintain the bone gain achieved [43]. Maximum treatment duration of 2 years is recommended because preclinical studies showed the development of osteosarcoma in rats [42]. Asymptomatic hypercalcemia, occasional nausea, dizziness, leg cramps, and headache were associated with teriparatide use. Teriparatide is contraindicated in clinical situations with high risk of osteosarcoma, such as children and adolescents, Paget's disease, bone metastasis, skeletal irradiation, or unexplained elevations of alkaline phosphatase.

17.8 Strontium Ranelate

Strontium ranelate contains two atoms of strontium, which is a divalent cation, like calcium. It has a dual action, increasing bone formation and decreasing resorption, but its exact mechanism of action is still unclear. The SOTI (Spinal Osteoporosis Therapeutic Intervention) trial showed a fracture risk reduction of 49% in the first year of treatment with 2 g daily and of 41% during the 3-year study [44]. The TROPOS (TReatment Of Peripheral OSteoporosis) trial showed a reduction of 19% on non-vertebral fracture, and among women at high risk of hip fracture, the reduction for hip fracture was 36% [45]. The most common side effects were nausea, diarrhea, and mild and transient elevation in creatine kinase. It is contraindicated in patients at high risk of thromboembolic events, and many cases of hypersensitivity were described, with eosinophilia and systemic symptoms [46]. As strontium has a higher atomic number than calcium, it attenuates more X-rays than calcium does. This attenuation can result in an overestimation of BMD that requires an adjustment for bone strontium content [47].

17.9 New Osteoporosis Targets and New Mechanisms of Action

17.9.1 Cathepsin K Inhibitors: Odanacatib

Cathepsin K is a lysosomal enzyme produced by the osteoclast to break down the bone matrix during resorption process, and odanacatib (ODN) is a specific inhibitor of this enzyme. The phase II study showed that women receiving odanacatib for 5 years gained BMD in spine and hip, with larger reductions in bone resorption than in bone formation markers. Discontinuation of ODN resulted in reversal on these effects, with fast bone loss. Treatment with ODN for up to 5 years was generally well tolerated [48].

17.9.2 Anti-sclerostin Antibodies

Sclerostin is a protein produced almost exclusively by osteocytes, and its function is to prevent the Wnt signaling in osteoblasts. The activation of Wnt pathway in the cell membrane of osteoblasts strongly induces bone formation. New monoclonal antibodies against sclerostin have been developed and are new promising therapeutic goal for osteoporosis.

Conclusions

Osteoporosis is a very common clinical situation, with an expected trend to and increasing incidence in the next decades due to the worldwide aging of the population. Bone loss and fractures follow the decrease in estrogen levels in the postmenopausal period, which increases osteoclast activity and, subsequently, bone resorption. The adequacy of calcium intake and vitamin D status are priority measures before starting osteoporosis treatment with specific drugs, as well as encouraging physical activity and prevention of falls. Several drugs are already available with proven efficacy against fractures and excellent safety profiles, and others are in the process of being developed. The challenge today is to improve the detection of osteoporosis and convince healthcare professionals to refer at-risk patients for treatment, and, due to their different and specific mechanisms of action, it will be possible to customize the best therapeutic approach for each patient in order to optimize response to treatment both in terms of patient compliance and clinical response.

References

1. NIH consensus development panel on osteoporosis. Osteoporosis prevention, diagnosis and therapy. JAMA. 2001;285:785–95.
2. Kado DM, Browner WS, Palermo L, Nevitt MC, Genant HK, Cummings SR. Vertebral fractures and mortality in older women: a prospective study. Study of Osteoporotic Fractures Research Group. Arch Intern Med. 1999;159(11):1215–20.
3. Gold DT. The nonskeletal consequences of osteoporotic fractures. Psychologic and social outcomes. Rheum Dis Clin N Am. 2001;27:255–62.
4. Seeman E. Bone quality. Osteoporos Int. 2003;14(S5):3–7.
5. Migliaccio S, Falcone S, Spera G. Bone modeling and remodeling: from biology to clinical application. Aging Clin Exp Res. 2004;3:S20–2.
6. Migliaccio S, Brama M, Spera G. The differential effects of bisphosphonates, SERMS (selective estrogen receptor modulators), and parathyroid hormone on bone remodeling in osteoporosis. Clin Interv Aging. 2007;2(1):55–64.

7. Boivin G, Meunier PJ. Methodological considerations in measurement of bone mineral content. Osteoporos Int. 2003;14(Suppl 5):S22–7. discussion S27–8.
8. Adami S, Bertoldo F, Brandi ML, SIOMMMS, et al. Guidelines for the diagnosis, prevention and treatment of osteoporosis. Reumatismo. 2009;61(4):260–84.
9. Migliaccio S, Brama M, Malavolta N. Management of glucocorticoids-induced osteoporosis: role of teriparatide. Ther Clin Risk Manag. 2009;5(2):305–10.
10. Diez-Perez A. Bisphosphonates. Maturitas. 2002;43(Suppl):S19–26.
11. Taranta A, Brama M, et al. The selective estrogen receptor modulator Raloxifene modulates osteoblast and osteoclast activity in vitro. Bone. 2002;30:365–37.
12. Ettinger B, Black DM, et al. Reduction of vertebral fracture risk in post menopausal women with osteoporosis treated with raloxifene. Results from a 3-year randomized clinical trial. JAMA. 1999;282:637–45.
13. Chesnut CH 3rd, Silverman S, Andriano K, Genant H, Gimona A, Harris S, et al. A randomized trial of nasal spray salmon calcitonin in postmenopausal women with established osteoporosis: the prevent recurrence of osteoporotic fractures study. PROOF Study Group. Am J Med. 2000;109(4):267–76.
14. Migliaccio S, Fornari R, Greco EA, Di Luigi L, Lenzi A. New therapeutical horizons in the management of postmenopausal osteoporosis. Aging Clin Exp Res. 2013;25(Suppl 1):S117–9.
15. Hodsman AB, Bauer DC, Dempster DW, Dian L, Hanley DA, Harris ST, Kendler DL, McClung MR, Miller PD, Olszynski WP, Orwoll E, Yuen CK. Parathyroid hormone and teriparatide for the treatment of osteoporosis: a review of the evidence and suggested guidelines for its use. Endocr Rev. 2005;26(5):688–703.
16. Khosla S. Update on estrogens and the skeleton. J Clin Endocrinol Metab. 2010;95(8):3569–77.
17. Wells G, Tugwell P, Shea B, Guyatt G, Peterson J, Zytaruk N, et al. Meta-analyses of therapies for postmenopausal osteoporosis. V. Meta-analysis of the efficacy of hormone replacement therapy in treating and preventing osteoporosis in postmenopausal women. Endocr Rev. 2002;23:529–39.
18. North American Menopause Society. Management of osteoporosis in postmenopausal women: 2006 position statement of the North American Menopause Society. Menopause. 2006;13:340–67.
19. Johnell O, Scheele WH, Lu Y, Reginster JY, Need AG, Seeman E. Additive effects of raloxifene and alendronate on bone density and biochemical markers of bone remodeling in postmenopausal women with osteoporosis. J Clin Endocrinol Metab. 2002;87(3):985–92.
20. Siris ES, Harris ST, Eastell R, Zanchetta JR, Goemaere S, Diez-Perez A, Continuing Outcomes Relevant to Evista (CORE) Investigators, et al. Skeletal effects of raloxifene after 8 years: results from the continuing outcomes relevant to Evista (CORE) study. J Bone Miner Res. 2005;20(9):1514–24.
21. Barrett-Connor E, Mosca L, Collins P, Geiger MJ, Grady D, Kornitzer M, Raloxifene Use for The Heart (RUTH) Trial Investigators, et al. Effects of raloxifene on cardiovascular events and breast cancer in postmenopausal women. N Engl J Med. 2006;355(2):125–37.
22. Watts NB, Diab DL. Long-term use of bisphosphonates in osteoporosis. J Clin Endocrinol Metab. 2010;95(4):1555–65.
23. Schnitzer T, Bone HG, Crepaldi G, Adami S, McClung M, Kiel D, et al. Therapeutic equivalence of alendronate 70 mg once-weekly and alendronate 10 mg daily in the treatment of osteoporosis. Alendronate Once-Weekly Study Group. Aging (Milano). 2000;12(1):1–12.
24. Black DM, Cummings SR, Karpf DB, Cauley JA, Thompson DE, Nevitt MC, et al. Randomised trial of effect of alendronate on risk of fracture in women with existing vertebral fractures. Fracture Intervention Trial Research Group. Lancet. 1996;348(9041):1535–41.
25. Cummings SR, Black DM, Thompson DE, Applegate WB, Barrett-Connor E, Musliner TA, et al. Effect of alendronate on risk of fracture in women with low bone density but without vertebral fractures: results from the Fracture Intervention Trial. JAMA. 1998;280(24):2077–82.
26. Pols HA, Felsenberg D, Hanley DA, Stepán J, Muñoz-Torres M, Wilkin TJ, et al. Multinational, placebo-controlled, randomized trial of the effects of alendronate on bone density and fracture

risk in postmenopausal women with low bone mass: results of the FOSIT study. Fosamax International Trial Study Group. Osteoporos Int. 1999;9(5):461–8.

27. Black DM, Schwartz AV, Ensrud KE, Cauley JA, Levis S, Quandt SA, Cummings SR, FLEX Research Group, et al. Effects of continuing or stopping alendronate after 5 years of treatment: the Fracture Intervention Trial Long-term Extension (FLEX): a randomized trial. JAMA. 2006;296(24):2927–38.
28. Reginster J, Minne HW, Sorensen OH, Hooper M, Roux C, Brandi ML, et al. Randomized trial of the effects of risedronate on vertebral fractures in women with established postmenopausal osteoporosis. Vertebral Efficacy with Risedronate Therapy (VERT) Study Group. Osteoporos Int. 2000;11(1):83–91.
29. McClung MR, Geusens P, Miller PD, Zippel H, Bensen WG, Roux C, Hip Intervention Program Study Group, et al. Effect of risedronate on the risk of hip fracture in elderly women. Hip Intervention Program Study Group. N Engl J Med. 2001;344(5):333–40.
30. Chesnut IIICH, Skag A, Christiansen C, Recker R, Stakkestad JA, Hoiseth A, Oral Ibandronate Osteoporosis Vertebral Fracture Trial in North America and Europe (BONE), et al. Effects of oral ibandronate administered daily or intermittently on fracture risk in postmenopausal osteoporosis. J Bone Miner Res. 2004;19(8):1241–9.
31. Miller PD, McClung MR, Macovei L, Stakkestad JA, Luckey M, Bonvoisin B, et al. Monthly oral ibandronate therapy in postmenopausal osteoporosis: 1-year results from the MOBILE study. J Bone Miner Res. 2005;20(8):1315–22.
32. Delmas PD, Adami S, Strugala C, Stakkestad JA, Reginster JY, Felsenberg D, et al. Intravenous ibandronate injections in postmenopausal women with osteoporosis: one-year results from the dosing intravenous administration study. Arthritis Rheum. 2006;54(6):1838–46.
33. Black DM, Delmas PD, Eastell R, Reid IR, Boonen S, Cauley JA, HORIZON Pivotal Fracture Trial, et al. Once-yearly zoledronic acid for treatment of postmenopausal osteoporosis. N Engl J Med. 2007;356(18):1809–22.
34. Lyles KW, Colón-Emeric CS, Magaziner JS, Adachi JD, Pieper CF, Mautalen C, HORIZON Recurrent Fracture Trial, et al. Zoledronic acid in reducing clinical fracture and mortality after hip fracture. N Engl J Med. 2007;357:1799–809.
35. Black DM, Reid IR, Boonen S, Bucci-Rechtweg C, Cauley JA, Cosman F, et al. The effect of 3 versus 6 years of zoledronic acid treatment of osteoporosis: a randomized extension to the HORIZON-Pivotal Fracture Trial (PFT). J Bone Miner Res. 2012;27(2):243–54.
36. Boonen S, Ferrari S, Miller PD, Eriksen EF, Sambrook PN, Compston J, et al. Postmenopausal osteoporosis treatment with antiresorptives: effects of discontinuation or long-term continuation on bone turnover and fracture risk--a perspective. J Bone Miner Res. 2012;27(5):963–74.
37. Rizzoli R, Reginster JY, Boonen S, Bréart G, Diez-Perez A, Felsenberg D, et al. Adverse reactions and drug-drug interactions in the management of women with postmenopausal osteoporosis. Calcif Tissue Int. 2011;89(2):91–104.
38. Daroszewska A. Prevention and treatment of osteoporosis in women: an update. Obstet Gynaecol Reprod Med. 2012;22(6):162–9.
39. Cummings SR, San Martin J, McClung MR, Siris ES, Eastell R, Reid IR, FREEDOM Trial, et al. Denosumab for prevention of fractures in postmenopausal women with osteoporosis. N Engl J Med. 2009;361(8):756–65.
40. Bone HG, Chapurlat R, Brandi ML, Brown JP, Czerwinski E, Krieg MA, et al. The effect of three or six years of denosumab exposure in women with postmenopausal osteoporosis: results from the FREEDOM extension. J Clin Endocrinol Metab. 2013;98(11):4483–92.
41. Bone HG, Bolognese MA, Yuen CK, Kendler DL, Miller PD, Yang YC, et al. Effects of denosumab treatment and discontinuation on bone mineral density and bone turnover markers in postmenopausal women with low bone mass. J Clin Endocrinol Metab. 2011;96(4):972–80.
42. Neer RM, Arnaud CD, Zanchetta JR, Prince R, Gaich GA, Reginster JY, et al. Effect of parathyroid hormone (1-34) on fractures and bone mineral density in postmenopausal women with osteoporosis. N Engl J Med. 2001;344(19):1434–41.
43. Black DM, Greenspan SL, Ensrud KE, Palermo L, McGowan JA, Lang TF, PaTH Study Investigators, et al. The effects of parathyroid hormone and alendronate alone or in combination in postmenopausal osteoporosis. N Engl J Med. 2003;349(13):1207–15.

44. Meunier PJ, Roux C, Seeman E, Ortolani S, Badurski JE, Spector TD, et al. The effects of strontium ranelate on the risk of vertebral fracture in women with postmenopausal osteoporosis. N Engl J Med. 2004;350(5):459–68.
45. Reginster JY, Seeman E, De Vernejoul MC, Adami S, Compston J, Phenekos C, et al. Strontium ranelate reduces the risk of nonvertebral fractures in postmenopausal women with osteoporosis: treatment of peripheral osteoporosis (TROPOS) study. J Clin Endocrinol Metab. 2005;90(5):2816–22.
46. Reginster JY, Kaufman JM, Goemaere S, Devogelaer JP, Benhamou CL, Felsenberg D, et al. Maintenance of antifracture efficacy over 10 years with strontium ranelate in postmenopausal osteoporosis. Osteoporos Int. 2012;23(3):1115–22.
47. Nielsen SP, Slosman D, Sørensen OH, Basse-Cathalinat B, De Cassin P, Roux C, et al. Influence of strontium on bone mineral density and bone mineral content measurements by dual X-ray absorptiometry. J Clin Densitom. 1999;2(4):371–9.
48. Langdahl B, Binkley N, Bone H, Gilchrist N, Resch H, Rodriguez Portales J, et al. Odanacatib in the treatment of postmenopausal women with low bone mineral density: five years of continued therapy in a phase 2 study. J Bone Miner Res. 2012;27(11):2251–8.

Surgical Therapy: Vertebro-Cifoplastic: – Pros and Cons

18

Umberto Tarantino, Giuseppina Resmini, Alessando Provenza, Eleonora Piccirilli, Maurizio Feola, and Riccardo Iundusi

18.1 Introduction

The prevalence of osteoporosis increases with increasing age of the population. Osteoporosis can lead to osteoporotic vertebral compression fractures (VCFs), being the most serious complaint for elderly people worldwide, followed by hip, wrist, and ankle fractures [1]. Osteoporotic VCFs are known as low-energy fractures or insufficiency fractures because the fragility of the bone is the main cause to injury with minimal or no trauma. In fact, we can define an osteoporotic fracture if it occurs in a person as a result of little or no trauma, the equivalent of a fall from standing position or lower [2]. In the United States, there are approximately 700,000 and in Europe 450,000 cases of osteoporotic VCFs every year although only one-third are diagnosed [3]. Incidence is doubled in menopausal women, and about 8% of women over 50 years of age and 27% of women over 80 years have VCFs [4]. The vertebra is compressed resulting in a reduction of its height and an abnormal increase of the curvature of the spine with kyphosis. Vertebral fractures may be symptomatic or asymptomatic. Symptomatic, or clinical, vertebral fractures cause either sufficient pain for the patient to bring them to the attention of a health professional or a measurable loss of height. Vertebral body height may be measured at posterior, middle, and anterior parts of the vertebra. Genant's semiquantitative method is the most accepted technique to classify the changes in vertebral body in terms of reductions in overall height and also indicates fracture severity. Then, vertebral bodies can be classed as normal (grade 0), mildly deformed (grade 1,

U. Tarantino · E. Piccirilli · M. Feola · R. Iundusi
Orthopaedic and Traumatology, University of Rome "Tor Vergata", University Hospital "Policlinico Tor Vergata", Rome, Italy

G. Resmini (✉) · A. Provenza
Section of Orthopaedic and Traumatology, ASST Bergamo Ovest Hospital, Treviglio, Bergamo, Italy

A. Lenzi, S. Migliaccio (eds.), *Multidisciplinary Approach to Osteoporosis*,
https://doi.org/10.1007/978-3-319-75110-8_18

reduction between 20 and 25% in anterior, middle, and/or posterior height and a reduction of area of 10–20%), moderately deformed (grade 2, reduction between 25 and 40% in anterior, middle, and/or posterior height and a reduction of area of 20–40%), and severely deformed (≥40% reduction in any height and area) [5]. Another classification for vertebral fracture is the Magerl one [6] based on purely morphological criteria; it is the most widely used system. It distinguishes three types of fracture (A = pure compression, B = distraction, C = translation or rotation), three groups and three subgroups, using the AO codes. Its interest lies in its good predictive value, with vertebral instability increasing from type A to type C. The most important consequence of VCFs is the acute pain, which may be persistent. The pain is exacerbated by movement and reduced by rest and may therefore limit mobility. Also, the risk of pain and disability increases progressively with the number and severity of vertebral deformities. In some patients, the acute pain is followed by chronic pain with progressive loss of height, kyphosis, and impairment of daily activities. Many studies have shown that the quality of life, assessed with QUALEFFO tests, is worse in the presence of a VCF, and these are accompanied by sleep disorders, psychiatric problems, impaired mobility, pulmonary complications, and increased mortality rates [7–9]. An important consequence after the first vertebral fracture is certainly the risk of developing new vertebral fractures that increases five to ten times [10]. Vertebral fractures can be linked to the risk of having fragility refractures also to other sites like the femur, wrist, and humerus [11, 12].VCFs commonly occur in the mid-thoracic, low thoracic, and high lumbar areas and mostly at the thoracolumbar junction, especially T12 and L1 [13]. Historically, surgical treatment is indicated for patients with VCFs and neurological deficits or spinal instability. Since the surgery entails for these elderly patients with VCFs and comorbidities greater health risk, conservative treatment that consists a short period of bed rest to avoid complications caused by immobilization and external brace is recommended. Pain medication with oral analgesic and narcotics which can be effective for fracture pain are also indicated, while nonsteroidal anti-inflammatory drugs (NSAIDs) may relieve pain associated with inflammation and muscle spasm [14]. Anti-osteoporosis medications with vitamin D should be prescribed to reduce the risk of further vertebral fractures, also reducing risk of fall. Conservatively treated VCFs are cured with partial relief of pain and quality of life within 2–12 weeks [15]. However, conservative treatment with long periods of inactivity can lead these elderly patients to pneumonia, bedsores, venous thromboembolism, new VCFs, and sometimes death. Furthermore, narcotic analgesics may lead to debilitating side effects, in particular cognitive impairment, nausea, and constipation, while NSAIDs are associated with gastrointestinal side effects such as nausea, gastritis, and ulcers. Unfortunately, these side effects tend to be more pronounced in frail older people.

Open surgery with internal fixation may be performed in patients whose pain does not resolve with conservative management, but the high morbidity and the high costs of surgical treatment related to VCFs make it a duty to find alternative, more effective, and less invasive treatments than open surgery. During the past 30 years, two kinds of minimally invasive spine surgical treatment have been increasingly used. Currently, the two main minimally invasive techniques are percutaneous vertebroplasty (PVP) and kyphoplasty (PKP) [16]. Both procedures are based on the injection of a bone cement of polymethyl methacrylate (PMMA) into the fractured vertebra for the mechanical stabilization of VCFs and for pain relief. Percutaneous vertebroplasty is an injection of PMMA bone cement into the vertebral body via a needle using a transpedicular or extrapedicular approach, with monolateral or bilateral approach. It may be performed under general anesthesia, although more commonly the procedure is performed under local anesthesia [17]. Deramon and Galibert introduced for the first time PVP for the treatment of painful hemangioma in 1984 [18]: the result was so gratifying in pain relief that many other surgeons use and extended the indications for PVP including osteoporotic compression fractures, traumatic compression fractures, and painful vertebral metastases [17]. Lieberman et al. in 2001 described the initial outcome and efficacy of a new minimally invasive spine procedure in the treatment of painful VCFs, kyphoplasty [19], biomechanically developed by Reiley and Belkoff [20]. The basic ideas behind PKP were to treat kyphosis deformity and restore vertebral size: PKP is a technique that involves the introduction of inflatable bone tamps into the vertebral body. Once inflated, the bone tamps restore the vertebral body back toward its original height while creating a cavity that can be filled with bone cement.

The inflation of the device via a radiopaque liquid restores the vertebral size and helps to correct the kyphotic deformity. The balloon is deflated and replaced by a cement made of PMMA. PVP and PKP are clearly advantageous compared to conservative treatment or open surgery in terms of pain and function. In older patients, percutaneous vertebral augmentation may promote early mobilization and reduce analgesic intake [21].

The analgesic effect of bone cement injection into the vertebra may result from the fixing of microfractures and the decrease of the mechanical stresses associated with the body weight and mobility. Furthermore, nerve endings are destroyed by the cytotoxic and exothermic action during the polymerization of the bone cement, reducing the pain. However, the benefits and shortcomings of these two techniques are still debated such as height restoration and bone cement leakage [22]. The maximum number of vertebrae augmentable per session should be three, although extensive augmentation to more than three vertebral levels per session has been shown as feasible [23].

Conventional radiographs are usually the first technique used to study patients with suspected vertebral fracture in osteoporotic patients. A 20% vertebral body height loss or 4 mm of vertebral height reduction constitutes the diagnosis of a vertebral compression fracture. But in many cases of osteoporotic vertebral fractures, morphologic changes may require time for their development. Therefore, the absence of a fracture on X-ray in an osteoporotic patient does not rule it out, and when symptoms persist, a magnetic resonance imaging (MRI) should be performed. In order to identify the VCFs with or without vertebral deformities and degree of edema, assess its age, define its anatomy, assess the posterior wall of the vertebral body, and exclude other causes of back pain, MRI is a requisite to screen all patients who are considered for planning medical, PVP, PKP, or open surgical treatment [24]. The presence of a pattern of bone marrow edema is associated with a good clinical short-term success relieving pain [25]. However, CT scanning or bone scintigraphy may be used instead when MRI is unsafe (e.g., in patients with pacemakers). CT equipment is also required if there are any doubts regarding the integrity of the posterior vertebral wall [26].

18.2 Technical Issues

PVP is performed under radiological guidance using fluoroscopy. It is usually performed using local anesthesia of the skin, subcutaneous tissue, and the periosteum of the vertebral body into which the needle is to be introduced; sometimes conscious sedation is an addiction. The patient is clearly positioned prone. A small skin incision is made and a disposable bone biopsy needle or trocar needle is placed centrally in the vertebral body using an image-guided safe access route. This may be done bilaterally or monolaterally through the pedicle, obliquely across one pedicle, or laterally oblique through the base of the pedicle. Under constant screening with X-ray image intensifier, it is advanced through the pedicle into the vertebral body; an orthopedic hammer can be useful in case of sclerotic cortical bone. The cement is then injected very slowly, again under constant fluoroscopic screening.

In unilateral approach, rotating the trocar tip, the cement can be spread throughout the vertebral body. In bilateral approach to achieve optimal vertebral filling, two trocars may be used, one on either side of the midline. The procedure may last from 15 min to 1 h, depending on the number of vertebrae being treated and the experience of the surgeon. Computed tomography (CT) scanning could be indicated at the end of the procedure to assess the distribution of cement and identify any complications [27].

PKP is a variant of PVP in which one or two balloon-like devices are inserted bilaterally into the vertebral body, through a transpedicular approach. A small balloon catheter surrounded by a metal stent is inserted into the vertebral body using a minimally invasive percutaneous approach under radiographic guidance and either local or general anesthetic. The balloon catheter is then inflated with liquid, under pressure, to create a cavity in which the stent is expanded. Balloons are slowly inflated until they reach their highest achievable volume, in order to restore vertebral body height. The balloons are then deflated and removed, leaving a cavity which is filled with PMMA bone cement; because of the existence of the cavity, the cement may be injected at a lower pressure than that used for PVP. The injected cement hardens within 1 h, and the patient may then be mobilized [17].

PVP and PKP are traditionally performed using PMMA to which a radiopaque substance such as barium, tantalum, or tungsten sulfate has been added to facilitate visualization during the procedure when polymerization of methyl methacrylate monomers to PMMA polymers occurs. It is prepared by mixing a liquid component containing the monomer, accelerator, and inhibitor with a powder containing the polymer, radio-opacifier, and initiator. It is cheap and easy to manipulate and gives the appropriate stiffness and strength to the vertebral body. However, there are no osteoinductive or osteoconductive properties and, therefore, no integration with host bone over time. Its stiffness may promote mechanical overload to adjacent vertebral bodies [28]. PMMA appears to have analgesic properties quite apart from those caused by the effect of the stability provided by the cement within the weakened vertebrae. The reason for such analgesic properties remains unclear, but one possibility is that it destroys or damages local nerve endings as a result of both the toxic effects of the free monomers of PMMA and the heat caused by the cement polymerization [29].

18.3 Criteria for Treatment

The National Institute for Health and Care Excellence guidance indicates that PVP and PKP should be limited to patients whose pain is refractory to more conservative treatment for PKP; there is an additional requirement that they should have continued vertebral collapse and severe pain [30, 31]. Recent guidance from the Cardiovascular and Interventional Radiology Society of Europe (CIRSE) states that PVP is indicated in patients with "painful osteoporotic VCFs refractory to medical treatment." It defines failure of medical treatment as "minimal or no pain relief with the administration of physician-prescribed analgesics for 3 weeks or achievement of adequate pain relief with only narcotic dosages that induce excessive intolerable sedation, confusion, or constipation." In case of painful patients at high risk of complications resulting from immobility (e.g., thrombophlebitis, DVT, pneumonia, or pressure ulcer), CIRSE guidelines further note that PVP may be considered at the beginning.

Contraindications

The CIRSE guidelines list the following absolute contraindications to PVP:

- Asymptomatic vertebral body compression fracture
- Patient improving on medical treatment
- Osteomyelitis, discitis, or active systemic infection
- Uncorrectable coagulopathy
- Allergy to bone cement or opacification agents
- Prophylaxis in osteoporotic patients

Relative contraindications in osteoporotic patients include:

- Radicular pain
- Tumor extension into the vertebral canal or cord compression
- Fracture of the posterior column and increased risk of cement leak
- Vertebral collapse >70% of body height (needle placement might be difficult)
- Spinal canal stenosis and asymptomatic retropulsion of a fracture fragment causing significant spinal canal compromise
- Patients with more than five metastases or diffuse metastases
- Lack of surgical backup and monitoring facilities

These contraindications appear to be equally applicable to PKP.

18.4 Clinical Evidences of PVP and PKP

PVP and PKP are therapeutic alternatives for patients in whom conservative treatment failed. They are minimally invasive procedures and seem to determine a rapid and sustained pain relief with a better quality of life. Although many studies have shown good clinical outcomes and improved quality of life after PVP and PKP, there is an ongoing debate on which of these two procedures can provide the most important efficacy and safety.

Analgesic effect of these techniques can be related to some factors, such as the thermal effect of the cement that produces the ablation of C-nociceptive fibers, the mechanical stabilization of the fracture, and the height restoration of the vertebral body [32]. Compared with medical treatments, short-term pain relief and long-term beneficial effects after PVP seem to be significantly superior [33]. Recent studies demonstrated that most patients who had favorable clinical results with conservative treatment for 3 weeks after the fracture also had successful clinical results at 1 year. If the patient failed conservative treatment, percutaneous cement augmentation also showed excellent results at 1 year after the trauma. However, the long conservative treatment period of 3 weeks has been criticized by other authors [34].

A follow-up survey indicated that patients who underwent percutaneous vertebroplasty were significantly more satisfied with given treatment than patients who underwent conservative treatment. In addition, lower rate of complications was observed in percutaneous vertebroplasty group [35].

Postoperative pain relief in osteoporotic VCFs has been shown in the literature using PVP and PKP, which was measured by the VAS pain scale. However, many studies showed that the follow-up point at which the difference becomes really insignificant varies after 3, 6, or 12 months [36]. Improvement in VAS score was not statistically significant between PVP and PKP groups. The potential reason for the similar pain scores is that clinical heterogeneity was induced by a double blind, the duration of illness, types of fractures, gender differences, and insufficient sample size bias [37]. Moreover, the natural history for spontaneous pain reduction is 3 months [38].

In this context, the results from a recent meta-analysis are focused on the timing in case of significant VAS reduction and showed that PKP has significantly lower VAS scores in the short-term follow-up, but at long-term follow-up, results were comparable [39].

Compared with medical treatments, two prospective controlled studies evaluated and compared the efficacy and safety of PKP and found better long-term pain relief and superior functional outcome up to 3 years [40, 41]. It was shown that both PKP and PVP can restore kyphosis. According to this meta-analysis, the angle of postoperative kyphosis was significantly improved in the short- and long-term follow-up in the PKP group. Patients who underwent PKP had a higher kyphosis angle improvement if compared with patients who underwent PVP, and there was a slight loss of kyphosis angle correction between the short- and long-term follow-up. As reported in previous studies, the improvement in kyphosis angle with PKP and PVP has been attributed in part to the lying position that patients assume during the operation and in part to the failure of the two end plates of the fractured vertebra. PKP corrects the kyphotic deformity through the expansion of a balloon, and this seems to be more beneficial to restore the vertebral size and correct the kyphotic deformity compared to PVP. A further advantage of PKP is the creation by the inflatable balloon of a cavity, which allows to inject larger quantities of cement compared to PVP [42]. Mechanical stabilization of the vertebral body relies on quantity and localization of the injected cement. The filling of 16–30% of the volume could recover the vertebral stiffness partially at the pre-fracture state, and this would be enough to obtain clinical healing [43]. Cadaveric studies have shown that kyphoplasty had greater recovery of vertebral height than vertebroplasty [44]. However, clinical studies are contradictory. Some authors found greater height restoration with kyphoplasty, but others did not find differences between both techniques [45]. Some studies found no better pain resolution with height restoration and do not consider this factor mandatory in order to achieve pain control [46].

Meta-analysis of published papers shows fair to good evidence that in patients with osteoporotic VCF outcomes on physical disability, general health and pain relief are better with PVP and PKP than with medical management within the first 3–6 months after intervention [47]. There is fair evidence that by the first or second year after intervention, PVP provides a similar degree of pain control and physical function as that obtained with optimal medical management. PKP seems to be superior to PVP according to short-term pain relief, kyphosis angle correction, and cement leakage.

A recently presented preliminary 1-year results of the multicenter randomized controlled Fracture Reduction Evaluation (FREE) study confirmed in the kyphoplasty group a significant improvement of the quality of life and VAS scale pain scores and function after 1 month controlled against nonsurgical treatment. These treatment effects diminished dramatically until the 12-month follow-up but were still significantly better than nonsurgical treatment for quality of life [40].

Controversy remains regarding whether a unilateral or a bilateral approach is superior, and there are no large studies comparing these two approaches. A recent meta-analysis tried to find if there is an evidence to suggest a benefit in clinical outcome of a unilateral kyphoplasty or bilateral kyphoplasties, but no clinically important differences were found between them. Only considering less operation time and less cost, a unilateral percutaneous kyphoplasty could be considered an advantageous method. [48]

Women with preexisting VCFs have a four times increased risk of subsequent vertebral fracture, but these fractures seem to be not different between the PKP and PVP groups [49]. There is insufficient evidence whether PKP results in greater pain relief 1 and 2 years after intervention [50].

18.5 Complications of PVP and PKP

International literature is unanimous about the low rate of complications associated with PVP and PKP when treating osteoporotic VCFs [43]. The cement leakage is one of the most common complications associated with PKP and PVP. Leakage occurs when the cement is not wholly contained by the fractured vertebra but escapes through either the fracture or the track created by the needle. Systematic reviews provided that little cement leakage is found after PVP and PKP by the standard X-ray imaging, whereas high rates are observed with computed tomography [51]. There are many routes by which cement may leak from a vertebra: paravertebral leakage, venous leakage, or leakage into the spinal canal and intervertebral foramen. Injury of the surrounding soft tissues is mainly due to the high temperature of polymerization of PMMA. The most sensitive structures are neural tissues, spinal cord, and nerve roots. Fortunately, most of the extravasations are to the disc or paravertebral tissues, hence asymptomatic. Transient radicular symptoms have been described in up to 3–4% of the patients, and only isolated cases of paraplegia after these procedures have been reported, most of them due to failure of technical issues. The monomers that do not contribute to the polymerization have systemic cardiopulmonary effects. Pulmonary embolism can be due not only to the cement but also to the fat from the bone marrow extruded into the venous system by the high-pressure cement injection or by inflating the balloons [52]. Although all of the included studies reported the incidence of cement leakage, no cases of spinal stenosis and pulmonary embolism due to cement leakage were reported. The Food and Drug Administration (FDA) states that PMMA is contraindicated in the presence of active or incompletely treated infection at the site where the cement is to be applied. It also notes that hypotensive reactions have been noted between 10 and 165 s after its application; as these have lasted from 30 s to over 5 min, and some have progressed to cardiac arrest, the FDA recommends that patients should be monitored carefully for any changes in blood pressure during and immediately following the application of the cement. Other reported adverse events include pyrexia due to allergy to the cement. In addition, the FDA notes that the heat released while the cement is hardening in situ may damage the bone or other tissues surrounding the implant [53].

In a systematic review of the literatures, the risk of experiencing new VCFs increased after PVP and PKP. Retrospective and prospective studies found an incidence of recompression of 12.5–36.8% after PVP and PKP [54, 55]. From the standpoint of vertebrae, adjacent recompression occurred more frequently than distant levels, and it demonstrated a remarkable propensity of refractures within three levels above or below preexisting fractures [56]. The exact mechanism for refracture is still unclear. Several authors indicate that the cemented vertebra can change the biomechanics of the spine with increased stresses and strains and therefore may increase the incidence of new adjacent VCFs. The greater height of the collapsed vertebra increases the tension of the soft tissues around it and can lead to an increase of the load on other vertebrae, especially adjacent [57]. Other authors also suggest that a wedge-shaped fracture increases the flexion bending moment due to the upper body weight, and thus a higher muscle force in the erector spinae is required to balance the spine, which results in a higher spinal load and a higher intradiscal pressure [58]. The erector spinae are a long muscle, and thus its force affects intradiscal pressure not only at adjacent levels but also the whole region.

Conclusion

PVP and PKP are two minimally invasive spine augmentation procedures which can increase bone strength as well as reduce the pain produced by VCFs, and both techniques depend on PMMA cement injection into the fractured vertebra for mechanical fixation. The advantage of PVP and PKP in comparison to conservative treatment including bed rest, painkillers, and bracing or open surgery has been well established in terms of pain and functional outcome. PVP and PKP produce immediate pain relief, and when compared with conservative management at least at 1 year, PVP and PKP are superior on clinical improvement with reduction in the use of analgesic drugs. Furthermore, PKP can restore the vertebral height in VCFs. Anyhow some studies report that there are no statistically significant differences in the vertebral height restoration and kyphosis angle correction of between PKP and PVP.

Cement leakage and new VCFs at the adjacent level are the most common complications. Cement leakage is more frequent in PVP [59]. Leakage into the disc space is more frequent in cases of cortical defect of the end plate or vertebral cleft than intrasomatic collapse, but there is no statistically significant correlation between intradiscal leakage and fracture severity, kyphosis angle, treated level, age, and sex of the patient [60]. High-viscosity PMMA significantly reduces the risk of leakage and related complications, and lower amount of cement is required [61].

According to the literature, the "domino" effect is present in both PVP and PKP but with different results probably depending on the heterogeneous characteristics of the patients studied. Hierholzer et al. reported 16% of new symptomatic VCFs after PVP but without considering new asymptomatic VCFs [62]. Klazen et al. reported 19.7% of new VCFs following PVP, but no statistically significant difference on the incidence of subsequent vertebral fractures between vertebroplasty and conservative treatment was found [63]. Different studies reported a higher incidence (15–25%) of consequent vertebral fracture after PKP compared with PVP; consequent fractures occur more frequently at the adjacent level to the treated vertebra [64–66].

From a biomechanical point of view, 2 ml of bone cement is sufficient to reinstate the bone strength of the vertebral body [67], but it has been calculated that the minimum dose of cement required to restore the resistance is about 16% of the vertebral volume, while the quantity necessary to restore vertebral hardness is 30%; then, as the vertebral bodies have different volumes depending on the segment concerned, it must take into account the level to be treated. Injection of large amounts of cement in order to obtain a better result is not needed; according to Kaufmann et al., there was no significant association between the volume of the cement injected and the clinical outcomes of postprocedure pain and medication use [68]. PMMA can cause adverse reactions during the polymerization (exothermic reaction) and have toxic effects. Within the vertebral body, the PMMA becomes a stranger inert body with disappearance of metabolic bone turnover, and for this reason new biocompatible, biodegradable, bioactive, and osteoconductive cements are the subject of numerous biomechanical and clinical investigations [69–73].

The ideal cement should be absorbable, nontoxic, with low polymerization temperature, biomechanically similar to the bone, and bioactive. The appropriate treatment of osteoporotic vertebral fractures requires understanding the effect of the disease on the material and structural properties of the bone tissue and the fracture healing process [74].

The careful reviewing of valid scientific publications shows that both vertebro- and kyphoplasty are effective and safe as minimally invasive procedures in the treatment of symptomatic vertebral collapse, but before using such procedures, it is important to keep in mind that the percutaneous interventional cementation methods do not treat the underlying metabolic bone fragility condition. They should be performed only after at least 3 weeks of unuseful conservative treatment, and they have better results when applied to antiosteoporotic therapy and physiotherapy. PVP and PKP are not free from complications and should be performed in multi-specialist centers with the presence of a multidisciplinary team (fracture unit), requiring an adequate informed consent of the patient as there are no absolute international guidelines based on evidence criteria.

Toolbox for Guidance

- Vertebro- and kyphoplasty are effective and safe as minimally invasive procedures in the treatment of symptomatic vertebral fractures, but they do not deal with the poor bone quality condition affecting osteoporotic patients (*grade A recommendation*).
- Vertebroplasty and kyphoplasty have better long-term pain relief and superior functional outcome up to 3 years if compared to conservative treatment (bed rest, painkillers, and bracing), and they should be performed only after at least 3 weeks of unuseful conservative treatment (*grade A and B recommendation*).
- The most frequent complications after vertebroplasty and kyphoplasty are cement leakage and new vertebral fractures at the adjacent level (*grade A recommendation*).
- These treatments should be always integrated with antiosteoporotic therapy and physical exercise if it is possible (*grade A and B recommendation*).

Case 1: L4 bone cement vertebroplasty for VCF in a 49-year-old glucocorticoid-induced osteoporotic woman

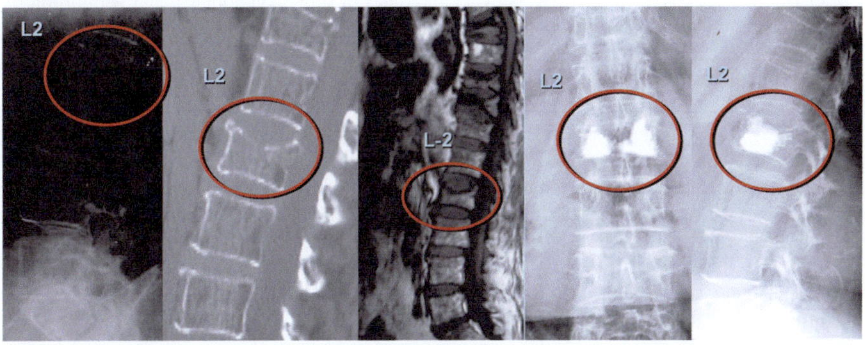

Case 2: L2 kyphoplasty (Vessel-X®) for VCF in a 65-year-old woman with multiple myeloma

References

1. Silverman SL. The clinical consequences of vertebral compression fracture. Bone. 1992;13(Suppl 2):S27–31.
2. Consensus development conference: diagnosis, prophylaxis, and treatment of osteoporosis. Am J Med. 1993;94:646–50.
3. Dennison E, Cooper C. Epidemiology of osteoporotic fractures. Horm Res. 2000;54(Suppl 1):58–63.
4. Bonnick SL. Osteoporosis in men and women. Clin Cornerstone. 2006;8:28–39.
5. Genant HK, Wu CY, van Kuijk C, Nevitt MC. Vertebral fracture assessment using a semiquantitative technique. J Bone Miner Res. 1993;8:1137–48.
6. Magerl F, Aebi M, Gertzbein SD, Harms J, Nazarian S. A comprehensive classifi-cation of thoracic and lumbar injuries. Eur Spine J. 1994;3(4):184–201.
7. Miyakoshi N, Itoi E, Kobayashi M, Kodama H. Impact of postural deformities and spinal mobility on quality of life in postmenopausal osteoporosis. Osteoporos Int. 2003;14(12):1007–12.
8. David C, Confavreux CB, Mehsen N, Paccou J, Leboime A, Legrand E. Severity of osteoporosis: what is the impact of co-morbidities? Joint Bone Spine. 2010;77(Suppl 2):S103–6.
9. Lombardi I Jr, Oliveira LM, Mayer AF, Jardim JR, Natour J. Evaluation of pulmonary function and quality of life in women with osteoporosis. Osteoporos Int. 2005;16(10):1247–53.

10. Lindsay R, Silverman SL, Cooper C, Hanley DA, Barton I, Broy SB, Licata A, Benhamou L, Geusens P, Flowers K, Stracke H, Seeman E. Risk of new vertebral fracture in the year following a fracture. JAMA. 2001;285:320–3.
11. Gallacher SJ, Gallagher AP, McQuillian C, Mitchell PJ, Dixon T. The prevalence of vertebral fracture amongst patients presenting with non-vertebral fractures. Osteoporos Int. 2007;18(2):185–92.
12. Ledlie JT, Renfro M. Balloon kyphoplasty: one-year outcomes in vertebral body height restoration, chronic pain, and activity levels. J Neurosurg. 2003;98:36–42.
13. Hansen L, Petersen KD, Eriksen SA, Langdahl BL, Eiken PA, Brixen K, Abrahamsen B, Jensen JE, Harsløf T, Vestergaard P. Subsequent fracture rates in a nationwide population-based cohort study with a 10-year perspective. Osteoporos Int. 2015;26(2):513–9.
14. Prather H, Hunt D, Watson JO, Gilula LA. Conservative care for patients with osteoporotic vertebral compression fractures. Phys Med Rehabil Clin North Am. 2007;18:577–91.
15. Brown CJ, Friedkin RJ, Inouye SK. Prevalence and outcomes of low mobility in hospitalized older patients. J Am Geriatr Soc. 2004;52:1263–70.
16. Garfin SR, Yuan HA, Reiley MA. New technologies in spine: kyphoplasty and vertebroplasty for the treatment of painful osteoporotic compression fractures. Spine. 2001;26:1511–5.
17. Hargunani R, Le Corroller T, Khashoggi K, Murphy KJ, Munk PL. Percutaneous vertebral augmentation: the status of vertebroplasty and current controversies. Semin Musculoskelet Radiol. 2011;15:117–24.
18. Galibert P, Deramond H, Rosat P, Le Gars D. Preliminary note on the treatment of vertebral angioma by percutaneous acrylic vertebroplasty. Neurochirurgie. 1987;33:166–8.
19. Lieberman IH, Dudeney S, Reinhardt MK, Bell G. Initial outcome and efficacy of "kyphoplasty" in the treatment of painful osteoporotic vertebral compression fractures. Spine (Phila Pa 1976). 2001;26(14):1631–8.
20. Belkoff SM, Mathis JM, Fenton DC, Scribner RM, Reiley ME, Talmadge K. An ex vivo biomechanical evaluation of an inflatable bone tamp used in the treatment of compression fracture. Spine (Phila Pa 1976). 2001;26(2):151–6.
21. Weninger P, Schultz A, Hertz H. Conservative management of thoracolumbar and lumbar spine compression and burst fractures: functional and radiographic outcomes in 136 cases treated by closed reduction and casting. Arch Orthop Trauma Surg. 2009;129:207–19.
22. Chandra RV, Yoo AJ, Hirsch JA. Vertebral augmentation: update on safety, efficacy, cost effectiveness and increased survival? Pain Phys. 2013;16:309–20.
23. Mailli L, Filippiadis DK, Brountzos EN, Alexopoulou E, Kelekis N, Kelekis A. Clinical outcome and safety of multilevel: clinical experience and results. Cardiovasc Intervent Radiol. 2013;36:183–91.
24. Cuénod CA, Laredo JD, Chevret S, Hamze B, Naouri JF, Chapaux X, Bondeville JM, Tubiana JM. Acute vertebral collapse due to osteoporosis or malignancy: appearance on unenhanced and gadolinium-enhanced MR images. Radiology. 1996;199:541–9.
25. Garfin SR, Buckley RA, Ledlie J. Balloon kyphoplasty for symptomatic vertebral body compression fractures results in rapid, significant, and sustained improvements in back pain, function, and quality of life for elderly patients. Spine (Phila Pa 1976). 2006;31:2213–20.
26. Gangi A, Sabharwal T, Irani FG, Buy X, Morales JP, Adam A, et al. Quality assurance guidelines for percutaneous vertebroplasty. Cardiovasc Intervent Radiol. 2006;29:173–8.
27. Kamath S, Venkatanarasimha N, Silver DAT. Percutaneous vertebroplasty. CPD J Radiol Update 2007; 6:82–96 and National institute for health and care excellence interventional procedures programme. Interventional procedure overview of percutaneous vertebroplasty (methyl methacrylate). London: NICE; 2003.
28. Blattert TR, Jestaedt L, Weckbach A. Suitability of a calcium phosphate cement in osteoporotic vertebral body fracture augmentation: a controlled, randomized, clinical trial of balloon kyphoplasty comparing calcium phosphate versus polymethylmethacrylate. Spine (Phila Pa 1976). 2009;34:108–14.
29. Kamath S, Venkatanarasimha N, Silver DAT. Percutaneous vertebroplasty. CPD J Radiol Update. 2007;6:82–96.

30. National Institute for Health and Care Excellence. Interventional procedure guidance 12: percutaneous vertebroplasty. London: NICE; 2003.
31. National Institute for Health and Care Excellence. Interventional procedure guidance 166: Balloon kyphoplasty for vertebral compression fractures. London: NICE; 2006.
32. Grohs JG, Matzner M, Trieb K, Krepler P. Minimal invasive stabilization of osteoporotic vertebral fractures: a prospective nonrandomized comparison of vertebroplasty and balloon kyphoplasty. J Spinal Disord Tech. 2005;18:238–42.
33. Grados F, Depriester C, Cayrolle G, Hardy N, Deramond H, Fardellone P. Long-term observations of vertebral osteoporotic fractures treated by percutaneous vertebroplasty. Rheumatology (Oxford). 2000;39:1410–4.
34. Lee HM, Park SY, Lee SH, Suh SW, Hong JY. Comparative analysis of clinical outcomes in patients with osteoporotic vertebral compression fractures (OVCFs): conservative treatment versus balloon kyphoplasty. Spine J. 2012;12:998–1005.
35. Yang EZ, Xu JG, Huang GZ, Xiao WZ, Liu XK, Zeng BF, Lian XF. Percutaneous vertebroplasty versus conservative treatment in aged patients with acute osteoporotic vertebral compression fractures: a prospective randomized controlled clinical study. Spine (Phila Pa 1976). 2016;41(8):653–60.
36. Rousing R, Hansen KL, Andersen MO, Jespersen SM, Thomsen K, Lauritsen JM. Twelve-months follow-up in forty-nine patients with acute/semiacute osteoporotic vertebral fractures treated conservatively or with percutaneous vertebroplasty: a clinical randomized study. Spine (PhilaPa 1976). 2010;35:478–82.
37. Shi-Ming G, Wen-Juan L, Yun-Mei H, et al. Percutaneous vertebroplasty and percutaneous balloon kyphoplasty for osteoporotic vertebral compression fracture: a metaanalysis. Indian J Orthop. 2015;49(4):377–87.
38. Cummings SR, Melton LJ. Epidemiology and outcomes of osteoporotic fractures. Lancet. 2002;359:1761–7.
39. Wang H, Sribastav SS, Ye F, et al. Comparison of percutaneous vertebroplasty and balloon kyphoplasty for the treatment of single level vertebral compression fractures: a meta-analysis of the literature. Pain Physician. 2015;18(3):209–22.
40. Wardlaw D, Cummings SR, Van Meirhaeghe J, Bastian L, Tillman JB, Ranstam J, Eastell R, Shabe P, Talmadge K, Boonen S. Efficacy and safety of balloon kyphoplasty compared with non-surgical care for vertebral compression fracture (FREE): a randomised controlled trial. Lancet. 2009;373:1016–24.
41. Kasperk C, Grafe IA, Schmitt S, Nöldge G, Weiss C, Da Fonseca K, Hillmeier J, Libicher M, Sommer U, Rudofsky G, Meeder PJ, Nawroth P. Three-year outcomes after kyphoplasty in patients with osteoporosis with painful vertebral fractures. J Vasc Interv Radiol. 2010;21:701–9.
42. Röllinghoff M, Siewe J, Zarghooni K, Sobottke R, Alparslan Y, Eysel P, et al. Effectiveness, security and height restoration on fresh compression fractures–a comparative prospective study of vertebroplasty and kyphoplasty. Minim Invasive Neurosurg. 2009;52:233–7.
43. Molloy S, Mathis JM, Belkoff SM. The effect of vertebral body percentage fill on mechanical behavior during percutaneous vertebroplasty. Spine (Phila Pa 1976). 2003;28(14):1549–54.
44. Hiwatashi A, Yoshiura T, Yamashita K, Kamano H, Dashjamts T, Honda H. Morphologic change in vertebral body after percutaneous vertebroplasty: follow-up with MDCT. AJR Am J Roentgenol. 2010;195:W207–12.
45. Hiwatashi A, Westesson PL, Yoshiura T, Noguchi T, Togao O, Yamashita K, Kamano H, Honda H. Kyphoplasty and vertebroplasty produce the same degree of height restoration. AJNR Am J Neuroradiol. 2009;30:669–73.
46. Feltes C, Fountas KN, Machinis T, Nikolakakos LG, Dimopoulos V, Davydov R, Kassam M, Johnston KW, Robinson JS. Immediate and early postoperative pain relief after kyphoplasty without significant restoration of vertebral body height in acute osteoporotic vertebral fractures. Neurosurg Focus. 2005;18:e5.
47. Klazen CA, Lohle PN, de Vries J, Jansen FH, Tielbeek AV, Blonk MC, Venmans A, van Rooij WJ, Schoemaker MC, Juttmann JR, Lo TH, Verhaar HJ, van der Graaf Y, van Everdingen

KJ, Muller AF, Elgersma OE, Halkema DR, Fransen H, Janssens X, Buskens E, Mali WP. Vertebroplasty versus conservative treatment in acute osteoporotic vertebral compression fractures (Vertos II): an open-label randomised trial. Lancet. 2010;376(9746):1085–92.
48. Huang Z, Wan S, Ning L, Han S. Is unilateral kyphoplasty as effective and safe as bilateral kyphoplasties for osteoporotic vertebral compression fractures? A meta-analysis. Clin Orthop Relat Res. 2014;472:2833–42.
49. Taylor RS, Fritzell P, Taylor RI. Balloon kyphoplasty in the measurement of vertebral compression fractures: an update systematic review and meta-analysis. Eur Spine J. 2007;16(8):1085–100.
50. McGirt MJ, Parker SL, Wolinsky JP, Witham TF, Bydon A, Gokaslan ZL. Vertebroplasty and kyphoplasty for the treatment of vertebral compression fractures: an evidenced based review of the literature. Spine J. 2009;9:501–8.
51. McCall T, Cole C, Dailey A. Vertebroplasty and kyphoplasty: a comparative review of efficacy and adverse events. Curr Rev Musculoskelet Med. 2008;1:17–23.
52. Choe DH, Marom EM, Ahrar K, Truong MT, Madewell JE. Pulmonary embolism of polymethyl methacrylate during percutaneous vertebroplasty and kyphoplasty. AJR Am J Roentgenol. 2004;183(4):1097–102.
53. FDA. Class II special controls guidance document: Polymethylmethacrylate (PMMA) bone cement: guidance for industry and FDA. 2011. URL: www.fda.gov/medicaldevices/deviceregulationandguidance/guidancedocuments/ucm072795.html.
54. Kim YY, Rhyu KW. Recompression of vertebral body after balloon kyphoplasty for osteoporotic vertebral compression fracture. Eur Spine J. 2010;19:1907–12.
55. Tanigawa N, Komemushi A, Kariya S, et al. Radiological follow-up of new compression fractures following percutaneous vertebroplasty. Cardiovasc Intervent Radiol. 2006;29:92–6.
56. Johannes H, Heiko F, Kerstin Wet al. Incidence of symptomatic vertebral fractures in patients after percutaneous vertebroplasty. Cardiovasc Intervent Radiol. 2006;29:92–6.
57. Micael NT, Susan MR, Frank MP, et al. Altered disc-pressure profile after an osteoporotic vertebral fracture in a risk factor for adjacent vertebral body fracture. Eur Spine J. 2008;17:1522–430.
58. Rohlmann A, Zander T, Bergmann G, et al. Spinal loads after osteoporotic vertebral fractures treated by vertebroplasty or kyphoplasty. Eur Spine J. 2006;15:1255–64.
59. Eck JC, Nachtigall D, Humphreys SC, Hodges SD. Comparison of vertebroplasty and balloon kyphoplasty for treatment of vertebral compression fractures: a meta-analysis of the literature. Spine J. 2008;8(3):488–97.
60. Hiwatashi A, Ohgiya Y, Kakimoto N, Westesson PL. Cement leakage during vertebroplasty can be predicted on preoperative MRI. AJR Am J Roentgenol. 2007;188(4):1089–93.
61. Anselmetti GC, Zoarski G, Manca A, Masala S, Eminefendic H, Russo F, Regge D. Percutaneous vertebroplasty and bone cement leakage: clinical experience with a new high-viscosity bone cement and delivery system for vertebral augmentation in benign and malignant compression fractures. Cardiovasc Intervent Radiol. 2008;31(5):937–47.
62. Hierholzer J, Fuchs H, Westphalen K, Baumann C, Slotosch C, Schulz R. Incidence of symptomatic vertebral fractures in patients after percutaneous vertebroplasty. Cardiovasc Intervent Radiol. 2008;31(6):1178–83.
63. Klazen CA, Venmans A, de Vries J, van Rooij WJ, Jansen FH, Blonk MC, Lohle PN, Juttmann JR, Buskens E, van Everdingen KJ, Muller A, Fransen H, Elgersma OE, Mali WP, Verhaar HJ. Percutaneous vertebroplasty is not a risk factor for new osteoporotic compression fractures: results from VERTOS II. AJNR Am J Neuroradiol. 2010;31(8):1447–50.
64. Campbell PG, Harrop JS. Incidence of fracture in adjacent levels in patients treated with balloon kyphoplasty: a review of the literature. Curr Rev Musculoskelet Med. 2008;1(1):61–4.
65. Taylor RS, Taylor RJ, Fritzell P. Balloon kyphoplasty and vertebroplasty for vertebral compression fractures: a comparative systematic review of efficacy and safety. Spine (Phila Pa 1976). 2006;31(23):2747–55.
66. Frankel BM, Monroe T, Wang C. Percutaneous vertebral augmentation: an elevation in adjacent-level fracture risk in kyphoplasty as compared with vertebroplasty. Spine J. 2007;7(5):575–82.

67. Belkoff SM, Mathis JM, Jasper LE, Deramond H. The biomechanics of vertebroplasty. The effect of cement volume on mechanical behavior. Spine (Phila Pa 1976). 2001;26(14):1537–41.
68. Kaufmann TJ, Trout AT, Kallmes DF. The effects of cement volume on clinical outcomes of percutaneous vertebroplasty. AJNR Am J Neuroradiol. 2006;27(9):1933–7.
69. Zheng Z, Luk KD, Kuang G, Li Z, Lin J, Lam WM, Cheung KM, Lu WW. Vertebral augmentation with a novel Vessel-X bone void filling container system and bioactive bone cement. Spine (Phila Pa 1976). 2007;32(19):2076–82.
70. Bae H, Shen M, Maurer P, Peppelman W, Beutler W, Linovitz R, Westerlund E, Peppers T, Lieberman I, Kim C, Girardi F. Clinical experience using Cortoss for treating vertebral compression fractures with vertebroplasty and kyphoplasty: twenty four-month follow-up. Spine (Phila Pa 1976). 2010;35(20):E1030–6.
71. Rauschmann M, Vogl T, Verheyden A, Pflugmacher R, Werba T, Schmidt S, Hierholzer J. Bioceramic vertebral augmentation with a calcium sulphate/hydroxyapatite composite (Cerament SpineSupport): in vertebral compression fractures due to osteoporosis. Eur Spine J. 2010;19(6):887–92.
72. Tomita S, Molloy S, Jasper LE, Abe M, Belkoff SM. Biomechanical comparison of kyphoplasty with different bone cements. Spine (Phila Pa 1976). 2004;29(11):1203–7.
73. Belkoff SM, Mathis JM, Deramond H, Jasper LE. An ex vivo biomechanical evaluation of a hydroxyapatite cement for use with kyphoplasty. AJNR Am J Neuroradiol. 2001;22(6):1212–6.
74. Ekman EF. The role of the orthopaedic surgeon in minimizing mortality and morbidity associated with fragility fractures. J Am Acad Orthop Surg. 2010;18(5):278–85.

Rehabilitation Therapy After Surgery in Osteoporotic Patients

19

Francesca Gimigliano, Alessandro de Sire, Antimo Moretti, Claudio Curci, and Giovanni Iolascon

19.1 Introduction

The most serious complication of osteoporosis is the fragility fracture. These fractures can cause increased long-term morbidity, functional limitation, decreased health-related quality of life (HRQoL), and mortality [1]. In many cases, a surgical approach with subsequent rehabilitative treatment is required. The main objectives of surgery and postoperative rehabilitation are to restore pre-fracture functioning and to prevent and treat complications like thrombosis, muscular contractures, and immobility syndrome [2]. The process ends when the patient is able to return to a full functional activity level, recovering his/her previous activities, whenever possible.

The foundation of a successful rehabilitation program is the development of an individual rehabilitation plan based on the results of a comprehensive evaluation (see Chap. 9).

The aim of this book chapter is to describe the postsurgical rehabilitative approach to the most common fragility fractures (see Table 19.1).

F. Gimigliano (✉)
Department of Mental and Physical Health and Preventive Medicine, University of Campania "Luigi Vanvitelli", Naples, Italy

A. de Sire · A. Moretti · C. Curci · G. Iolascon
Department of Medical and Surgical Specialties and Dentistry, University of Campania "Luigi Vanvitelli", Naples, Italy

A. Lenzi, S. Migliaccio (eds.), *Multidisciplinary Approach to Osteoporosis*,
https://doi.org/10.1007/978-3-319-75110-8_19

Table 19.1 Post-surgical rehabilitative approach to the most common fragility fractures

	Functioning	Functional assessment	Rehabilitative intervention
Vertebral fractures	Back pain	Numerical Rating Scale (NRS) Spine Pain Index (SPI) Brief Pain Inventory (BPI)	Short-term bed rest Pain killers Physical therapies Back brace
	Decreased pulmonary function	Spirometry	Respiratory exercises
	Reduced muscle strength	Manual Muscle Testing (MMT)	Back extensors strenghtening
	Depression	Geriatric Depression Scale (GDS)	Psychotherapy Anti-depressive drugs
	Decreased Health-Realted Quality of Life (HRQoL)	The 36-Item Short Form Health Survey (SF-36)	
	Limitation in Activities of Daily Living (ADL)		
Hip fractures	Pain	NRS Harris Hip Score Western Ontario and McMaster Universities Osteoarthritis Index (WOMAC)	Pain killers Physical therapies
	Reduced Range Of Motion (ROM)	Goniometric assessment Harris Hip Score Western Ontario and McMaster Universities Osteoarthritis Index (WOMAC)	Exercises for restoring ROM
	Reduced muscle strength	MMT	Muscle strengthening (progressive increasing load)
	Reduced balance	Berg Balance Scale Performance-Oriented Mobility Assement (POMA) (Tinetti Test)	Balance training Falls prevention
	Walking disability	4-meter gait speed (4MGS)	Gait training
	Delirium	Delirium Assessment Scale (DAS)	
	Depression	GDS	Psychotherapy Anti-depressive drugs
	Decreased HRQoL	SF-36	
	Limitation in ADL		
Wrist fractures	Pain	NRS BPI	Pain killers Physical therapies
	Edema	Clinical assessment	Reduction of swelling
	Reduced ROM	Goniometric assessment	Exercises for restoring ROM
	Reduced muscle strength	MMT	Muscle strengthening
	Decreased HRQoL		
	Limitation in ADL	The Disabilities of the Arm, Shoulder and Hand (DASH) Score	

Table 19.1 (continued)

	Functioning	Functional assessment	Rehabilitative intervention
Proximal humerus fractures	Pain	NRS BPI	Pain killers Physical therapies
	Edema		Reduction of swelling
	Reduced ROM	Goniometric assessment	Exercises for restoring ROM
	Reduced muscle strength	MMT	Muscle strengthening
	Decreased HRQoL		
	Limitation in ADL	DASH Score	
Ankle fractures	Pain	Foot and Ankle Outcome Score (FAOS)	Pain management
	Edema	Clinical assessment	Reduction of swelling
	Reduced ROM	Goniometric assessment	Exercises for restoring ROM
	Reduced muscle strength	MMT	Muscle strengthening (progressive increasing load)
	Reduced balance	Berg Balance Scale POMA	Balance training
	Walking disability	FAOS 4MGS	Gait training
	Decreased HRQoL	FAOS	
	Limitation in ADL	FAOS	

19.2 Vertebral Fractures

Vertebral fragility fractures are defined as fractures that occurred in the absence of a trauma or following a fall from a standing position or a lower height [3]. They are the most common type of osteoporotic fractures [4]. The incidence of vertebral fractures increases with age in both men and women and seems to be greater in women than men across all ages [5]. The prevalence is underestimated because it has been calculated that only the 30% of vertebral fragility fractures come to clinical attention due to pain or height loss [6]. A vertebral fracture represents a major risk for subsequent vertebral fractures. This mechanism is called "vertebral fracture cascade." In the first year after sustaining a vertebral fracture, the risk of a second vertebral fracture increases by four to seven times, while the presence of more than one vertebral fracture rises this risk exponentially [7].

Lumbar spine and the dorsolumbar passage are the most interested sites [8]. The symptoms are significant and include back pain [9–11], decreased pulmonary function (one study demonstrated a decrease in vital capacity of 9% for every vertebral fracture) [12], decreased HRQoL, depression, and loss of self-esteem [13]. Acute vertebral fracture is usually characterized by disabling pain and muscle spasm. Pain usually persists for several months [10].

The spinal deformity index (SDI), based on the morphometric analysis, is a useful tool to classify vertebral fragility fractures and to define the specific treatment [14, 15].

The treatment of spine fractures is generally conservative including short-term bed rest and pain relief (acetaminophen, nonsteroidal anti-inflammatory drugs, and narcotics) [16]. Back bracing (i.e., spinal orthoses or corsets) might be also considered at this stage to immobilize the fracture site, to reduce loads on fractured vertebrae, and to improve spinal alignment, thus favoring the healing process and pain management [17, 18]. Rehabilitation is also aimed to reduce pain and improve mobility. The use of pain management techniques (ultrasounds, hydrotherapy, ice, heat, early mobilization, stretching exercises to decrease muscle spasm, and a gentle strengthening exercise program) in the acute phase after vertebral fracture might be beneficial.

The indications for surgery depend on patients' general conditions, age, fracture pattern and stability, involvement of the spinal cord, bone quality, severity of pain, and timing [2]. The surgical possibilities are vertebro-kyphoplasty with cement, vertebral stabilization, and/or spinal stabilization with or without fusion [8]. In any case rehabilitation should start soon after surgery. Short-term goals are to reduce hyper-kyphosis and respiratory problems. Therefore, breathing exercises and back extensors' strengthening exercises are proposed along with postural training and instructions on how to lift objects [19]. Back extensors' strengthening exercises should start with low impact and with short lever arms with a progressive increase of the load. Bending of the spine or flexion exercises, especially in combination with twisting, should be avoided [20]. Tai chi and hydrotherapy are also recommended.

Long-term outcomes are the increase of the global muscular strength and mobility of the vertebral column and the improvement of balance during postural changes and walking.

19.3 Hip Fractures

Hip fractures are the most common fractures that require hospitalization [21]. Mortality of individuals who sustain a hip fracture increases significantly (33% at 1 year) [22], and those who survive do not regain their pre-fracture level of functioning and independence in their daily activities [23]. Most of the guidelines for the management of hip fracture recommend that surgeons perform hip fracture surgery within 24 h after the injury. Early surgery is associated with better functional outcome, shorter hospital stay, and lower rates of complications and mortality.

There are three different types of hip fractures, considering the involvement of the upper femur area: intracapsular, intertrochanteric, and subtrochanteric fracture. Open reduction and internal fixation are usually reserved to very young patients. Stable intertrochanteric fractures are typically treated with sliding hip screw fixation. Unstable fractures are treated with an intramedullary nail because it provides the buttress for the proximal fragment [24]. In elderly, the gold standard for hip fractures is the arthroplasty (hemi or total), usually associated with optimal functional outcomes after surgery [25].

In any case, patients should undergo an intensive and multidisciplinary rehabilitation program to regain the pre-fracture functional status [26]. Rehabilitation, in fact, has to start immediately after hip fracture surgery and should be tailored to the patient needs.

In general, the aims of the postsurgical rehabilitation management of hip fractures are (1) to reduce pain, (2) to improve functioning, (3) to regain an adequate level of functional activity and social participation, and (4) to improve HRQoL. Even though the scientific community agrees on these aims, there are still some open issues such as the ideal rehabilitative setting and the best timing for starting the loading exercises.

The individual rehabilitation plan includes three distinct periods of recovery, with different locations:

1. Acute phase—from the time of fracture to 5–7 days postoperatively, usually conducted in an orthopedic department
2. Subacute—after 5 days up to 90 days postoperatively, in a rehabilitative setting or at home
3. Post-acute—90 days postoperatively up to 1 year after fracture, at home

If during the acute postoperative period there is a general consensus on what kind of rehabilitation should be performed, less agreement exists regarding the optimal rehabilitative care of patients in the subacute period. This period can vary in length, depending upon the pre-fracture clinical and functional conditions of the patient, the type of surgery, and peri- and postoperative patient's conditions. In the post-acute phase, the choice of the best rehabilitation setting is still controversial. Patients generally prefer home-based rehabilitation; on the other hand in a rehabilitation clinic, a more comprehensive technical and methodological approach can be applied.

One of the specific aims of rehabilitation soon after surgery is to prevent cardiovascular and pulmonary complications. Therefore, lower limb pumping exercises and deep breathing exercises are proposed; both activities should be continued until patients start walking. An early mobilization (within 24 h) might avoid prolonged bed rest and prevent complications such as deep vein thrombosis. Oldmeadow et al. showed that patients who started an early ambulation (within 48 h after surgery) compared to a delayed ambulation (over 48 h postsurgery) were able to walk for greater distances, were more independent during transfers, and were more frequently discharged home rather than to a rehabilitation facility [27].

In the first 3 days after surgery, it is also mandatory to maintain muscular strength and endurance of the upper extremities and of the non-operated lower limb, to prevent muscle atrophy of the operated limb, to regain active mobility and voluntary control of the operated limb, and to prevent muscular contractions. Strengthening exercises for the knee extensors, started 2–3 days after surgery, are feasible and effective with improvements in functional outcomes [28]. The rehabilitative approach should include a progressive increasing load on the operated hip, from low load exercises (i.e., submaximal quad sets, bicycle with no resistance) in an early phase to a moderate-high load (i.e., stairs, resistance training) in a late phase [29]. It is also necessary to work on balance and correct potential walking deviations. It is paramount to teach the patients how to avoid risky movements that might dislocate the operated hip and to apply all necessary environmental changes to their houses, including those aimed to reduce the risk of falls. If we consider that more than the 95% of all hip fractures occur during a fall, fall risk reduction must be a very important part of the rehabilitative project of all patients who sustained a hip fracture [30]. A recent Cochrane review concluded that group and home-based exercise programs and home safety interventions are successful in reducing the rate of falls and the overall risk of falling [31]. El-Khoury et al. said that exercise programs aimed to prevent falls in elderly also seem to be useful in preventing fall injuries as well, including fractures [32].

The “F balance” is a theory that can be useful for clinicians in making decision process when approaching patients with a hip fracture. It consists of a balance between the achievement of the optimal function and obtained controlling forces (i.e., exercises of mobilization) and improving form (i.e., strength, endurance, balance), against the risk of tissue damage (failure). The “F balance” focuses the attention on the “feel” of the patient that should always be the main objective of the rehabilitative treatment [33].

Pain management is crucial. It should start as soon as possible, ideally in the ambulance going to the hospital, and should continue throughout the process of care (see Fig. 19.1).

It is also important to consider the patient cognitive status. Iolascon et al. have recently analyzed the possible stressful events that might be responsible for the high rate of delirium in those patients who experienced a hip fracture [34]. Among others, the accident itself, the transfer to the hospital, the clinical and radiological examinations, the type of anesthesia and surgery, the administration of opioids, the sleep deprivation, and the pain that is not always properly treated were identified as having a key role in the development of delirium [35]. Delirium usually appears within the first 48 h after surgery; prodromic symptoms such as disorientation, difficulty in concentration, short-term and/or long-term memory impairment, and an underlying somatic illness are frequently observed [36]. It is important to identify promptly these symptoms and to apply a multifactorial intervention program, such as the one proposed by Björkelund et al., which consists of supplementation of oxygen and intravenous fluid, accurate monitoring of vital signs, adequate pain management, daily screening of the delirium, reduction in drug assumption, and modification in perioperative management [34, 37].

Nutrition is another important component in the management of elderly fractured patients [38]. Bell et al. reported a state of malnutrition in 48% of patients who sustained a hip fracture [39]. Moreover, serum albumin levels lower than 3 g/dL were associated with poor recovery after a fragility fracture [40].

Magaziner et al. evaluating community-dwelling hip fracture patients at baseline, at 1 and at 2 years after sustaining the fracture, demonstrated that, when

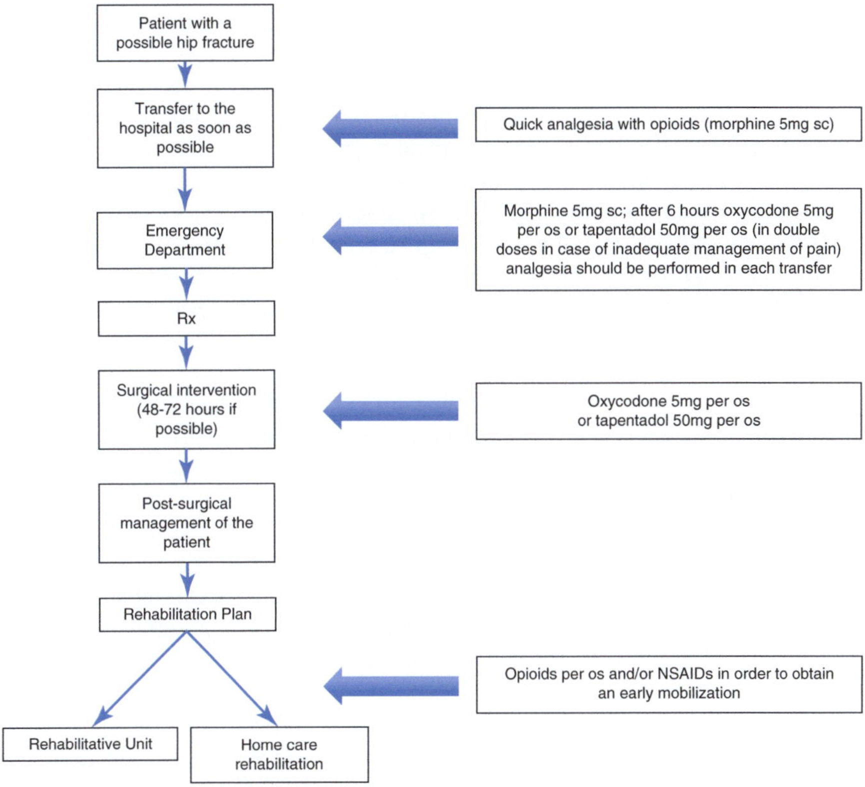

Fig. 19.1 Operational flow-chart for the management of patients with hip fracture

compared to age, sex, and pre-fracture walking ability matched controls, they presented a significant decline in functioning. In fact, over 50% presented a walking disability (unable to walk across a room—3 m), and about 39% had disability in transferring and 18% in personal grooming [23]. In another paper from the same research group, a difference in performance-based functioning of older women 2 years after the hip fracture when compared to age-matched women without hip fracture was demonstrated. Those who sustained a hip fracture had slower walking speeds [41]. The rate of recovery of activities of daily living (ADL) varies over time. Activities such as ambulation, chair/bed transfers, self-care, and bladder control usually recover during the first 6 months. Others such as bathing, dressing, and climbing stairs take longer to recover, usually over 12 months. Moreover the likelihood of returning to pre-fracture status is greatest for activities such as grooming, feeding, bowel and bladder control, and even for using the toilet, bathing, dressing, ambulation, transfers, and stair climbing [42]. After 2 years from the hip fracture, also the HRQoL, measured by the 36-Item Short Form Health Survey (SF-36), remained decreased [43].

19.4 Wrist Fractures

Wrist fractures are the third most common fragility fractures. Women are four to six times more likely to sustain a distal radius fracture than men [44]. Its overall incidence is increasing and the highest is around the age of 50 [45].

Fractures of the distal radius generally occur as a consequence of a fall onto the outstretched hand from a standing position. The typical fracture pattern is the dorsal displacement of the distal radius that might be accompanied by comminution of the radius and lesion of the ulnar side of the wrist or of the scapholunate ligament. Nondisplaced fractures are considered stable and are usually treated conservatively with a short arm cast for 4–6 weeks, while displaced distal radius fractures need to be reduced and then splinted [46].

Restoring motion and reducing swelling are key points in the rehabilitative treatment of wrist fractures. Older patients are susceptible to stiffness of the upper limb joints and to severe hand edema. The patient must be instructed to elevate the hand and on how to use the sling. If symptoms and signs such as pain, stiffness swelling, and changes in skin temperature occur, a complex regional pain syndrome must be investigated and its treatment started as soon as possible [24].

If the orthopedic surgeon decides to go for surgery, there are several options such as a percutaneous fixation with a Kirschner wire (K-wire), a closed reduction and stabilization with an external fixator [47], an open reduction and internal fixation, or combinations thereof.

Rehabilitation usually starts after cast removal or surgery. The general goals are the reduction of edema, increasing the range of motion (ROM), and muscular strengthening [24]. Wound care and pain management are also important to be performed. A program of home-based exercise should be followed by patients including shoulder, elbow, forearm, wrist, and digit movements. Specific hand exercises include tendon gliding (for flexor digitorum profundus, flexor digitorum superficialis), metacarpophalangeal flexion and extension, and thumb extension and opposition [48]. It is also recommended to perform other exercises such as gripping, rolling, pinching, scraping, and full flexion and extension of extrinsic muscles [49]. When the hand and forearm strength is regained, patients will start using again their upper limb in their ADLs.

Existing literature seems to be in favor of early mobilization [50, 51]. However, there are still concerns about the best timing at which wrist motion should be started after the reduction is obtained. Most of the authors agree that the early mobilization of the wrist and fingers might prevent complications.

19.5 Proximal Humerus Fractures

Proximal humerus fractures represent the 36.3% of the fragility fractures that require hospitalization ([21]). They usually occur after a fall from a standing position on the outstretched arm or directly on the shoulder [52]. The fracture might be complicated by neurovascular injuries, in particular the impairment of the axillary nerve or of the brachial plexus [24]. Therefore, an accurate neurological examination should be performed and documented in all these patients.

These fractures are usually treated conservatively in the elderly, unless there is an unstable or displaced fracture that requires surgical approach. The conservative treatment foresees the use of a sling or shoulder immobilizer for about 2 weeks followed by a careful mobilization of the wrist and elbow and then after 3–4 weeks of the shoulder itself [53]. Early mobilization is paramount to prevent muscle contractions and reduce the edema [54]. The sling should be discontinued as early as their pain allows.

The surgical treatment usually consists of open reduction with internal fixation or arthroplasty [8]. After surgery, exercises aimed to enhance shoulder ROM should start as soon as possible. In particular, Codman exercises can be started during the first week. Patients should be instructed to avoid above chest level activities until the fracture callus is evident. The complete functional recovery of the shoulder is not expected. Even though the limited use of the upper extremity can compromise some activities of daily living, it is possible to teach the patient alternative movements to carry out such actions as scapular plane motion can supply the loss of glenohumeral movements that include hand-to-head function [24].

19.6 Ankle Fractures

The incidence and severity of ankle fractures in elderly patients have been recently increasing [55]. Clinical studies reported that the incidence rises until 65 years old, and then there is a plateau or a decrease [56].

Nondisplaced fractures are usually immobilized with a splint or a cast for 4–6 weeks [57]. In case of displaced fractures, surgical stabilization is generally needed. Although early studies recommended that a conservative approach should be always pursued in the elderly, recent studies are in favor of the surgical intervention [56]. However, the best treatment of ankle fractures in older people is still debated, because of their instability, low bone quality, weak soft tissue integrity, and weight-bearing limitations [24].

The aims of the management of ankle fracture are to reduce pain, to improve ankle mobility and balance, and to recover the ADLs and pre-fracture functional levels, avoiding the complications of immobilization and bed rest.

Rehabilitation should start as soon as the cast is removed or after the surgical treatment. The proposed programs generally include stretching, manual therapy, proprioceptive exercises, mobilization, strengthening exercises, and balance and gait training [58].

There are poor evidences on the effects of rehabilitation in the management of ankle fractures. A Cochrane systematic review assessed the effects of rehabilitation during or after the period of ankle immobilization. The authors concluded that starting the weight bearing during the immobilization period and wearing a sling that can be removed to allow ankle exercises might improve the outcome after ankle fracture [59].

References

1. Piscitelli P, Brandi M, Cawston H, Gauthier A, Kanis JA, Compston J, Borgström F, Cooper C, McCloskey E. Epidemiological burden of postmenopausal osteoporosis in Italy from 2010 to 2020: estimations from a disease model. Calcif Tissue Int. 2014;95(5):419–27.
2. Gimigliano F, Iolascon G, Riccio I, Frizzi L, Gimigliano R. Post-surgical rehabilitative approach to fragility fractures. Aging Clin Exp Res. 2013;25(Suppl 1):S23–5.
3. CG146. Osteoporosis: fragility fracture risk: osteoporosis: assessing the risk of fragility fracture. National Clinical Guideline Centre (UK). London: Royal College of Physicians (UK). 2012. https://www.nice.org.uk/guidance/cg146/evidence/full-guideline-pdf-186818365. Accessed 17 May 2018.
4. Burge R, Dawson-Hughes B, Solomon DH, Wong JB, King A, Tosteson A. Incidence and economic burden of osteoporosis-related fractures in the United States, 2005–2025. J Bone Miner Res. 2007;22(3):465–75.
5. Papaioannou A, Kennedy CC, Ioannidis G, Sawka A, Hopman WM, Pickard L, Brown JP, Josse RG, Kaiser S, Anastassiades T, Goltzman D, Papadimitropoulos M, Tenenhouse A, Prior JC, Olszynski WP, Adachi JD. The impact of incident fractures on health-related quality of life: 5 years of data from the Canadian Multicentre Osteoporosis Study. Osteoporos Int. 2009;20(5):703–14.
6. Wiktorowicz ME, Goeree R, Papaioannou A, Adachi JD, Papadimitropoulos E. Economic implications of hip fracture: health service use, institutional care and cost in Canada. Osteoporos Int. 2001;12(4):271–8.
7. Lunt M, O'Neill TW, Felsenberg D, Reeve J, Kanis JA, Cooper C, Silman AJ. Characteristics of a prevalent vertebral deformity predict subsequent vertebral fracture: results from the European Prospective Osteoporosis Study (EPOS). Bone. 2003;33(4):505–13.
8. Pietri M, Lucarini S. The orthopaedic treatment of fragility fractures. Clin Cases Miner Bone Metab. 2007;4(2):108–16.
9. Ettinger B, Black DM, Nevitt MC, Rundle AC, Cauley JA, Cummings SR, Genant HK. Contribution of vertebral deformities to chronic back pain and disability. The Study of Osteoporotic Fractures Research Group. J Bone Miner Res. 1992;7(4):449–56.
10. Fink HA, Ensrud KE, Nelson DB, Kerani RP, Schreiner PJ, Zhao Y, Cummings SR, Nevitt MC. Disability after clinical fracture in postmenopausal women with low bone density: the fracture intervention trial (FIT). Osteoporos Int. 2003;14(1):69–76.
11. Matthis C, Weber U, O'Neill TW, Raspe H. Health impact associated with vertebral deformities: results from the European Vertebral Osteoporosis Study (EVOS). Osteoporos Int. 1998;8(4):364–72.
12. Harrison RA, Siminoski K, Vethanayagam D, Majumdar SR. Osteoporosis- related kyphosis and impairments in pulmonary function: a systematic review. J Bone Miner Res. 2007;22(3):447–57.
13. Gold DT. The nonskeletal consequences of osteoporotic fractures. Psychologic and social outcomes. Rheum Dis Clin N Am. 2001;27(1):255–62.
14. McCloskey EV, Spector TD, Eyres KS, Fern ED, O'Rourke N, Vasikaran S, Kanis JA. The assessment of vertebral deformity: a method for use in population studies and clinical trials. Osteoporos Int. 1993;3:138–47.
15. Sauer P, Leidig G. Spine deformity index versus other objective procedures in vertebral fractures identification in patients with osteoporosis: a comparative study. J Bone Miner Res. 1991;6:227–35.
16. Kendler DL, Bauer DC, Davison KS, Dian L, Hanley DA, Harris ST, McClung MR, Miller PD, Schousboe JT, Yuen CK, Lewiecki EM. Vertebral fractures: clinical importance and management. Am J Med. 2016;129(2):221.e1–10.
17. Pfeifer M, Begerow B, Minne HW. Effects of a new spinal orthosis on posture, trunk strength, and quality of life in women with postmenopausal osteoporosis: a randomized trial. Am J Phys Med Rehabil. 2004;83(3):177–86.

18. Stadhouder A, Buskens E, Vergroesen DA, Fidler MW, de Nies F, Oner FC. Nonoperative treatment of thoracic and lumbar spine fractures: a prospective randomized study of different treatment options. J Orthop Trauma. 2009;23(8):588–94.
19. Bonner FJ Jr, Sinaki M, Grabois M, Shipp KM, Lane JM, Lindsay R, Gold DT, Cosman F, Bouxsein ML, Weinstein JN, Gallagher RM, Melton LJ III, Salcido RS, Gordon SL. Health professional's guide to rehabilitation of the patient with osteoporosis. Osteoporos Int. 2003;14(Suppl 2):S1–22.
20. Sinaki M, Mikkelsen BA. Postmenopausal spinal osteoporosis: flexion versus extension exercises. Arch Phys Med Rehabil. 1984;65(10):593–6.
21. Tarantino U, Capone A, Planta M, D'Arienzo M, Letizia Mauro G, Impagliazzo A, Formica A, Pallotta F, Patella V, Spinarelli A, Pazzaglia U, Zarattini G, Roselli M, Montanari G, Sessa G, Privitera M, Verdoia C, Corradini C, Feola M, Padolino A, Saturnino L, Scialdoni A, Rao C, Iolascon G, Brandi ML, Piscitelli P. The incidence of hip, forearm, humeral, ankle, and vertebral fragility fractures in Italy: results from a 3-year multicenter study. Arthritis Res Ther. 2010;12(6):R226.
22. Roche J, Wenn RT, Sahota O, Moran CG. Effect of comorbidities and postoperative complications on mortality after hip fracture in elderly people: prospective observational cohort study. BMJ. 2005;331(7529):1374.
23. Magaziner J, Fredman L, Hawkes W, Hebel JR, Zimmerman S, Orwig DL, Wehren L. Changes in functional status attributable to hip fracture: a comparison of hip fracture patients to community-dwelling aged. Am J Epidemiol. 2003;157(11):1023–31.
24. Mears SC, Kates SL. A guide to improving the Care of Patients with fragility fractures, edition 2. Geriatr Orthop Surg Rehabil. 2015;6(2):58–120.
25. Healy WL, Iorio R. Total hip arthroplasty: optimal treatment for displaced femoral neck fractures in elderly patients. Clin Orthop Relat Res. 2004;429:43–8.
26. Fagerson TL. Diseases and disorders of the hip. In: Fagerson TL, editor. The hip handbook. Boston: Butterworth-Heinemann; 1998.
27. Oldmeadow LB, Edwards ER, Kimmel LA, Kipen E, Robertson VJ, Bailey MJ. No rest for the wounded: early ambulation after hip surgery accelerates recovery. ANZ J Surg. 2006;76(7):607–11.
28. Kronborg L, Bandholm T, Palm H, Kehlet H, Kristensen MT. Feasibility of progressive strength training implemented in the acute ward after hip fracture surgery. PLoS One. 2014;9(4):e93332.
29. Overgaard J, Kristen MT. Feasibility of progressive strength training shortly after hip fracture surgery. World J Orthop. 2013;4(4):248–58.
30. Parkkari J, Kannus P, Palvanen M, Natri A, Vainio J, Aho H, Vuori I, Järvinen M. Majority of hip fractures occur as a result of a fall and impact on the greater trochanter of the femur: a prospective controlled hip fracture study with 206 consecutive patients. Calcif Tissue Int. 1999;65:183–7.
31. Gillespie LD, Robertson MC, Gillespie WJ, Sherrington C, Gates S, Clemson LM, Lamb SE. Interventions for preventing falls in older people living in the community. Cochrane Database Syst Rev. 2012;9:CD007146. https://doi.org/10.1002/14651858.CD007146.pub3.
32. El-Khoury F, Cassou B, Charles MA, Dargent-Molina P. The effect of fall prevention exercise programmes on fall induced injuries in community dwelling older adults: systematic review and meta-analysis of randomised controlled trials. BMJ. 2013;347:f6234.
33. Magee DJ, Zachazewski JE, Quillen WS. Pathology and intervention in musculoskeletal rehabilitation. 2nd edition. Elsevier; 2016. ISBN: 978-0-323-31072-7.
34. Iolascon G, Cervone M, Gimigliano R, Di Pietro G, Gimigliano F. Neuropsychiatric disorders in hip fracture. Clin Cases Miner Bone Metab. 2011;8(3):49–53.
35. Bitsch M, Foss N, Kristensen B, Kehlet H. Pathogenesis of and management strategies for postoperative delirium after hip fracture: a review. Acta Orthop Scand. 2004;75(4):378–89.
36. de Jonghe JF, Kalisvaart KJ, Dijkstra M, van Dis H, Vreeswijk R, Kat MG, Eikelenboom P, van der Ploeg T, van Gool WA. Early symptoms in the prodromal phase of delirium: a

prospective cohort study in elderly patients undergoing hip surgery. Am J Geriatr Psychiatry. 2007;15(2):112–21.
37. Björkelund KB, Hommel A, Thorngren KG, Gustafson L, Larsson S, Lundberg D. Reducing delirium in elderly patients with hip fracture: a multi-factorial intervention study. Acta Anaesthesiol Scand. 2010;54(6):678–88.
38. Roberts KC, Brox WT. AAOS clinical practice guideline: management of hip fractures in the elderly. J Am Acad Orthop Surg. 2015;23(2):138–40.
39. Bell JJ, Bauer JD, Capra S, Pulle RC. Quick and easy is not without cost: implications of poorly performing nutrition screening tools in hip fracture. J Am Geriatr Soc. 2014;62(2):237–43.
40. Pioli G, Barone A, Giusti A, Oliveri M, Pizzonia M, Razzano M, Palummeri E. Predictors of mortality after hip fracture: results from 1-year follow-up. Aging Clin Exp Res. 2006;18(5):381–7.
41. Fredman L, Magaziner J, Hawkes W, Hebel JR, Fried LP, Kasper J, Guralnik J. Female hip fracture patients had poorer performance-based functioning than community-dwelling peers over 2-year follow-up period. J Clin Epidemiol. 2005;58(12):1289–98.
42. Alarcón T, González-Montalvo JI, Gotor P, Madero R, Otero A. Activities of daily living after hip fracture: profile and rate of recovery during 2 years of follow-up. Osteoporos Int. 2011;22(5):1609–13.
43. Hallberg I, Rosenqvist AM, Kartous L, Löfman O, Wahlström O, Toss G. Health-related quality of life after osteoporotic fractures. Osteoporos Int. 2004;15(10):834–41.
44. Centers for Disease Control and Prevention (CDC). Incidence and costs to medicare of fractures among Medicare beneficiaries aged greater than or equal to 65 years—United States, July 1991–June 1992. MMWR Morb Mortal Wkly Rep. 1996;45(41):877–83.
45. Brogren E, Petranek M, Atroshi I. Incidence and characteristics of distal radius fractures in a southern Swedish region. BMC Musculoskelet Disord. 2007;8:48.
46. Roth KM, Blazar PE, Earp BE, Han R, Leung A. Incidence of displacement after nondisplaced distal radial fractures in adults. J Bone Joint Surg Am. 2013;95(15):1398–402.
47. Lin C, Sun JS, Hou SM. External fixation with or without supplementary intramedullary Kirschner wires in the treatment of distal radial fractures. Can J Surg. 2004;47(6):431–7.
48. Katarincic JA. Fractures of the wrist and hand. Occup Med. 1998;13(3):549–68.
49. Weinstock TB. Management of fractures of the distal radius: therapist's commentary. J Hand Ther. 1999;12(2):99–102.
50. Bennett GL, Leeson MC, Smith BS. Intramedullary fixation of unstable distal radius fractures. A method of fixation allowing early motion. Orthop Rev. 1989;18(2):210–6.
51. Raskin KB. Management of fractures of the distal radius: surgeon's perspective. J Hand Ther. 1999;12(2):92–8.
52. Jo MJ, Gardner MJ. Proximal humerus fractures. Curr Rev Musculoskelet Med. 2012;5(3):192–8.
53. Court-Brown CM, Garg A, McQueen MM. The translated two part fracture of the proximal humerus. Epidemiology and outcome in the older patient. J Bone Joint Surg Br. 2001;83(6):799–804.
54. Hertel R, Hempfing A, Stiehler M, Leunig M. Predictors of humeral head ischemia after intracapsular fracture of the proximal humerus. J Shoulder Elb Surg. 2004;13(4):427–33.
55. Kannus P, Palvanen M, Niemi S, Parkkari J, Jarvinen M. Increasing number and incidence of low-trauma ankle fractures in elderly people: Finnish statistics during 1970-2000 and projections for the future. Bone. 2002;31(3):430–3.
56. Strauss EJ, Egol KA. The management of ankle fractures in the elderly. Injury. 2007;38(Suppl 3):S2–9.
57. Salai M, Dudkiewicz I, Novikov I, Amit Y, Chechick A. The epidemic of ankle fractures in the elderly—is surgical treatment warranted? Arch Orthop Trauma Surg. 2000;120(9):511–3.
58. Beckenkamp PR, Lin CC, Herbert RD, Haas M, Khera K, Moseley A. EXACT: exercise or advice after ankle fracture. Design of a randomised controlled trial. BMC Musculoskelet Disord. 2011;12:148.
59. Lin CW, Donkers NA, Refshauge KM, Beckenkamp PR, Khera K, Moseley AM. Rehabilitation for ankle fractures in adults. Cochrane Database Syst Rev. 2012;11:CD005595. https://doi.org/10.1002/14651858.CD005595.pub3. Review

Index

A

Acidosis
- metabolic, 186, 189, 194
- renal tubular, 185, 186

Acromegaly, 87–89, 93
Activating transcription factor 4 (ATF4), 8, 11
Adipokines, 11, 144, 148
Adiponectin, 143, 145, 146
Advanced glycation end products (AGEs), 49, 157–159
Adynamic bone disease, 191, 197, 204, 205
AGEs, *see* Advanced glycation end products (AGEs)
Aldosterone, 107–109, 117–120
Alkaline phosphatase (ALP), 7, 11, 51, 52, 87, 109, 157, 160, 163, 169, 186, 190, 192–195, 214, 228, 291
ALP, *see* Alkaline phosphatase (ALP)
Androgens, 30, 48, 107, 108, 110–114, 117, 118, 120, 143, 166, 190, 227, 231, 247
Ankylosing spondylitis, 238–240
Antiresorptive drugs, 196, 231
Aromatase, 30, 48, 110, 111, 143, 166, 227
Arterial stiffness, 213
ATF4, *see* Activating Transcription Factor 4 (ATF4)
Atherosclerosis, 212–219, 245, 246

B

Back pain, 53, 68, 240, 299, 314, 315
Balance assessment, 64–65
Balanced diet, 260, 268
Balance training, 280–282, 314, 315
bALP, *see* Bone specific-alkaline phosphatase (bALP)
Biopsy
- bone, 79, 81, 192, 196, 205, 300

Biphosphonates (BP), 218, 219, 244–245, 248, 249
BMP, *see* Bone morphogenetic protein (BMP)
Bone
- biopsy, 79, 81, 192, 196, 205, 300
- formation, 3, 9–12, 14–15, 25, 34, 47, 52, 75–77, 79, 80, 83–85, 87, 90–92, 114, 119, 132, 133, 136–141, 143–147, 153, 155–157, 161, 164–168, 188, 190, 191, 193, 197, 198, 199, 212, 214, 216, 218, 224, 225, 227, 228, 230, 237–240, 242, 244, 245, 265, 266, 285, 286, 291, 292
- histomorphometry, 90, 195, 197, 200, 201
- mineral density, 9, 10, 14, 25–40, 46–50, 52, 53, 62, 77, 80, 84, 86, 88–93, 107, 108, 111–120, 135, 144, 154, 155, 156, 158, 161, 162, 166–171, 195, 199–202, 212, 213, 214, 217, 218, 219, 225, 228–232, 237–248, 260, 265, 266, 268, 269, 271, 278, 280, 286–292
- mineralization, 14, 85, 189, 214, 218, 219, 264, 271
- remodeling, 2, 38, 48, 80, 84, 85, 90, 93, 114, 131, 138, 139, 144, 145, 148, 195, 198, 217, 225, 230, 238, 242, 245, 260, 262, 279, 285, 290
- resorption, 2, 3, 5, 9, 10, 14–16, 25, 27, 31, 52, 75–77, 79, 80, 83, 84, 86, 87, 92, 111, 114, 119, 132, 133, 135, 138, 143, 145, 146, 153, 155, 157–159, 161, 163–168, 189, 190, 193, 195, 197, 201, 205, 215, 217, 219, 224, 225, 227, 228, 229, 231, 232, 237, 238, 242, 244, 245, 259, 265, 285, 286, 292
- turnover, 25, 26, 32, 52, 75, 77, 79, 80, 86, 87, 88, 90, 91, 93, 113, 115, 119, 134, 137, 138, 146, 158, 161, 169, 188–190, 193, 195–198, 205, 215, 217, 228, 232, 237, 285, 287, 289, 306
- volume, 10, 82, 145, 148, 170, 196–201

Bone-adipose axis, 144, 148

A. Lenzi, S. Migliaccio (eds.), *Multidisciplinary Approach to Osteoporosis*, https://doi.org/10.1007/978-3-319-75110-8

Bone anabolic drugs, 232
Bone markers, 52, 77, 216, 230, 291
Bone marrow mesenchimal stem cells (BMMSCs), 147, 148
Bone mass peak, 25, 26, 260, 265, 267
Bone mineral density (BMD), 9, 10, 14, 25–40, 46–50, 52, 53, 62, 77, 80, 84, 86, 88–93, 107, 108, 111–120, 135, 144, 154, 155, 156, 158, 161, 162, 166–171, 195, 199–202, 212, 213, 214, 217, 218, 219, 225, 228–232, 237–248, 260, 265, 266, 268, 269, 271, 278, 280, 286–292
Bone morphogenetic protein (BMP), 9, 33, 84, 214
Bone quality, 25, 26, 46, 49, 92, 109, 112, 115, 120, 156, 158, 160, 163, 170–171, 196, 200, 201, 216, 223, 240, 241, 243, 306, 316, 321
Bone remodelling, 2, 38, 48, 80, 84, 85, 90, 93, 114, 131, 138, 139, 144, 145, 148, 195, 198, 217, 225, 230, 238, 242, 245, 260, 262, 279, 285, 290
Bone specific-alkaline phosphatase (bALP), 186, 193, 195, 214, 215
Bone turnover, 25, 26, 32, 52, 75, 77, 79, 80, 86, 87, 88, 90, 91, 93, 113, 115, 119, 134, 137, 138, 146, 158, 161, 169, 188–190, 193, 195–198, 205, 215, 217, 228, 232, 237, 285, 287, 289, 306

C

Calcifications
- ectopic, 184, 190, 194
- vascular, 187, 189, 196, 199, 200, 202, 212–216, 218, 219

Calcimimetics, 203
Calcium
- sensing receptor (CaSR), 75, 188, 203, 204
- serum, 51, 52, 88, 192, 194, 202
- urinary, 51, 52, 91, 186, 262, 270

Calcium ion, 261
Chronic kidney disease (CKD), 119, 183–196, 199–202, 205, 215
Chronic kidney disease-mineral and bone disorder (CKD-MBD), 184, 190, 193, 195, 196, 199
Chronic renal failure (CRF), 183–190, 194, 201, 203, 246
CKD, *see* Chronic kidney disease (CKD)
CKD-MBD, *see* Chronic kidney disease-mineral and bone disorder (CKD-MBD)
Clinical evaluation, 45–50, 62, 78, 191, 194
Collagen type I alpha I, 30–31, 160
Cortical bone, 1, 2, 77, 78, 80, 83, 86, 88, 91, 112, 119, 132, 133, 135–138, 140, 161, 163, 170, 225, 226, 227, 300
Cortisol, 51, 52, 93, 107–110, 112, 113, 116, 117, 120, 139
CRF, *see* Chronic renal failure (CRF)
Cross-talk, 144, 148, 201
C-telopeptide of type 1 collagen (CTX), 52, 87, 168, 169, 193, 195
CTX, *see* C-telopeptide of type 1 collagen (CTX)

D

Dairy products, 264, 268, 270, 271
Denosumab, 116, 204, 205, 219, 231, 245, 248, 249, 290–291
Density
- bone mineral, 9, 10, 14, 25–40, 46–50, 52, 53, 62, 77, 80, 84, 86, 88–93, 107, 108, 111–120, 135, 144, 154, 155, 156, 158, 161, 162, 166–171, 195, 199–202, 212, 213, 214, 217, 218, 219, 225, 228–232, 237–248, 260, 265, 266, 268, 269, 271, 278, 280, 286–292

Dent's disease, 185, 186
Depression, 64, 242, 314, 315
Diabetic complications, 160–161, 169
Dipeptidyl peptidase-4 (DPP-4), 160, 167
Disability and health, 59
Disability assessment, 65–66
DPP-4, *see* Dipeptidyl peptidase-4 (DPP-4)

E

Efficacy, 48, 50, 53, 89, 205, 218, 244, 286, 287, 288, 290, 291, 292, 299, 302
Epidemiology, 212, 223–224
Estrogen receptor alpha (*ERα)*, 28–30, 130–132, 228
Estrogens, 26, 28, 29, 30, 46, 47, 85, 110, 111, 113, 114, 120, 129–133, 137–139, 143, 144, 147, 148, 189, 190, 211, 214–217, 223, 225, 227, 228, 286, 292
Exercise, 11, 47, 48, 90, 156, 160, 268, 277–282, 306, 314–318, 320, 321
Exercise prescription, 280

F

Falls prevention, 314
Fanconi syndrome, 186
Fat mass, 90, 143, 144
FGF23, *see* Fibroblast Growth Factor 23 (FGF23)
Fibroblast Growth Factor 23 (FGF23), 2, 13, 14, 184–189, 191, 192, 193, 195, 196, 201, 204, 218
Food proteins, 265, 268
Fracture risk assessment (FRAX), 49, 50, 89, 201, 230, 247, 248
Fragility fractures, 25–32, 40, 46, 47, 53, 59, 60, 62, 64, 68, 80, 92, 107, 113, 119, 143, 154, 164, 166, 168, 170, 224, 237, 267, 269, 313, 314, 315, 316, 318, 320
FRAX, *see* Fracture risk assessment (FRAX)

G

Gait training, 314, 315, 321
Genome-wide association, 119
Glucagon-like peptide-1 (GLP-1), 159, 160, 167
Glucocorticoids, 48, 50, 51, 53, 85, 90–93, 108–110, 114–117, 139, 201, 212, 229, 230, 232, 237
Glucose toxicity, 156–158

H

Hcy, *see* Homocysteine (Hcy)
Health-related quality of life (HRQoL), 68–69, 313, 314, 315, 317, 319
Histomorphometry, 79, 87, 90, 197, 200, 201
Homeostasis, 2, 3, 10, 11, 27, 39, 83, 84, 111, 129, 134, 143, 144, 145, 146, 148, 184, 219, 237, 268, 269, 271, 285
Homocysteine (Hcy), 158, 217, 218, 266, 271
HRQoL, *see* Health-related quality of life (HRQoL)
Hypercalciuria
- idiopathic, 51, 186
- X-linked recessive hypophosphatemic rickets with, 185, 186

Hyperinsulinaemia and Insulin Resistance, 155–156
Hyperparathyroidism
- secondary hyperparathyroidism in CKD (SHP), 184, 187, 191, 192, 193, 194, 198, 199, 202, 203, 204, 205

Hypopituitarism, 89, 91

I

Idiopathic osteoporosis, 27, 223, 224, 225, 228–229
IGF-1, *see* Insulin-like growth factor-1 (IGF–1)
IL-6, *see* Interleukin-6 (IL-6)
Incretin system, 153, 159–160, 167
Inflammation, 6, 7, 146, 147, 153, 161, 189, 215, 237, 238, 239, 241, 244, 245, 248, 269, 298
Insulin deficiency, 153, 155–156
Insulin-like growth factor-1 (IGF–1), 3, 10, 86, 135, 137, 140, 141, 156, 166, 168, 169, 225, 227, 228, 229
Interleukin-6 (IL-6), 11, 132, 138, 143, 145, 146, 161, 214, 237, 238, 242, 245, 287, 321
International classification of functioning, disability and health (ICF), 59
Irisin, 11, 163

K

Klotho, 13, 14, 186–188, 192, 193, 195, 196, 201
Kyphoplasty (PKP), 299–307

L

Leptin, 143, 145, 146
Lifestyle, 25, 26, 213, 225, 229, 249, 259, 260, 268, 270, 277
LIGHT, 6
Lipocalin-2 (LCN2), 11
Lipoprotein receptor-related protein 5 (LRP5), 8, 14, 26–27, 39
Lipoprotein receptor-related protein 6 (LRP6), 8, 26–27
LRP5, *see* Lipoprotein receptor-related protein 5 (LRP5)
LRP6, *see* Lipoprotein receptor-related protein 6 (LRP6)

M

Macro nutrients, 265
Marrow adiposity, 148, 153, 162
Mechanical loading, 278
Mediterranean diet (MeDi), 264, 265, 268–269
Men
- epidemiology, 223–224
- pathophysiology, 224–230, 232

Menopause, 26, 28, 47, 129–141, 144, 147, 148, 201, 212, 214, 217, 219, 237, 247, 248, 262, 286
Mesenchymal stem cells (MSCs), 7, 40, 144–148, 156, 157, 230
Metformin, 163–166
Micro nutrients, 260, 261, 265, 267, 268
Mineralization
in CKD-MBD (*see* TMV classification)
Mineral metabolism, 12, 26, 184, 187, 188, 190
MSCs, *see* Mesenchymal stem cells (MSCs)
Muscle power assessment, 63
Muscle strength assessment, 63
Muscle strengthening, 314, 315

N
Nephrolithiasis, 185, 186
X-linked recessive n., 185, 186
Neuropeptide Y (NPY), 145
Nitric Oxide (NO), 216, 219

O
Obesity, 143–148, 161, 213, 259, 270
Osteoblastogenesis, 7–11, 76, 84, 85, 110, 117, 132–134, 137–140, 145, 148, 155–157, 165, 188, 193, 203, 230, 242
Osteoblasts (OBs), 2, 7, 9, 27, 32, 34, 38, 46, 48, 49, 76, 77, 84–87, 92, 109, 111, 114, 117, 119, 131, 132, 133, 135, 137, 144–148, 155–157, 159, 160, 162, 163, 165, 188, 190, 192, 193, 195–198, 204, 214, 215, 218, 219, 224, 227, 228, 230, 232, 238, 242, 246, 259, 265, 266, 285, 286, 291, 292
Osteocalcin (OCN), 2, 14, 84, 87, 109, 114, 117, 144, 146, 156, 184, 190, 195, 215, 216, 218, 228, 230, 265
Osteoclastogenesis, 3–7, 10, 11, 76, 84, 86, 111, 117, 120, 132–134, 137, 139, 140, 145, 146, 155, 157, 158, 161, 162, 193, 219, 230, 238, 286, 290
Osteoclasts (OCs), 2–4, 27, 31, 32, 35, 37, 48, 49, 76, 77, 84, 85, 86, 87, 111, 114, 131, 132, 137, 145, 146, 155, 157–161, 166, 186, 188–190, 193, 195, 197, 198, 203, 205, 215, 216, 219, 224, 227, 228, 231, 237, 238, 242, 259, 285–287, 291, 292
Osteocytes, 2, 7, 11–15, 76, 92, 109, 111, 114, 119, 131, 132, 133, 135, 137, 139, 140, 157, 160, 166, 167, 228, 242, 292
Osteocytogenesis, 12–15
Osteomalacia, 14, 47, 48, 52, 55, 186, 189, 191, 194, 197, 198, 199, 203, 264
Osteopontin (OPN), 2, 7, 11, 144, 146, 193, 214, 215
Osteoporosis, 4, 25, 45, 59, 76, 83, 109, 135, 143, 159, 185, 211, 223, 237, 259, 277, 285, 297, 309 and CKD, 215
Osteoprotegerin (OPG), 4, 32, 35, 36, 84, 86, 133, 146, 163, 193, 195, 214, 238
Osterix (OSX), 7, 11, 157, 161

P
Pain, 53, 61, 66–69, 240, 242, 245, 281, 287, 289, 297–303, 305, 306, 314–318, 320, 321
Pain management, 315, 316, 318, 320
Parathyroid hormone (PTH), 3, 75, 80–81, 85, 88, 161, 186, 187, 190, 193, 215, 225, 232, 262, 270
Pathophysiology, 40, 92, 155–163, 184, 195, 212–218, 224–230, 232
Peroxisome Proliferator-Activated Receptor γ (PPAR γ), 137, 139
Pharmacological therapy, 285–292
Phosphate
binders, 202, 203
serum, 52, 85, 194, 202
PINP, 193, 195
Pituitary hormones, 90–93
PKP, *see* Kyphoplasty (PKP)
Polymorphism, 27–34, 36, 38, 110, 116, 117, 161
Prevention, 48, 93, 199, 204, 231, 239, 244, 248, 249, 260, 265, 266, 269, 277, 278, 288, 292, 314
Primary osteoporosis, 112, 113, 224–226, 229, 232
Proteinuria, 183, 186
Japanese idiopathic low molecular weight, 185, 186
Psoriatic arthritis, 238, 240–241
Puberty, 26, 46, 47, 83, 110, 111, 120, 129–141, 169, 260, 261, 278

R
Raloxifene (RLX), 212, 219, 286, 287
Range of Motion (ROM), 61–62, 314, 320

RANK-L, *see* Receptor Activator of NF-κB Ligand (RANKL)
Receptor Activator of NF-κB (RANK), 4, 5, 32, 37, 76, 133, 146, 163, 195, 237, 238, 245, 248, 287
Receptor Activator of NF-κB Ligand (RANKL), 3–8, 10, 11, 13, 15, 32, 35, 37, 76, 84, 86, 114, 132, 133, 138, 139, 146, 155, 158, 161, 163, 167, 186, 204, 205, 214–216, 219, 228–230, 237, 238, 240, 242, 245, 246, 248, 286, 290
Recommended nutrient intake, 264
Remodeling, 131, 138, 139, 144–146, 148, 191, 195, 196, 197, 198, 201, 216, 217, 225, 230, 259, 260, 262, 285–287, 290
Renal osteodystrophy (ROD), 184, 186, 188, 190–192, 195, 196, 198, 201–202, 204
Renal tubular disorders, 185
Resistance exercise, 280, 281
Resistin, 143, 145
Rheumatic diseases, 237–249
Rheumatoid arthritis (RA), 6, 51, 201, 229, 237, 240–245
Rickets
  X-linked recessive hypophosphatemic, 185, 186
  X-linked recessive hypophosphatemic with hypercalciuria, 185, 186
Risk of fragility fracture, 269
Rosiglitazone, 164, 166
Runt domain-containing transcription factor (Runx2), 7, 11, 32, 38, 109, 157, 161

S
Sarcopenia, 62, 93, 162, 238, 264, 278
Sclerostin, 8, 11, 13, 14, 31–33, 76, 157, 161, 166–169, 184, 188, 191, 192, 193, 196, 218, 230, 242, 292
Secondary osteoporosis, 48, 51, 87, 92, 113, 225, 229–230
Semaphorins, 10
Seronegative spondyloarthropathies (SnSp), 237–239
Sex steroids, 88, 111, 115, 129–140, 189, 278
SGLT2 Inhibitors, 168
SIBLINGs, 184, 193, 196
Skeletal tissue, 1–15, 107, 119, 129–141, 167, 259, 260
Statins, 219
Sufonylureas, 164–165
Systemic lupus erythematosus (SLE), 237, 245–249

T
Teriparatide, 116, 204, 205, 232, 245, 248, 249, 291
Thiazolidinediones, 48, 165–168
TMV classification, 191
Trabecular bone, 1, 9, 10, 46, 77–81, 86, 88, 90, 109, 112, 114, 115, 118, 119, 132, 135–138, 140, 145, 148, 158, 160, 161, 170, 199, 200, 224, 225, 239
Transforming growth factor beta (TGF-β1), 31–32
TRAP, 158, 163, 168, 193, 195, 269, 299
Treatment, 10, 11, 49, 50, 52, 53, 76, 79–81, 88, 89, 91, 92, 112–119, 157, 163–167, 199, 212, 218, 219, 228–232, 237–239, 241–245, 247, 248, 249, 260, 265, 286–292, 298, 299, 301–303, 305, 306, 313, 316, 320, 321
Tumor necrosis factor α (TNFα), 4, 5, 132, 133, 143, 161, 214, 217, 237, 238
Turnover
  in CKD-MBD (*see* TMV classification)
Type 1 Diabetes (T1D), 49, 153, 154
Type 2 Diabetes, 49, 154–157

U
Uremia, 187, 188, 186. *See also* Chronic kidney disease (CKD)
Uremic toxins, 189, 190

V
Vascular calcification, 187, 189, 196, 199, 200, 202, 212, 214–216, 218
Vertebral compression fracture (VCFs), 297–299, 301–305
Vertebral fracture, 10, 31, 48, 49, 53, 55, 60, 79, 112, 116, 154, 212, 244, 287, 288, 290, 291, 298, 299, 303, 305, 315, 316
Vertebral Fracture Assessment (VFA), 53, 244
Vertebroplasty, 303, 305–307
Vitamin D
  calcitriol, 187, 188
  cholecalciferol, 203, 204
  paricalcitol, 203, 204
  analogues, 204, 216, 219
  receptor, 27–28, 204, 215, 246

Vitamin K, 215, 218, 265, 271
Volume
Bone volume in CKD-MBD (*see* TMV classification)
Bone volume in histomorphometry, 79, 191

W
Weight-bearing exercise, 278
Wnt/β-catenin, 10, 76, 148, 157, 218, 238, 245, 248
canonical pathway, 10, 148
WNT signaling, 8, 14, 15, 27, 40, 85, 110, 120, 148, 168, 188, 230, 292

MIX
Papier aus verantwortungsvollen Quellen
Paper from responsible sources
FSC® C105338

If you have any concerns about our products,
you can contact us on
ProductSafety@springernature.com

In case Publisher is established outside the EU,
the EU authorized representative is:
Springer Nature Customer Service Center GmbH
Europaplatz 3, 69115 Heidelberg, Germany

Printed by Libri Plureos GmbH
in Hamburg, Germany